T0323510

Practical Primer of Dermatology

Studying for boards is straightforward, but clinical competence relies on experience, and this guide is designed to accelerate that.

It's amazing how much one can know and still not know what to do. This is likely, at least in part, due to the fact that many existing resources are not usually oriented toward the practical aspects of patient care. For instance, a book might say, for traction alopecia, a patient should adopt looser hairstyles, but it might not explain how to counsel a patient on what they need to communicate to their loctician to achieve lower tension. While acing exams and having a strong knowledge fund are necessary, they alone are not sufficient; one could spend all day memorizing the properties and minutiae of sutures, be able to answer every test question about them correctly, and yet still not know what to do when a knot repeatedly slips in a tight area. Boards answers don't always necessarily hold in real-world contexts either; obtaining a DIF specimen perilesionally for bullous pemphigoid (classic exam answer) wouldn't be the appropriate site if there were no bullae. The list of examples of conventional information failing to translate to successful clinical practice is endless.

This book provides practical pearls to fill these gaps and emphasizes the areas that are the most crucial for trainees to prioritize early on. It is a compilation of insights from several well-recognized leaders in dermatology and dermatologic surgery. *Practical Primer of Dermatology* is written in a succinct, conversational style and is a perfect read for residents, medical students, and non-dermatology physicians.

Series in Dermatological Treatment

About the Series

Published in association with the *Journal of Dermatological Treatment*, the *Series in Dermatological Treatment* keeps readers up-to-date with the latest clinical therapies to improve problems with the skin, hair, and nails. Each volume in the series is prepared separately and typically focuses on a topical theme. Volumes are published on an occasional basis, depending on the emergence of new developments.

Practical Ways to Improve Patient Adherence
Daniel J. Lewis and Steven R. Feldman

Atlas of Genital Dermoscopy
Giuseppe Micali and Francesco Lacarrubba

Hair Disorders: Diagnosis and Management
Alexander C. Katoulis, Dimitrios Ioannides, and Dimitris Rigopoulos

Techniques in the Evaluation and Management of Hair Disease
Rubina Alves and Juan Grimalt

Retinoids in Dermatology
Ayse Serap Karadag, Berna Aksoy, and Lawrence Charles Parish

Facial Skin Disorders
Ronald Marks

Dermatologic Reactions to Cancer Therapies
Gabriella Fabbrocini, Mario E. Lacouture, and Antonella Tosti

Acne Scars: Classification and Treatment, Second Edition
Antonella Tosti, Maria Pia De Padova, Gabriella Fabbrocini, and Kenneth Beer

Phototherapy Treatment Protocols, Third Edition
Steven R. Feldman and Michael D. Zanolli

Dermatoscopy in Clinical Practice: Beyond Pigmented Lesions, Second Edition
Giuseppe Micali and Francesco Lacarrubba

Nail Surgery
Bertrand Richert, Niton Di Chiacchio, and Eckart Haneke

Abdominal Stomas and Their Skin Disorders, Second Edition
Callum C. Lyon and Amanda Smith

Practical Primer of Dermatology: A High Yield Guide for Residents
Matthew L. Hrin

For more information about this series, please visit: www.crcpress.com/Series-in-Dermatological-Treatment/book-series/CRCSERDERTRE.

Practical Primer of Dermatology

A High Yield Guide for Residents

Matthew L. Hrin, MD

Dermatology Resident, Class of 2026
Wake Forest University School of Medicine
Winston-Salem, North Carolina, USA

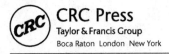

CRC Press

Taylor & Francis Group

Boca Raton London New York

CRC Press is an imprint of the
Taylor & Francis Group, an **informa** business

Designed cover image: Shutterstock

First edition published 2025
by CRC Press
2385 NW Executive Center Drive, Suite 320, Boca Raton, FL 33431

and by CRC Press
4 Park Square, Milton Park, Abingdon, Oxon, OX14 4RN

CRC Press is an imprint of Taylor & Francis Group, LLC

© 2025 Matthew L. Hrin

ISBN: 978-1-032-88468-4 (hbk)
ISBN: 978-1-032-88465-3 (pbk)
ISBN: 978-1-003-53794-6 (ebk)

DOI: 10.1201/9781003537946

Typeset in Palatino
by Apex CoVantage, LLC

Contents

Preface xi

Acknowledgments xii

1 Foundations 1
    1.1 Basics of Evaluating Lesions 1
    1.2 Basics of Clinical-Pathologic Correlation 2
    1.3 Basic Management 3
        1.3.1 Topical Corticosteroids (TCSs) 5
        1.3.2 Systemics 5
        1.3.3 Package Inserts 6
    1.4 Basic Procedures 6
        1.4.1 Biopsies 6
            1.4.1.1 Shave 6
            1.4.1.2 Punch 7
        1.4.2 Liquid Nitrogen (LN2) 7
        1.4.3 Intralesional Triamcinolone (Kenalog) (ILK) 8

2 Outpatient 9
    2.1 General Dermatology—Rashes 9
        2.1.1 Papulosquamous 9
            2.1.1.1 Psoriasiform 9
            2.1.1.2 Pityriasiform 12
            2.1.1.3 Lichenoid 16
        2.1.2 Eczematous 17
            2.1.2.1 Acute vs. Subacute vs. Chronic 18
            2.1.2.2 Intrinsic Atopic Dermatitis (AD) 18
            2.1.2.3 Contact Dermatitis 20
            2.1.2.4 Seborrheic Dermatitis 22
            2.1.2.5 Intertrigo 23
            2.1.2.6 Dyshidrotic 23
            2.1.2.7 Periorificial 23
            2.1.2.8 Eyelid/Orbital 24
            2.1.2.9 Ear 24
            2.1.2.10 Areolar 24
            2.1.2.11 Asteatotic (Eczema Craquelé) 24
            2.1.2.12 Stasis Dermatitis 24
            2.1.2.13 Lichen Simplex Chronicus (LSC) and Prurigo
                     Nodularis (PN) 25
        2.1.3 Vesiculobullous 25
            2.1.3.1 Bullous Pemphigoid (BP) 26
            2.1.3.2 Pemphigus Vulgaris 28
            2.1.3.3 Pemphigus Foliaceus 29
            2.1.3.4 Mucous Membrane (Cicatricial) Pemphigoid
                     (MMP) 30
            2.1.3.5 Linear IgA Bullous Dermatosis (LABD) 31
            2.1.3.6 Bullous Arthropod Assault (Bug Bites and Stings) . . . 31
            2.1.3.7 Porphyria Cutanea Tarda (PCT) 31
            2.1.3.8 Dermatitis Herpetiformis 31

            2.1.3.9 Hailey–Hailey 32
            2.1.3.10 Grover's 32
   2.1.4 Vascular 32
            2.1.4.1 Urticaria 32
            2.1.4.2 Vasculitis 34
            2.1.4.3 Vasculopathy 37
            2.1.4.4 Capillaritis (Pigmented Purpuric Dermatoses) 37
            2.1.4.5 Mastocytoses 38
            2.1.4.6 Urticaria Multiforme 38
            2.1.4.7 Regional Erythemas 38
   2.1.5 Pigmentary 40
            2.1.5.1 Hyperpigmentation 40
            2.1.5.2 Hypo- or Depigmentation 43
   2.1.6 Infectious 47
            2.1.6.1 Bacterial 47
            2.1.6.2 Fungal 48
            2.1.6.3 Viral 53
            2.1.6.4 Infestations 56
   2.1.7 Dermal 59
            2.1.7.1 Granulomatous 59
            2.1.7.2 Neutrophilic 65
            2.1.7.3 Lymphocytic 69
            2.1.7.4 Depositional 69
   2.1.8 Panniculitides 71
            2.1.8.1 Erythema Nodosum (EN) 71
   2.1.9 Acne, Rosacea, Papillomatoses, Keratotic, and
          Follicular Disorders 71
            2.1.9.1 Acne 71
            2.1.9.2 Rosacea 77
            2.1.9.3 Acrochordon (Skin Tag) 78
            2.1.9.4 Acanthosis Nigricans 79
            2.1.9.5 Corn 79
            2.1.9.6 Porokeratosis 79
            2.1.9.7 Keratosis Pilaris (KP) 79
            2.1.9.8 Folliculitis 80
            2.1.9.9 Pseudofolliculitis Barbae 81
   2.1.10 Psychiatric 82
            2.1.10.1 Approach 82
            2.1.10.2 Management 84
   2.1.11 Undifferentiated Pruritus 86
  2.2 General Dermatology—Neoplasms 89
   2.2.1 Keratinocytic 89
            2.2.1.1 Malignant 89
            2.2.1.2 Benign 96
   2.2.2 Melanocytic 98
            2.2.2.1 Melanoma 98
            2.2.2.2 Congenital Melanocytic Nevus 103
            2.2.2.3 Epidermal Nevus 104
            2.2.2.4 Acquired Nevus 104
            2.2.2.5 Common Acquired Nevus 104
            2.2.2.6 Spitz Nevus 105

2.2.2.7 Nevus Spilus...................................105
2.2.2.8 Blue Nevus 105
2.2.2.9 Halo Nevus..................................105
2.2.2.10 Combined Nevus 105
2.2.3 Lentigines...105
2.2.3.1 Solar Lentigines 105
2.2.3.2 Lentigo Simplex 106
2.2.3.3 Cafe au Lait Macule (CALM) 106
2.2.3.4 Freckles (Ephelides)........................106
2.2.3.5 Melanotic Macule..........................106
2.2.3.6 Linear and Whorled Nevoid Hypermelanosis 106
2.2.4 Adnexal Tumors and Glandular Disorders 107
2.2.4.1 Hyperhidrosis...............................107
2.2.4.2 Sebaceous Hyperplasia 109
2.2.4.3 Nevus Sebaceus 110
2.2.4.4 Syringoma..................................110
2.2.4.5 Microcystic Adnexal Carcinoma (MAC) 110
2.2.5 Vascular Tumors.....................................111
2.2.5.1 Cherry Hemangioma..........................111
2.2.5.2 Infantile (Strawberry) Hemangioma............111
2.2.5.3 Pyogenic Granuloma.........................111
2.2.5.4 Venous Lake 111
2.2.5.5 Glomus Tumor 111
2.2.5.6 Malformations 112
2.2.5.7 Lymphangioma..............................112
2.2.5.8 Cutis Marmorata Telangiectasia Congenita.......113
2.2.6 Spindle Cell Tumors..................................113
2.2.6.1 Dermatofibroma (DF) 113
2.2.6.2 Dermatofibrosarcoma Protuberans (DFSP) 113
2.2.6.3 Keloid....................................114
2.2.7 Fat Tumors 115
2.2.7.1 Lipoma....................................115
2.2.7.2 Nevus Lipomatous Superficialis 115
2.2.8 Cysts 115
2.2.8.1 Milia......................................115
2.2.8.2 Epidermal Inclusion Cyst (EIC) 115
2.2.8.3 Pilar Cyst..................................116
2.2.8.4 Pilonidal Cyst 116
2.2.8.5 Pseudocyst.................................116
2.3 General Dermatology—Miscellaneous Complaints
and Conditions 117
2.3.1 Ingredient Labels for Cosmetic Products 119
2.4 Subspecialty Clinics..121
2.4.1 Complex Medical Dermatology and Connective
Tissue Diseases 121
2.4.1.1 Dermatomyositis (DM) 121
2.4.1.2 Lupus 125
2.4.1.3 Scleroderma................................127
2.4.1.4 Morphea...................................130
2.4.1.5 Eosinophilic Fasciitis (EF)....................132
2.4.1.6 Considerations in Skin of Color................133

2.4.2 Hair 133
    2.4.2.1 Evaluation 133
    2.4.2.2 Hair Medications 136
    2.4.2.3 Procedural Options 138
    2.4.2.4 Scarring Alopecias 139
    2.4.2.5 Non-Scarring Alopecias 145
    2.4.2.6 Hair Shaft Disorders 147
    2.4.2.7 Considerations in Skin of Color 148
2.4.3 Hidradenitis Suppurativa (HS) 152
    2.4.3.1 Evaluation 153
    2.4.3.2 Approach 153
    2.4.3.3 Management 153
2.4.4 Vulvar and Male Genital Derm 156
    2.4.4.1 Lichen Planus 157
    2.4.4.2 Lichen Sclerosus (LSA) 157
    2.4.4.3 Atrophic Vulvovaginitis 158
    2.4.4.4 Various Benign Vulvar Dermatoses 159
    2.4.4.5 Malignancies to Consider 159
    2.4.4.6 Considerations for Male Genital Dermatoses 160
2.4.5 Cutaneous T-Cell Lymphoma (CTCL) 161
2.4.6 Pediatric Dermatology 165

3 Inpatient (Calls/Consults) 167

3.1 General Principles 167
3.2 Differential Diagnosis Based on "Call" 168
  3.2.1 "Concern for SJS" 168
    3.2.1.1 Stevens–Johnson Syndrome (SJS)/Toxic
               Epidermal Necrolysis (TEN) 168
    3.2.1.2 Erythema Multiforme (EM) Major 170
    3.2.1.3 RIME (Reactive Infectious Mucocutaneous
               Eruption) 171
    3.2.1.4 Generalized Bullous Fixed Drug Eruption 172
    3.2.1.5 LABD (Linear IgA Bullous Dermatosis) 172
  3.2.2 "Concern for DRESS" 173
    3.2.2.1 Drug Reaction with Eosinophilia and
               Systemic Symptoms (DRESS)/Drug-Induced
               Hypersensitivity Syndrome (DIHS) 173
    3.2.2.2 Exanthematous Drug Reaction 174
    3.2.2.3 General Checklist for Drug Reactions 174
  3.2.3 "Concern for Bullous Pemphigoid" 175
    3.2.3.1 Bullous Pemphigoid 175
    3.2.3.2 Edema Bullae 176
    3.2.3.3 Coma Bullae 176
    3.2.3.4 Friction Blisters 176
    3.2.3.5 Post-Burn/Graft Blisters 176
    3.2.3.6 IV Infiltration vs. Extravasation 176
    3.2.3.7 LABD 177
  3.2.4 "Concern for Vasculitis" 177
    3.2.4.1 Vasculitis 177
    3.2.4.2 Vasculopathy 178
    3.2.4.3 Calciphylaxis 180

3.2.5 "Rule Out Child Abuse" 182
    3.2.5.1 Suspicious Things 182
    3.2.5.2 Obtaining History 183
    3.2.5.3 Physical Exam............................. 183
    3.2.5.4 Next Steps 183
3.2.6 Erythroderma Differential Diagnosis.................. 184
3.2.7 Acute Infections 186
    3.2.7.1 Angioinvasive Fungal Infections............... 186
    3.2.7.2 Bacterial Infections......................... 186
    3.2.7.3 Other..................................... 189
3.2.8 Pregnancy Dermatoses 189
3.2.9 Infantile and Neonatal Dermatoses.................... 191
3.2.10 Other Inpatient Entities 193
    3.2.10.1 Graft vs. Host Disease (GVHD) 193
    3.2.10.2 Acute Generalized Exanthematous Pustulosis
        (AGEP) 194
    3.2.10.3 Generalized Pustular Psoriasis (GPP)........... 195
    3.2.10.4 Localized Fixed Drug Eruption (FDE) 195
    3.2.10.5 Leukemia Cutis............................. 195
    3.2.10.6 Sweet Syndrome........................... 195
    3.2.10.7 Symmetrical Drug-Related Intertriginous and
        Flexural Exanthema (SDRIFE) 196
    3.2.10.8 Chemotherapy Reactions 196
    3.2.10.9 Severe Toxic Erythema of Chemotherapy 196
    3.2.10.10 Sudden Conjunctivitis, Lymphopenia, Rash,
        and Hemodynamic Changes (SCoRCH)........... 196
    3.2.10.11 Nutritional Dermatoses....................... 197
    3.2.10.12 Wounds 197

4 Medications, Phototherapy, and Wound Care 199

4.1 Topicals.. 199
4.2 Systemics 204
    4.2.1 Small Molecules 205
    4.2.2 Biologics 209
    4.2.3 Newer Therapies................................... 213
4.3 Phototherapy and Photodynamic Therapy (PDT)............... 217
    4.3.1 Phototherapy 217
    4.3.2 Blue Light Therapy (**aka** PDT)..................... 219
4.4 DIY Formulations Instructions.............................. 220
4.5 Wound Care and Wound Healing 221

5 Procedures... 226

5.1 General Principles... 226
    5.1.1 Numbing 227
    5.1.2 Cutting 228
    5.1.3 Suturing 229
        5.1.3.1 General Things.............................. 229
        5.1.3.2 Nomenclature Basics and Choosing
            Appropriate Sutures 230
        5.1.3.3 Closing (Primary)........................... 231

5.1.4   Hemostasis. 235
5.1.5   Peri-Operative Considerations 236
5.1.6   Bandaging + Post-Care. 236
5.2   Electrodesiccation and Curettage (EDC). 236
5.3   Incision & Drainage (I&D). 237
5.4   Excisions. 238
5.4.1   Benign Lesions 238
5.4.1.1   Epidermal Inclusion Cysts (EICs) 238
5.4.1.2   Lipomas 240
5.4.1.3   Pilar Cysts 240
5.5   Mohs 241
5.5.1   Closures and Basics of Flaps/Grafts .242
5.5.1.1   Second Intent. 242
5.5.1.2   Primary Closures 243
5.5.1.3   Grafts 243
5.5.1.4   Flaps 244

6   Cosmetics 246

6.1   Botox 246
6.2   Lasers and Energy-Based Devices 246
6.2.1   Basic Principles 246
6.2.2   Intense Pulsed Light (IPL). 249
6.2.3   PDL (Vbeam)—585 nm for Vascular Lesions. 251
6.2.4   Nd:YAG—532 nm for Black Ink 251
6.2.5   Non-Ablative Fractional Infrared—1927 nm 253
6.2.6   Radiofrequency (RF) Microneedling. 253

7   Post-Procedure Counseling. 255

7.1   Post-Operative Care Instructions. 255
7.2   Physician's Access Line (PAL) Calls from Patients 257
7.3   Scars 257

8   Miscellaneous Doctoring. 259

8.1   Documentation 259
8.2   Writing Manuscripts 261
8.3   Reviewing Manuscripts. 263
8.4   Being a Resident 266

Preface

Studying for boards is straightforward, but clinical competence relies on experience, and this guide is designed to accelerate that.

You probably know ketoconazole is a treatment for seborrheic dermatitis, but you may not be confident in how to manage/counsel a skin-of-color patient who can only wash their hair once monthly. You might be able to easily recognize Stevens–Johnson syndrome on an exam and know the HLAs but find yourself not entirely comfortable speaking with a primary team about a "concern for SJS" case when on-call. This is designed to guide you through those things. It has an inpatient chapter to help you navigate call/consults. There are FYI reminders to help you avoid embarrassment (for example, you can't get GVHD from autologous transplants [those are the ones you get from yourself], etc.). Other topics covered include understanding package inserts, critically analyzing literature, writing manuscripts, reviewing for journals, etc.

I write this assuming you already know the basics (describing lesions, etc.) and classic buzzwords (islands of sparing, etc.). I omitted those things to avoid diluting more fruitful stuff.

This guide is not exhaustive or comprehensive. It is a supplement designed to give you a good start. I aim to cover the ~20% of derm that comprises ~80% of clinic (perhaps not literally—but you get the point). I touch on a few uncommon conditions I've seen to share my experiences/exposures.

This is not a boards resource. There are great resources for that already. I encourage you to refer to those for genes/inheritance patterns, bugs/plants, contactants, and so on, which are important to know. You will notice that some things in this book are actually inconsistent with traditional board answers (for example, many patients with isolated discoid lesions have essentially 0% chance of progressing to SLE vs. the board answer [10–20%]—I will explain why later). I also try to point out caveats to knee-jerk board answers (for example, "should get immunofluorescence from lesional erythema in bullous pemphigoid when there is no blister" [you only get it perilesionally—the traditional board answer—when there is a blister]).

The treatment ladders are not formal, up-to-date, evidence-based recommendations; they are designed to be a good starting point for developing an intuition for management algorithms.

The percentages and numbers are rough estimates (mainly for counseling patients vs. writing papers); thus, you shouldn't cite these but refer to peer-reviewed research publications.

Dermpath/cosmetics/Mohs are not heavily represented.

This is not formal medical advice. You should independently verify diagnoses/dosages, etc. No responsibility/liability is assumed by any contributor (including me) for any injury or damage to persons. All rights reserved. No part of this may be reproduced/transmitted without written permission from the author/publisher except as permitted by US copyright law.

Reach out with questions/concerns/feedback. I'm a PGY-2 at the time of writing so of course still accumulating knowledge. I would love to hear if you've been taught things differently. E-mail: matthewhrin@virginia.edu.

Matthew L. Hrin, MD
Winston-Salem, NC, USA

Acknowledgments

Special thanks to the faculty at Wake Forest for inspiring me and affording me the opportunity to embark on this endeavor of pursuing mastery of what I envision to be my life's work. Forever indebted to them for their generosity in sharing their insights and for making Wake Forest a fun, pleasant, and productive place to learn. Most of the content is stuff I've learned from working with them in clinic and their lectures. They are the true authors.

- Christine S. Ahn, MD
- Zeynep M. Akkurt, MD
- Laura B. Doerfler, MD
- Steven R. Feldman, MD, PhD
- Neal D. Goldman, MD
- William W. Huang, MD, MPH
- Joseph L. Jorizzo, MD
- Maria C. Mariencheck, MD, PhD

- Amy J. McMichael, MD
- Angela G. Niehaus, MD
- Rita O. Pichardo, MD
- Kyle E. Robinson, MD
- Omar P. Sangueza, MD
- Lindsay C. Strowd, MD
- Sarah L. Taylor, MD, MPH

Several outside faculty have also graciously contributed tremendous insights:

- Crystal Aguh, MD
- Jeremy S. Bordeaux, MD, MPH
- Dirk M. Elston, MD
- Teri M. Greiling, MD, PhD
- Iltefat Hamzavi, MD
- Joanna Harp, MD
- John E. Harris, MD, PhD
- Christopher T. Kelly, MD
- John Koo, MD
- Payman Kosari, MD
- Shawn G. Kwatra, MD

- Frank Lacy, MD
- Avery H. LaChance, MD, MPH
- Jorge Larrondo, MD
- Kiran Motaparthi, MD
- Gilly Munavalli, MD
- Oluwakemi Onajin, MD
- Geoffrey A. Potts, MD
- Misha Rosenbach, MD
- Lucian G. Vlad, MD
- Gil Yosipovitch, MD

1 Foundations

1.1 BASICS OF EVALUATING LESIONS

For growths, you can have a solid ddx with a basic understanding of lesion morphologies and knowing what cells are in each layer.

- If it's a tumor with scaly sandpaper = epidermis (melanocytes, keratinocytes, etc.).

- If it looks like an orange peel = dermis (hair follicles, smooth muscle, blood vessels, elastic fibers, collagen—go through these tumors).

- If you can move skin over the lesion = subQ (fat).

- If it's fixed = could be sarcoma or something attached to deep fascia.

    Histology is usually reliable for tumors (more so than for rashes).

    For rashes, categorize by morphology/reaction pattern—see Chapter 2. In the beginning, would strive to at least get the category correct even if you're not yet familiar with specific diagnoses.

    Try to train your eye to appreciate subtleties in color, shape, and distribution. The following are just some examples to help you start to organize your thinking.

Color

- *Brown*: think melanin (such as pigment incontinence in inflammatory lesions), hemosiderin (such as in vascular lesions), lipofuscin (such as in sweat gland tumors or depositions from drugs).
    - Can also have "green" stuff that appears brown from myeloperoxidase.

- *Blue*: think cyanosis or Tyndall effect (optical scatter) from brown pigment (when brown is deep, it appears blue via refraction).
    - For example, hidrocystomas appear bluish because they have brown lipofuscin that is deep.

- *Pink*: think mild inflammation.

- *Red*: oxygenated heme; think intense inflammation and/or damage (extravasated blood).

- *Purple*: deoxygenated heme; usually implies tissue/vessel damage (extravasated blood) from intense inflammation.

- *Black*: implies death or dying tissue (ischemia, necrosis).

- *Plum*: think lymphoma, leukemia cutis, Merkel, other tumors.

- *Yellow* or *orange*: think lipids (carotenoids), elastotic tissue.

- *Yellow-green*: think about heme components breaking down into bilirubin (yellow) and biliverdin (greenish)—would suggest a chronic vascular process with RBC extravasation, giving rise to hemoglobin breakdown.

- *Shiny*: think surface atrophy (seeing reticular vessels in the lesion [due to the atrophy] and not the adjacent non-lesional skin may also be a clue).

DOI: 10.1201/9781003537946-1

SHAPE

- *Angulated/geometric*: think exogenous.

- *If the ends are broader (dumbbell-shaped)*: think about tumors, such as a keloid (inflammatory things don't really tend to be expansile at the ends).

  - Most tumors also ablate skin markings, whereas rashes can lichenify (accentuate skin markings—which can be from rubbing/chaffing—not just scratching).

- *If livedo patterned*: think vascular (though could also include rare occlusive neoplasms, such as angioendotheliomatous or intravascular lymphoma something).

Distribution is not only where it is on the body; also ask yourself if the lesions are along skin lines, etc.

For pigmented lesions, dermoscopy is critical. Best to learn via pics and repetition. Would start looking dermoscopically primarily at stuff that you already know clinically (for example, SKs, DFs, angiomas, etc.) and building a foundation from that.

1.2 BASICS OF CLINICAL-PATHOLOGIC CORRELATION

You need to transition away from thinking like an internist (in terms of lab tests) and start thinking clinical-pathologically.

Must understand the factors that influence a biopsy's potential to be insightful (these are super basic examples; more details throughout book).

1. *Site/lesion selection*

   a. For example, identify representative lesions, know where the pathology is (don't take a DIF sample from a blister for suspected bullous pemphigoid).

2. *Biopsy technique*

   a. For example, don't do a shave biopsy if looking for a pathology that is subQ.

3. *Quality and handling of specimen obtained*

   a. For example, if shave too superficially (insufficiently), might not capture representative histologic findings; don't crush punch specimens with the forceps.

4. *Disease evolution*

   a. For example, LCV

      i. If you biopsy a lesion that's too young, you'll just see lymphocytes that haven't yet organized themselves into the disease.

      ii. If you biopsy a lesion that's too old, might just see extravasated RBCs.

      iii. Biopsying 24 hours after lesion onset (when it's just becoming purpuric) gives you the best chance of seeing an LCV's characteristic histology.

5. *Influences from prior therapies*

   a. For example, if biopsy after patient received days of IV methylprednisolone (Solumedrol), might not see very many inflammatory cells (path might read "no evidence of LCV").

While clinical-pathologic discrepancies are generally avoidable with appropriate selection of lesions, biopsies obviously aren't always perfect. But you need to at least appreciate and account for these factors when interpreting reads and realize that your clinical impression takes precedence over the path (which is just an additional piece of info—despite it often being viewed as a slam-dunk confirmatory test by patients). Should view antibody reports/tests the same way—they don't single-handedly establish disease designations.

Other specialties might also tend to rest their hat on the histologic diagnosis (since they don't have path training/exposure and the way they conceptualize their illnesses is different). So there is utility in biopsying even classic presentations (particularly if instituting systemic treatment). Biopsy-proving conditions can also sometimes help with insurance approvals.

1.3 BASIC MANAGEMENT

Cures are hard to come by; for the most part, doctors control diseases until they go away (with the exception of some cancers, infections that aren't viruses, the stuff that is cut out, etc.). Some basic principles:

- Know what you're treating; epidermal surface problems like eczema are going to respond much faster than deep granulomatous processes, for instance. For example, you can't really call a GA treatment a failure if you only tried it for one month.

- Localized problems warrant localized solutions.

  - For example, if a psoriasis patient is on risankizumab (Skyrizi) and has two resistant plaques, improve their topical regimen (don't switch their biologic for that).

- An effective med needs to both be strong enough and reach the site of the pathology.

  - Think about this when you read (and especially review) literature. For example, you should question how PO diltiazem could impact calcinosis cutis if there aren't any blood vessels to take it to the pathology (the calcium bricks are in the soft tissue). Similarly, there are no vessels that could whisk the calcium away if something like topical sodium thiosulfate were applied to the skin (and that's if you assume it even makes it to the site of the pathology in any meaningful/relevant way).

- Always match treatment duration with disease duration.

  - For example, prednisone for an atopic is a no-no; it's a 2-week solution for a chronic problem.

- Suppress diseases and keep them quiet (no roller coasters, promptly and proactively address flares if they occur—especially with dose reductions, discontinuation trials; basically want to make the body forget how to organize the disease). This lends best odds of yielding sustained remissions.

■ Make sure patients are confident in knowing what they're supposed to do (and what not to do), and try to get read on their preferences. Some appreciate complexity, but most probably prefer simplicity, and the way you explain things matters (probably easier if you say "Apply every other day on even numbered dates" than to say "Apply 3–4 times per week").

■ Follow a therapeutic ladder.

• For skin-limited LCV that is just red dots, may not need any treatment; if bothersome or joint pains, etc., can consider dapsone/colchicine. Maybe MTX and slow prednisone taper for ulcerative spots; if have renal disease, perhaps IV methylprednisolone (Solumedrol), pulsed cyclophosphamide, etc.

• Basically, don't give isotretinoin for a solitary comedone, and don't give OTC BPO for acne fulminans.

■ If you exhaust a treatment ladder, reconsider an alternative diagnosis and/ or brainstorm meds that are mechanistically rational (in other words, meds with mechanisms of action that mirror the problem, for example, dapsone or colchicine for neutrophilic processes, retinoids to renew the epithelial surface for keratotic disorders, etc.).

■ Need to learn to recognize when not to treat.

• Distinguish tissue infections vs. surface organisms. Don't chase bacteria growing from soup. If you culture a deep ulcer and it grows fecal organisms like *E. coli*, probably doesn't warrant antibiotics, unless there's cellulitic/lymphangitic change, fevers, etc. All wounds have bacterial biofilms and colonization.

– Another example: eczema skin—97% of atopics have staph colonization, and 60% of that is MRSA. Don't give anti-MRSA antibiotics; otherwise, they'll have MRSA their whole life (and likely super-MRSA). Just reduce colonization with SSD so they don't get styes.

• You may also apply this ideology in stuff like DM when you taper their prednisone and they start reporting "weakness" ("concern for muscle flaring"), which a lot of times is actually just wear/tear arthritis (and other age-related stuff) resurfacing. Many patients love prednisone and the way it makes them feel, so important to recognize when to say no—more on this later.

■ Don't just put on Band-Aids. Seek and address the underlying issue. Heavily emphasize identifying the "why" and the "what" (to do) will fall into place.

• If they have LSC in an L4/L5 distribution, don't just send them out on clobetasol and hydroxyzine (Atarax); address the neuropathy. Otherwise, they will never get better.

Lab monitoring/dosing for meds is covered later (so if you're at the VA and don't have reliable internet or something, you can pull up that section). Will also cover tips for documentation relevant to obtaining insurance approvals (your prior auth teams will appreciate you).

1.3.1 Topical Corticosteroids (TCSs)

Should know at least one TCS from each category (low, medium, high potency).

- For example: hydrocortisone 2.5%, triamcinolone (TAC) 0.1%, clobetasol 0.05%

- OTC hydrocortisone is 1% (even though it's called Cortisone 10—*FYI*). Relative strengths to that:

- *Mild*: hydrocortisone 2.5% (2.5×), desonide (4×)—cannot go stronger than 4× on face or will risk resistant acne that takes >8 weeks anti-inflammatory antibiotics to resolve.

- *Mid*: TAC (15×).

- *Mid-upper*: fluocinonide (150×).

  - *FYI*: Different from fluocinolone, which is basically TAC strength.

- *Super potent*: clobetasol (1,600×).

Generally, inflammatory reactions need TAC strength at the site of the pathology (15×).

Axillae and groin/folds have natural occlusion which increases potency 10×.

If lesions are thick, almost like it starts as clobetasol, then becomes fluocinonide as it works its way through, then it's TAC where the action is (what you want).

That may not literally happen, but that's the way you should think about it.

For example: Wouldn't want to use weak TCSs for a dermal disorder (such as GA, morphea, or even stuff like vitiligo) because will likely cause epidermal atrophy before it makes any meaningful impact in the dermis. Pulsing clobetasol (BID only on weekends) is probably best for dermal issues.

Should also consider the baseline condition of patient's skin; probably want to err on side of weaker TCSs for radiation dermatitis skin, for example.

Develop judgment for how much to give.

A 30 g tube covers an adult only once (a half-sized adult twice, a quarter-sized adult 4×). So no matter how small a person, an atopic isn't going to get better with one 30 g tube. Give them a 1 lb (454 g) jar for the body, 60 g tube for face, and ask if prefers ointment (like a Vaseline); most people prefer creams.

While TCSs don't cause rebound flares, you shouldn't treat on/off (non-dermatologists frequently prescribe 5 days on, 5 days off, etc.—don't do that, makes roller coaster). Just treat by feel (only to sandpaper areas) until clear. Avoid systemic steroids, which cause rebound (generalizes diseases, basically makes poison ivy look like chickenpox).

1.3.2 Systemics

Pharmacists may tell patients to take certain meds 1 hour before and 2 hours after a meal. Warn patients of this and tell them to just take 5 min before meal with big glass of water (otherwise, patients may set alarm and take 2 AM or something ridiculous). The absorption difference is probably negligible, and you will titrate based on way patients take it, anyway. Simple regimens are easier to adhere to.

1.3.3 Package Inserts

Written by pharma company/FDA lawyers. Much of it is ludicrous.

All topicals have to state what would happen if you ate it. But you'd have to eat more than 60 g clobetasol QW to experience systemic side effects. Thus, 95% of the package insert doesn't apply. There are two realistic side effects: steroid acne/rosacea and skin thinning. Avoid these by telling patients never to apply to face and only use on thickened rashes; if it's thick, it won't thin.

For systemic meds, a good amount of "potential side effects" are manifestations of the disease they're used to treat or are issues that exist at baseline in that patient population. For instance, isotretinoin doesn't cause depression, but acne patients may be depressed. Weekly MTX won't cause pulm fibrosis, but untreated/undertreated AICTDs can progress to involve the lungs, and sometimes MTX is blamed for that.

Equally as relevant and important to acknowledge that MTX at chemo doses can indeed cause pulm fibrosis, and its package insert relates to it in the context of it being used as chemotherapy. So of course there are legitimate things on package inserts that are important to counsel patients on. Just make sure you know what is realistic and what is not (and why), and communicate that with patients before asking them to take it. Goes without saying, but you should always avoid equivocality when counseling patients on side effects (for example, you should say "You must not get pregnant" rather than "You can't get pregnant" when using isotretinoin).

1.4 BASIC PROCEDURES

Setup is key. Never assume everything you need has already been laid out (for example, if on blood thinner and anticipating needing cautery/pressure dressing, then make sure it's all on the tray; if you're doing a punch, make sure you have needle drivers, sutures, pickups, scissors).

Always have gauze near the site, and anticipate where the blood, etc., is going to drip. Don't ruin patients' clothes.

1.4.1 Biopsies

When numbing, aim superficial (especially for older people, who have thin dermis); if you inject in subQ, they won't get numb. Should almost look like a bleb from a TB skin test (in other words, you really don't need much anesthetic; if you feel like you're injecting a lot without success, you're probably too deep).

Drysol hurts—don't get it in their eyes (and don't use for procedures where you don't use numbing, like cutting off skin tags or something).

Obviously, know what you're looking for, which will dictate site selection. If it's a tumor, get the thick part and avoid necrotic tissue. If an ulcer, get the edge and adjacent skin—not just the center, where the path will just show "ulcer." For vesiculobullous conditions, know the particulars for where to get DIF. You want to get the most representative areas of the lesions (the most inflammation/activity). And don't biopsy crusty old eczema plaques, unless you're looking to rule out CTCL. Don't do punches for CTCL or melanoma, etc.

1.4.1.1 Shave

Natural tendency is to hold the blade with index finger and thumb (which many people do), but if you hold it with your middle finger and thumb, you can use your index finger to hold the specimen (and get better countertraction—which gives you better finishes, in my opinion). Also helps to make a conscious effort to change the angle of your wrist halfway through (most people come up too late). Sawing motion helps with thick skin.

If working in an area where it's tough to finesse instruments (for example, inside the ear), can use gradle scissors. Or can do a partial punch (don't punch all the way through) and snip off a piece of the tissue if want to be more precise.

If on scalp, can desiccate after taking the specimen to shrink the eventual scar (can let patients know they may have small scar, but it shouldn't create frank alopecia patch).

1.4.1.2 Punch

Don't squish the specimen. Best to grab it on the very side (forceps touching as little of the top edge of specimen as possible and right below it; avoid the center, and definitely don't grab it horizontally). If your forceps have huge teeth on them, can also try sticking a very small needle through to grip the tissue.

Good for tough spots (for example, lower conjunctiva—can take small 2 mm punch and let it second intent, for instance). Of course, also better than shaves if looking for deep pathologies.

Scalp punches are bloody (let the lidocaine with epinephrine sit for a few minutes, if possible). Usually will want two samples on scalp; try to get them right next to each other so it's basically just one wound (closes better; can do this for DIFs, too, when possible/appropriate). Use Drysol on Q-tip for scalp biopsies, and press it in biopsy site (to get both chemical and mechanical hemostasis). Figure-of-eight stitch works well (basically two interrupted sutures without cutting after the first); can use chromic gut. Nice to use absorbable sutures if patient lives far away (or can give them a suture removal kit to take home, if they're comfortable).

Telescope punch is what it sounds like (basically two punches to get deeper sample—fine to use the same size, although some people do a larger one on the first punch). Just make sure the pathology team/histotechnician knows it's intentional, so they don't throw away the fat. You can also push hard and keep turning to get a deep one-piece sample (some find it easier than trying to punch again in a hole, only for fatty areas—be mindful of structures).

For biopsies on legs, probably should apply a pressure dressing (although it looks like it won't bleed, it will when they start to walk).

1.4.2 Liquid Nitrogen (LN2)

Be precise. Usually better to pulse unless the lesion is huge.

Decrust things like hypertrophic AKs before spraying (crust gets in way of getting to the pathologic cells). Can use a curette. If not strong enough, can use a biopsy blade (should do this before intralesional chemotherapy for thick crusty SCCs, too).

If they're thick SKs, freeze more on the sides of them rather than just freezing the top of them.

Legs are slow to heal; be gentle with LN2, and warn about discoloration (melanocytes most sensitive to cold; keratinocytes second most). Generally best to avoid LN2 in skin of color (can instead use hyfrecation for most lesions [usually best to numb before hyfrecation]).

If LN2-ing the face, can use tongue depressor to shield eyes.

In general, want to spray SKs 2–3 rounds, AKs 1–2 rounds if thin, or 2–3 if thicker, or on leathery skin. Palmar warts are stubborn; need to spray more aggressively (~5–10 seconds). Genital warts hurt; would pulse until turns white and little bit around it (1 mm).

Make sure patients know LN2 will create a wound (not good to do before weddings, photoshoots). Healing period is ~2–3 weeks, and they will need to take care of the areas by applying Vaseline, cleaning with soap and water, keeping it covered until healed.

1.4.3 Intralesional Triamcinolone (Kenalog) (ILK)

Do not inject ILK deep (good way to start is to make it look like a PPD test—that way, the ILK will dissect down and won't get into fat/cause atrophy). If you choose to inject with syringe oriented straight up/down, make sure you have a strong sense of your depth. Always point bevel up (less painful for patient because easier to puncture skin).

ILK strengths:

- 2.5–3.3 mg/mL for acne

- 10 mg/mL for inflammatory stuff, like psoriasis or prurigo nodule

- 40 mg/mL for keloids (assuming your injecting high up)

Warn skin-of-color patients about hypopigmentation around the lesion (resolves over months).

If patients are fearful of needles, can try cool spray, such as Gebauer's Pain Ease (spray until skin turns white, then can insert needle) or EMLA cream (apply and occlude 30 minutes before injecting); however, these are better at numbing the surface (will still hurt when injected into the tissue). Can also mix the ILK with lidocaine to alleviate pain.

If you accidentally cause ILK atrophy:

- Flush with bacteriostatic normal saline.

- Use 30G needle, put 3–5 cc in there (enough to create a mound), and repeat Q1–2 weeks for 3–4 visits.

- Can also use the 30G needle to subcise.

- In path, you can see the steroid crystals in the fat; the saline basically flushes out those crystals that clog up the lymph vessels that cause the atrophy.

- Once done with that, can resurface as needed (microneedling + PRP, CO_2), but the saline alone helps a lot.

2 Outpatient

2.1 GENERAL DERMATOLOGY—RASHES
2.1.1 Papulosquamous
2.1.1.1 Psoriasiform

If you have psoriasiform lesions without pathognomonic features of psoriasis, it's best to call it "psoriasiform dermatitis" because Koebnerization eczema skin will present as a psoriasiform lesion.

While psoriasis used to be thought of as a Th1 condition (on the opposite end of the Th1/Th2 spectrum from AD), we now know it is Th17 (thus, it isn't necessarily bizarre to have them coexist like once believed). If ~7% of the population has AD, it's not surprising if ~7% of psoriasis patients have AD. Similarly, if ~2% of the population has psoriasis, it's not surprising if 2% of AD patients have psoriasis.

That said, an AD patient can have psoriasiform lesions without truly having coexistent psoriasis, and this is something you should consider when assessing patients and/or reviewing manuscripts (for example, if an AD patient stops dupilumab, itches/scratches their skin, and consequently develops psoriasiform lesions, it doesn't mean their dupilumab induced psoriasis). Psoriasis is if you have pathognomonic lesions.

2.1.1.1.1 Psoriasis

Exaggerated response to injury of the skin. Some patients will ask if it's autoimmune; some regard it as such, but no autoantigen identified. Probably what patients are getting at is they're wondering if it's like a lupus or Sjögren's-type of disease (which it obviously isn't). *An aside that may help*: the HLAs DR and DQ are MHC 2 HLAs (generally associated with autoantibody-mediated conditions), whereas HLAs A, B, and C are MHC 1 HLAs (generally associated with conditions that are NOT antibody-mediated, such as psoriasis [Cw6], Behçet's [B51]). This is because MHC 2 is expressed on macrophages and B-cells, which are trained to recognize and present antigens, and B-cells, of course, ultimately drive antibody production. Mainly bring this up to make connections with exam stuff and because it's relevant for therapy planning (for example, why rituximab [anti-CD20 antibody that targets B-cells] works for pemphigus but isn't really rational for psoriasis, etc.).

Ask about joint pain (important how you frame the question, or everyone will say they have it; ask if it's so bad it wakes them up [since characteristically worse in AM])—usually, it's hands, but can be back pain, too.

If has joint pain, an argument could be made for either manage vs. refer, but just make sure you address it (albeit most patients with psoriasis don't have psoriatic arthritis [PsA]; of the ones who do have PsA, most don't have progressive joint destruction, and of those who do, many won't really have significant change from therapy).

Five conditions go along with clinical picture of psoriasis + axial arthritis (knees, sacroiliac joints, spine, possibly shoulders): PsA, ankylosing spondylitis, enteropathic Crohn's, Reiter's, and undifferentiated spondyloarthropathy.

MANAGEMENT

There are generally two forms: mild (can put topicals on all spots) and moderate-severe (can't put topicals on all spots). Scale is the first to improve,

DOI: 10.1201/9781003537946-2

9

then thickness, then redness (thus central clearing can be an initial sign of response).

For Mild, Localized

TCSs are the most effective; some patients can melt their psoriasis in 2 weeks. Ixekizumab (Taltz) and bimekizumab (Bimzelx) appear to be the fastest biologics for psoriasis and take ~4–6 weeks; infliximab (Remicade) takes 3 months to do what clobetasol does in 2–4 weeks. People think TCSs are less effective probably because patients don't adhere well.

Tachyphylaxis (the *more* they use TCSs, the less they work) is debatable; some people think it happens because patients develop mutant steroid receptors or have them downregulated, but a more likely explanation is that they just don't stay consistent (the *less* they use TCSs, the less they work).

Might consider tapinarof cream (Vtama) for patients who resist the idea of TCSs.

Scalp is local and quite resistant; some think it's due to scratching/ Koebnerization and poor penetration through thick skin, but patients scratch all their psoriasis lesions and their diseased skin has poor barrier function (and further, the scalp has comparable penetration to the axilla), so those reasons don't really make sense. A more probable explanation for the "resistance" seen in scalp psoriasis is poor adherence (hard to get patients to apply meds consistently in their hair).

Some experts will say something like: descale the scalp with regular shampoo or psoriasis scalp oil (applied 8 hours before shower), salicylic acid/urea + ointment, then apply vitamin D lotion + superpotent TCSs; if that's not effective after 8 weeks (quite a long time), combine with UVB, or anthralin, or tar.

Which is quite complicated . . . and trying to explain such a drawn-out/ long-term and complicated treatment ladder up front is like telling an alcoholic to quit drinking for the rest of their life—it's overwhelming and makes it seem insurmountable (vs. asking them to apply a medicine for just 3 days to see if it works [or asking an alcoholic to abstain for a day at a time]).

Probably most realistic to just do clobetasol in a vehicle they're willing to use, involve other people (particularly anal-attentive family members, such as spouses), let them know putting it on may sting and is a sign it's working, and have a follow-up of some kind in 3–7 days (such as a phone call or message).

Palms/soles (pustular psoriasis or keratoderma) are also resistant—acitretin might work but is expensive, and they must not get pregnant while on it and for 3 years after if they have any EtOH exposure, such as from drinking or using cough medicine (EtOH esterifies acitretin to etretinate [which stays in body for much longer]).

Localized resistant disease needs a localized solution (avoid changing systemic treatments [just improve the topical regimen; switching systemics risks the generalized disease becoming uncontrolled]).

Avoid scratching (Koebnerization); 1 flake off today is 20 flakes 2 weeks later.

For Severe, Generalized

Probably start with IL23s (unless want fastest-acting, which are IL17s, which seem associated with IBD [good for joints, not good for bowels]).

Secukinumab + brodalumab were tested in patients with IBD, and in both placebo controlled trial studies, the drug groups did worse; so pretty convincing they at least exacerbate IBD.

However, IL17s directly causing IBD is more debatable than most might make it seem. Some might think that IL17s only exacerbate existing, subclinical involvement; you could imagine a patient with sacroiliitis, been on TNFs for that, but also has canker sores or PG (possible occult IBD), and the question is this: What did they have before the IL17 for their joints/psoriasis? Probably pred, MTX, TNFs, maybe ustekinumab (Stelara), or even risankizumab (Skyrizi)—all of which treat IBD; but then they switch to an IL17 (which doesn't cover their IBD), and they later get diagnosed when their latent IBD becomes clinically apparent (in other words, gets diagnosed "in association with starting an IL17"). While in some ways this isn't an unreasonable explanation, at the end of the day, if a patient develops symptomatic IBD on a drug, it is going to seem to them that it caused the IBD, and they won't be happy about it.

A reasonable approach is to screen whether they're appropriate for IL17s. *Ask*: What joints? Is it axial vs. peripheral arthritis? Do they have canker sores? Do they get neutrophilic dermatoses? If yes to any of those, then would probably be more careful with 17s. Perhaps even more relevant for HS, though access to alternatives can be hard if they don't have coexistent IL23 indication diagnoses.

Be familiar with dosing schedules (patients appreciate the convenience of shots further spread out).

Non-Targeted Systemics

Apremilast (Otezla) objectively works well 30% of time, usually causes GI upset (frequently treatment-limiting); no lab monitoring. Patients' subjective improvement may exceed the objective benefit.

Deucravacitinib (Sotyktu) works 60% of time (2× better than apremilast); no GI intolerance, but risk of HSV reactivation. Maybe try if fail a bunch of biologics (probably not good as first-line).

When ordering shingles vaccine, need to mention patient going on immunosuppressive therapy; only approved for healthy adults down to age 50, but if on immunosuppressives, then goes down to age 18.

MTX is cheap and accessible.

For GPP and erythrodermic psoriasis: IM MTX preferred over PO because GI absorption impaired. If using IM MTX for GPP, don't do full dose at once (will solve it all at once and can cause ulcerations; could do something like 2.5 mg QoD until perfect, then 2.5 mg QW).

Acitretin is much more expensive than MTX (can be ~$2k per year) and has a longer post-treatment period, during which women must not get pregnant (3 years if they've had any EtOH exposures, such as alcoholic drinks or cough medicines), then MTX (3–6 months).

Can do erythromycin 250 mg QD for 1 y for strep-induced guttate psoriasis (same with strep-induced LCV, and probably for other skin consequences of strep-mediated immune happenings [can also do penicillin VK 500 mg BID]).

See Medications section in Chapter 4.

Non-Pharmacologic Options

Many dermatologists think tanning beds don't work. Possibly due to selection bias (in other words, if ten patients go to tanning bed and tanning beds have 80% response rate, eight will clear and two won't, but it's only the two nonresponders that end up in dermatologists' offices). Same reason specialists tend to think PCPs never know what they're doing, because they only send us the ones they can't manage themselves.

Tanning beds are mostly UVA. UVB is 100× more effective at clearing psoriasis on a per joule basis, but also 100× more effective at burning people on a per joule basis; so you can give 100× more joules of UVA and psoriasis should get better. Tanning beds standard bulb in USA is 5% UVB, which is a lot; if you give 1 J of UVA (a standard dose for PUVA, but probably give more in tanning bed), 5% of that is 50 mJ—(for context, many light-skinned patients start around 10 mJ)—so you can get a lot of UVB from tanning beds.

2.1.1.2 Pityriasiform

2.1.1.2.1 Pityriasis Rosea (PR)

One-third of the world gets PR once.

Herald spot can resemble PIH; active smaller oval lesions (vs. EAC, which also has trailing scale but more circular) should be along skin lines. Lesions are in various stages of evolution. Starts with a macule, then develops a pin-point-like scale in the center of the macule, which becomes a collarette that expands; when the collarette touches the edge of the macule, then it resolves.

Time is the best medicine—have to wait ~8 weeks to resolve. If takes way longer, re-think diagnosis. Erythromycin probably doesn't actually expedite resolution. Some people think if you get an "almost sunburn," it might make it go away quicker (could use a light box, but going out in the sun until they get a little pink is obviously cheaper for them [remind them to put sunscreen on their face]).

Can use Sarna Sensitive if gets itchy (can use 20× daily without side effects), or hydroxyzine (Atarax).

2.1.1.2.2 Pityriasis Rubra Pilaris (PRP)

Often present erythrodermic—tough to know if mimicker.

Should make conscious effort to rule out CTCL (which can have anything, such as islands of sparing).

Although nutmeg grater on back of hands (rare) is pathognomonic for PRP, folliculotropic MF can resemble nutmeg grater papules (albeit are usually smoother, more infiltrated plaques).

Nuances to distinguish from erythrodermic psoriasis:

- PRP scale is fine/powdery (like wheat bran; constantly flakes off—patient may describe as "dust storm"), mostly on face/scalp (vs. psoriasis-adherent scale that builds up thick before flakes off).

- Most PRP patients get palmoplantar keratoderma (PPK) early in disease (oddly strikingly fluorescent yellow hard layer of hyperkeratotic skin on palms/soles; extensive painful fissuring) vs. psoriasis PPK, which is not waxy and more dry, flaky palms.

Griffiths categories aren't validated for predicting likelihood for spontaneous resolution/response to treatment, but probably helpful for morphologic description.

- *Type 1:* Some misinterpret as bad seb derm in beginning. Many clear within 3 years (but probably designated in hindsight—in other words, people probably see it clear then call it typical PRP; and if it doesn't clear, then they call it atypical PRP). As PRP clears, can get an erythema gyratum repens–like rash (but EGR is migratory, spreading over weeks; resolving PRP is little more fixed—important to differentiate so don't waste a full paraneoplastic EGR work-up).

- *Type 2*: More ichthyosiform, eczematous, more alopecia, less waxy, and more coarse lamellated keratoderma; traditionally thought of as longer-lasting but doesn't seem to be predictive of disease course.

- *Type 3*: Classical juvenile—looks like type I, but usually not as bad; less often erythrodermic, lighter pink/orange salmon color, less coalescent; 50% clear in 6 months, many take a few years, some never clear.

- *Type 4*: Circumscribed juvenile; can start anytime in childhood, get localized plaques over bony prominences (elbows, knees, over Achilles); 50% remit after 1 year, 32% at 3 years.

- *Type 5*: Called atypical juvenile—original description was familial lifelong, possible contractures/sclerodactyly. May have seen patients with congenital ichthyosis; now more used to describe familial PRP (CARD14 genetic variation, thus better described CAPE—"CARD14-associated papulosquamous eruption"). Some look like classic psoriasis, classic PRP, atypical PRP, and a few may have sclerodactyly, thus confusing, because can have classic morphology. Responds nicely to ustekinumab.

- *Type 6*: HIV-associated PRP. All adults should be screened, but this is a rare association; only a few case reports. Can be in well-controlled or poorly controlled CD4 counts.

- *Wong-type DM*: Basically DM + PRP; biopsy follicular papules looks like PRP; biopsy poikilodermatous rash on chest/shoulders looks like DM; can be either classical or amyopathic DM; unclear cancer associations.

MANAGEMENT

Usually ramps up over a few months, followed by a slow, gradual resolution.

Although 50% adults and children have spontaneous resolution off treatment within 3 years (minimum few months), be cautious of selling this as a positive thing (patients are very debilitated—some cannot tolerate even wearing clothes, can't grip things [lose fingerprints], can't walk [pain]).

They may stop sweating during disease course (unclear if common to other erythroderma things), but sweat function returns as they recover (and can be a sign of treatment response).

Should probably screen for HIV if diagnosing PRP. Possible referrals:

- Flaky scale can build up in auditory canal and impair hearing; may need ENT.

- They can get rhinorrhea (maybe 2/2 increased blood flow to skin), hair loss; subjective (not inflammatory erosive) joint pain is common (70–80%).

- Consider podiatry referral for keratoderma/nail dystrophy.

- Can get ectropion if facial erythema prolonged (skin is taut and pulls down eyelid). Exposure of eyes can cause scarring keratitis over time; refer to ophtho if ectropion.

■ Similar to other derm diseases, screen for depression. PRP often not fatal, but patients do unfortunately commit suicide; consider referral to psych.

PHARMACOLOGIC

Most PRP patients need systemic treatment; topicals don't work well.

Prednisone also doesn't work well either (one of very few inflammatory skin diseases that doesn't respond to prednisone—thus a potential diagnostic clue).

Of accessible meds, first-line treatment is acitretin, MTX.

However, biologics are much better first-line options if patients can get them.

IL17s or IL23 probably in right pathway (can expect 2/3 roughly to respond); response much slower than in psoriasis (which is like 75% better at 8 weeks), so don't stop the biologic too early.

■ *Ixekizumab*—maybe 2/3 improve by 50% in 24 weeks

■ *Secukinumab*—roughly 2/3 improve by 50% at 28 weeks

■ *Guselkumab*—similar response at 24 weeks

These are on psoriasis dosing.

For getting prior auths, sometimes will carry a diagnosis of psoriasis–PRP overlap; can also try arguing that they have a lot of genetic overlap.

For PPK, can start acitretin to give a head start, since it's the last thing to resolve even with biologics. Isotretinoin might even be more effective and also good to start while waiting for biologics to start working.

Phototherapy NOT good for PRP and will make worse in almost all patients (80–90% are actually photosensitive; burning and redness get worse when in sunlight).

Topicals/adjuncts:

■ OK to give sleep aids—start hydroxyzine, gabapentin; can even go up to mirtazapine, trazadone, or even zolpidem, but not in combination.

■ Can apply non-stop greasy thick emollients (Aquaphor, CeraVe cream, etc.) to try to recreate skin barrier.

■ Sauna suits may help seal in humidity (hot suits on Amazon have somewhat stylish options)—can wear day and night.

■ Urea cream for hands/feet.

■ Scuba socks—basically cushion and occlusion (vs. having to walk around with Saran Wrap), affordable.

■ DuoDERM for fissuring (cut into strips and wrap over fingers, cover all sides of feet).

2.1.1.2.3 *Pityriasis Versicolor*

Red, white, or brown, sometimes scaly.

Common, especially in active patients (more sweaty). Not due to poor hygiene. Usually not itchy.

KOH spaghetti and meatballs.

Many treatments, but culprit yeast is part of normal flora, so if killed, is really only temporary.

Skin won't be perfect for 3 months after killing the yeast.

Few options:

- Ketoconazole shampoo QD as bodywash (or alternate with OTC Selsun Blue or Head & Shoulders shampoo as bodywash). Let sit on skin for a few minutes before rinsing off.

- Can prescribe clotrimazole cream if they prefer.

- Fluconazole 150–300 mg QW for 1–4 weeks.

- Itraconazole 200 mg QD for 5–7 days (check LFTs).

2.1.1.2.4 Pityriasis Amiantacea

Like a cement that grabs hair.

Can be residual from having had cradle cap or in association with psoriasis, seb derm, AD, tinea capitis, and so on.

For young kids, ddx: of course Langerhans cell histiocytosis (LCH), cradle cap (if first few months of life), seb derm usually in puberty or older.

Can recommend OTC Dermasolve Psoriasis & Seborrheic Dermatitis Scalp Oil (from Amazon) to dissolve crusty plaques—leave on overnight, then wash with shampoo in AM.

After mostly dissolved, can treat inflammation with TCSs.

2.1.1.2.5 Pityriasis Lichenoides et Varioliformis Acuta (PLEVA) and Pityriasis Lichenoides Chronica (PLC) and Lymphomatoid Papulosis (LyP)

Benign T-cell lymphoproliferative disorder.

The spectrum (purely lymphocytic) includes PLEVA, PLC, LyP. Odd and fascinating continuum of illnesses.

PLEVA (acute):

- Somewhat bizarre disorder; not a vasculitis, but histologically almost essentially is (has an intense perivascular disease that makes RBCs extravasate), and also has a psoriasiform epidermis and apoptosis; so it crosses a lot of the disease spectrum. Some even say PR is the acute exanthematous form (though doesn't really seem like it [I saw a patient with biopsy-proven PLEVA who was tapering MTX, they came in because they thought they were "flaring" after a viral infection but actually had PR which self-resolved and the PLEVA never came back, so sort of goes against it being the same thing]).

- PLEVA is characterized clinically by recurrent red/brown papules, commonly ulcerated/crusted/vesicular, sometimes hemorrhagic.

- Self-resolves (leaves scars) and recurs on/off, lasts 1–3 years (more diffuse actually predicts shorter disease lifespan).

- Severe variant = febrile ulceronecrotic PLEVA—can clinically resemble entities on SCARs ddx. Can have GI/pulm/CNS involvement.

- PLC (chronic) has less crusty/vesicular/pustular and more scaly papules. Instead of scars, typically leaves hypopigmentation.

Management (typically initiate systemic treatment if symptomatic, if getting new lesions, if lesions are scaly/red, if flaring often):

- MTX typically to reduce flares to limit PLEVA scars and to give PLC a chance to resolve/remodel the color (usually melts PLEVA better than PLC; PLC might need concomitant phototherapy). Can do prednisone if severe.

- Wound care for ulcerations.

- There are also reports of anti-inflammatory antibiotics (tetracyclines, macrolides) being used.

LyP is a pure monoclonal colony of CD30+ cells, supposedly a marker of hematologic malignancy (probably is a marker but seems overstated [not the 20% the books say] because they don't necessarily get CD30+ lymphomas; they can obviously get CTCL, but also Hodgkin's disease, B-cell lymphoma so it's somewhat of an odd illness). It's probably a marker for a slight increased tendency to get lymphomas, but the lesions themselves are not malignant (in other words, in the LyP patients that get CTCL, it's not like the LyP lesions spill over and become CTCL; they're separate).

As an aside, small vs. large plaque parapsoriasis has a similar confusing relationship with CTCL that's honed in on and made somewhat confusing. Basically, there is true small plaque parapsoriasis (super rare; yellow digitate plaques/patches on trunk; never goes into CTCL), and there's "large plaque parapsoriasis," which is just CTCL from the beginning (large poikilodermatous CTCL patches).

2.1.1.3 Lichenoid

MMF/MTX good for undifferentiated lichenoid processes. JAKis may also make sense, since lichenoid interface stuff is heavily enriched with interferon signatures (activating JAK-STAT to destroy stuff at basal layer).

2.1.1.3.1 Lichen Planus (LP)

Common, but no on-label treatments.

Oral LP more common than skin LP (4% vs. 1% incidence), probably because dentists diagnose OLP and skin LP doesn't really require routine clinical inputs.

Skin LP:

- Several clinical variants. Characteristically itchy. Koebnerizes.

- Classic skin LP lasts ~1 year (vs. mouth + nails, which go longer); 50% get it back.

- If localized and recalcitrant or generalized, can consider MMF or MTX. **FYI**: Phototherapy doesn't tend to work very well (takes an average of 80 treatments vs. 36 treatments to clear psoriasis).

- For patients who self-resolve but later develop a restless epithelium (continually sprout KAs, etc.) (particularly chronic hypertrophic LP), can do acitretin—usually the small ones go away (acitretin protects against NMSCs because normalizes keratinocytes—used in transplant patients); for the remaining ones, can inject 5-FU, and if some are resistant/big, can do Mohs.

- **FYI**: Drug-induced LP not the same thing as a lichenoid drug reaction (which can occur months to years after culprit initiation).

Oral LP:

- Lasts 5–10 to 30–40 years.

- Doesn't really need DIF, but if you get it, needs to be lesional.

- About 50% of OLP patients have genital LP (so ask/look).

- First goal is no cancer; 7% of OLP patients get SCC supposedly but can prevent that by not allowing chronic erosions (always look/ask about erosions).

- Second goal is no teeth loss; look for gingival retraction.

- Can try TCSs first, such as Lidex gel (might have a bitter taste, but some patients get used to it). Should blot the area dry, then put the TCSs on (slides over wet mucosa; adheres to dry mucosa).

- Can also do ILK (more well tolerated if do on mucosa not attached to bone— such as the cheek—in contrast to attached mucosa, such as the gums).

- MTX and MMF are good systemic options. If have to use steroids, be aware that sometimes, when tapering them to 10 or 5 mg QD, patients develop canker sores (even when haven't had them since were kids; same thing happens in MMP + paraneoplastic pemphigus).

- Can always do tacrolimus swish/spit (see DIY section in Chapter 4).

Nail LP:

- Pterygium (when skin grows to nail bed) important to know about because can be a sign of scarring (vs. matrix streaking + pitting, which is OK and usually just cosmetic); nails will resolve eventually but don't want to scar.

- Tough to treat. ILK may be best but very painful. Systemics don't seem to work well, although acitretin may be better than MTX/MMF/HCQ. Like other nail disorders, have to address the inflammation/problem and then wait ~12 months +/– ~6 months to appreciate its impact or lack thereof.

Scalp LP (LPP)—see Hair section.

2.1.2 Eczematous

Eczema and *dermatitis* are synonymous ("eczematous dermatitis" is redundant).

Can be from outside (usually squares/triangles/checkmarks) or from inside (usually round borders).

From outside, eczema is a classic type 4 hypersensitivity reaction.

For example, ACD (85% of people are allergic to poison ivy). Langerhans cell processes an antigen, brings down to dermis, exposes to lymphocytes, which go to lymph node, recruit memory T-cells, then when re-exposed, lymphocytes go up and cause acute damage and spongiosis.

Another exogenous eczema is ICD (such as a diaper rash from leaving a stooly diaper on for too long—gets colonized with organisms).

From inside, eczema is due to cytokines. Includes intrinsic AD and many other IL4-responsive dermatoses: dyshidrotic eczema, nummular eczema, juvenile plantar dermatosis, asteatotic eczema (which are all essentially "AD not otherwise specified").

Important to distinguish from eczemas that are not IL4-responsive (ones that dupilumab won't work for): ACD, seb derm, and so on.

Staph is transient part of flora; if you check 100 people walking down the street, 25% will have staph; check again next week, a different 25% will have staph, etc. However, 97% of atopics have staph on their skin, and eczema skin is like fertilizer for infections (warts, styes—all it takes is rubbing their eye to get a stye), so give them 1 lb jar of SSD (to apply QW to body, face, eyelids). Apply TCSs in direction of hair follicles to prevent follicular colonization.

Look for areas of impetiginization/cellulitic change; may need antibiotics (for example, doxycycline).

Don't forget about true infectious stuff too on ddx. Dermatophytes/fungi can reside in stratum corneum and cause spongiosis like eczema (thus not surprising that tinea can clinically mimic eczema too, though it tends to be marginated with scale and superficial). Scabies living in the stratum corneum can also make eczematous changes.

Don't biopsy crusty old eczematous plaques if trying to differentiate AD vs. psoriasis; only reason to biopsy old plaques is if you're trying to rule out CTCL (or Hailey–Hailey, Darier's, etc.).

Although eczema has spongiosis (edema within and around epidermal cells) from lymphocytes that go up into the epidermis/produce damage and plaque psoriasis has neutrophils that go up into the epidermis and produce damage, chronic eczema looks psoriasiform, and the T-cell mixture in chronic eczema changes to mimic that of psoriasis. Thus, histology isn't helpful unless you have a virginal lesion (no therapy, no time to emerge and become psoriasiform).

Additionally, it's not unusual for the acral, inverse, erythrodermic, and guttate forms of psoriasis to have spongiosis (and typically lesions that are clinically straightforward are also histologically straightforward).

Because 10% of patients who present to PCPs have eczema, you can imagine how misleading biopsy reports can confuse non-dermatologists.

2.1.2.1 Acute vs. Subacute vs. Chronic

Eczema = edema in skin (spongiosis).

More acute = more pronounced spongiosis—correlates clinically:

- *Acute* (fluid so big makes blisters—such as poison ivy)

- *Subacute* (weepy because microvesicles go to surface and leak to make crust—such as stasis derm)

- *Chronic* (looks like tree bark—such as LSC)

2.1.2.2 Intrinsic Atopic Dermatitis (AD)

Prototypical eczema. Very common in kids, less so in adults (can reassure children/parents that most kids will eventually outgrow it and thus won't need treatment forever). Tends to run in families. Sometimes associated with hay fever (AKA allergic rhinitis) and asthma (this tendency is called atopic diathesis), so it's good to ask about. Some of the systemics for AD (dupilumab, etc.) will make those conditions better too. Usually, you know AD when you see it, but try to make a conscious effort to rule out stuff like scabies as well (especially since patients often scratch/manipulate their skin/have tried various treatments, so it can be hard to tell what the original lesions looked like). If not totally sold on a diagnosis, can look for more subtle things, such as hyperlinear palms (associated with keratin anomalies, such as AD and ichthyosis vulgaris), pityriasis alba lesions, diffuse xerosis, coexistent KP, which can help support an AD diagnosis.

MANAGEMENT

Some patients are more concerned with the discoloration, so explain that they must control eczema to control the post-inflammatory discoloration (or pityriasis alba, which is basically mild eczema) and that the sun doesn't tan eczema skin.

Patients may fear topical steroids, but patients must know that AD will never go away with moisturizers only. Can frame it as this: "TCSs are safe, eczema is not (magnet for staph germs, etc.)," or something. You might see patients referred for concern for TCS overuse due to hypopigmentation (particularly in skin of color), but it's usually just resolved eczema with post-inflammatory hypopigmentation (should still obviously look for striae, telangiectasias, and clarify how they were applying the TCSs and for how long). If it's just post-inflammatory hypopigmentation, you can basically say the factory sends color to 20 skin cells at a time, but if there is inflammation present, then the cells won't accept the color and it stays white. ILK has much more of a tendency to cause hypopigmentation in comparison to TCSs.

Worth reiterating here that a 30 g tube covers an adult only once (half-sized adult twice, quarter-sized adult 4×). No matter how small a person, an atopic isn't going to get better with one 30 g tube. Give them a 1 lb (454 g) jar for the body, 60 g tube for face. Ask if they prefer an ointment (like a Vaseline) vs. cream; most people prefer creams.

Example starter treatment program for mild AD:

1. TCSs for the inflammation—need constant regimen, avoid ups/downs in therapy.
   a. Mindful of site and amount needed—see TCSs section in Chapter 1.
      i. Hydrocortisone for face.
      ii. TAC for body (emphasize never to face).
      iii. Clobetasol for thickest/most resistant lesions (emphasize never apply to face/armpits/genitals/groin).
2. SSD cream QW–QD to prevent secondary impetiginization, styes.
3. Ceramide-containing moisturizer (CeraVe) QD in winter after bath.
   a. Regular moisturizers without ceramide (for example, Eucerin, Aquaphor) only improve barrier function for 1 hour (and that's just in dry skin, vs. inflammatory eczema, which is probably even less).
   b. Applying when skin damp is more effective because skin more absorbent in damp state.
4. Cool mist vaporizer

Consider systemics if more severe/extensive.

Never give prednisone to atopics (it's a 2-week solution for a chronic process); develop plan that matches duration of problem.

1. Dupilumab is a miracle drug; 85% of patients are 95% better in 8 weeks and super safe.
   a. No lab monitoring.
   b. Can follow Q 1 year if stable, basically just for prior auth renewal (some insurances are only doing 6 months at a time now, though).
   c. Failure if no response after 12 weeks.
      i. If people get worse with dupilumab, reconsider diagnosis (possible Th1 pathway stuff, like psoriasis, scabies, CTCL, which of course is often misdiagnosed as eczema early on).
   d. Doses seem low for children; adults tend to be perfect on adult dose. Kids usually need concomitant TCSs; dosing changes at age 6 (so know their weight).
      i. Dupilumab is an antibody, so overdosing doesn't matter as much because the antibody just gets chewed up (vs. meds like MTX that need kidneys to pee out, etc.); so just get the higher dose approved if you can.

e. If they recently discontinued dupilumab and aren't sure if they need it anymore, probably won't be able to tell for 8 weeks post-discontinuation whether they need it to maintain stability or not.

If they fail dupilumab, you can try JAKis (upadacitinib, abrocitinib). They do tend to pretty consistently clear with JAKis, but probably not as favorable because they're not targeted therapies like dupilumab and tralokinumab. Have to wonder about durability of responses and long-term safety. Should give Valtrex prophylaxis (eczema herpeticum risk).

Thick lesions take 3 months to thin; discoloration takes 1 year to normalize.

Hands tend to be worse in summer, but if patient struggles with flares in winter and also uses inhaler, consider dupilumab. Hand AD needs to be perfect for 3 months to remain perfect.

Warn them they may flare in winter (cold air doesn't carry water well).

2.1.2.3 Contact Dermatitis

Patients often refuse to believe that something they're applying is causing the rash (often will say they've been applying it forever without issue). While the cause may be unclear, there are several plausible explanations worth mentioning. Somehow an immune switch may have just gotten turned on (explain that our bodies change as we age). Manufacturers occasionally change ingredients (and of course don't tell anyone). Possibly also was allergic to something the whole time and it just became clinically apparent after repeated exposures.

Detergent being the culprit of contact derm is probably overstated; more often, the culprits are OTC lotions with parabens, etc. Always ask what they're putting on their skin. Both active and inactive ingredients are relevant. Explain "natural," "essential," "clean," are marketing terms; poison ivy is also "natural." Good place to start is to remove fragrances, things with propylene glycol, parabens, methylisothiazolinone (common culprits).

Terrible things:

- Cocoa/shea butter (has fragrances); the soapy feeling is from chemical additives.
- Oils—first they sooth, then they itch.

Safer options:

- CeraVe hydrating facial cleanser, Vanicream bodywash.
- Aquaphor or Vaseline is thick; CeraVe cream is thinner.

If suspect contact derm from eye drops, look below the nose (would go down through the nasolacrimal duct); if just confined to the eyes, then probably external contactant vs. something that goes directly into the eyes like drops. *FYI*: A lot of topical meds are fine to use past their expiration date, but old eye drops can be dangerous (*Pseudomonas* and *Aeromonas* love old aqueous solutions).

FYI: Prednisone tapers are terrible for contact derm; poison ivy clears in 14–18 days without treatment but with roller coaster from prednisone can last 3–4 months.

2.1.2.3.1 Allergic Contact Dermatitis (ACD)

About 20% of contact derms, type 4 hypersensitivity reaction (1–2 days after contact; thus, patients often at a loss for what it is).

And 6% of people who use Neosporin below the waist are allergic. (Thus, tell them not to use it. It's so old and frequently used that it's not even good against bacteria anyway. Use SSD if they have wounds.)

Most other allergens are 1/1,000 or 1/5,000 (topical Benadryl, topical -caines, nickel [ear piercings])—uncommon, but enough that you'll see these antigens cause issues.

Really have to stay up-to-date with contactants/irritants/allergens because the stuff manufacturers use in their products is always changing. In general, think about perfumes, makeup, soaps, shampoos/conditioners, hair dyes, sunscreens, moisturizers, essential oils, candles/humidifiers, lip balms, recreational activities (such as sports, helmets, goggles, gloves), occupation, etc.

Consider TCS-induced ACD (if looks like rash spreading beyond first rash).

MANAGEMENT

Set expectations; although the dogma (and board answer) is that ACD's lifespan is only ~3 weeks, recovery for ACD in practice seems much slower—often will take multiple months to clear (due to the resident memory T-cells hanging out in skin, waiting to cause problems). The meds are trying to quiesce the immune response to the allergen, so if can avoid the allergen, hope for ~30–50% improvement at 3 months; ups/downs are likely, but as long as overall trajectory is improvement, then you're on right track.

Look up cross-reactivities for TCSs—may have to adjust to a TCS you're not as familiar with.

Consider patch test—gives list of things with the contactant in it and list of alternatives. While it's the best test we have for detecting sensitivities to materials, it's not perfect, because the adhesives can cause irritation.

Usually best if the patient does the patch test at a dermatology office. The issue with referring to allergy is that they train for type 1 hypersensitivity reactions (RAS blood tests, things that cause asthma and hay fever, etc., and the way they patch test is only 45% predictive of contact derm).

FYI: You don't want to do patch testing in an atopic who is not clear (IgE levels may be elevated; thus, serum IgE and skin prick test [atopy patch] may not be reliable). This is of course different thinking than biopsy (when it's ideal for the disease to be flaring). And even if patients do come in with a clear back, they can still have reactions that are so big that it makes neighboring patches light up falsely (thus can't necessarily strongly believe a patient is positive for all allergens in a particular area).

Informal self-usage tests can be a practical, easy way to get started toward getting an answer—basically tell them to put small amounts of stuff they use (soaps, for instance) on arms twice daily and see if they react; if not, then it's safe.

Ask patient to send you picture of ingredients of culprits.

If the patient is absolutely miserable before patch testing and needs some sort of treatment: Can put on a low dose of MMF or MTX as long as they stop taking it a few days before the patch test is performed (albeit it's not really established whether MMF or MTX interferes with patch test results). Basically want to do the lowest possible dose to clear their back. We know prednisone up to 10 mg QD does not interfere with results, but you should avoid prednisone for contact derm. Would also avoid CsA. Although dupilumab doesn't cause false negatives (according to papers), remember that dupilumab doesn't work for contact derm so it would only really help if they have underlying endogenous AD (ask if skin is irritable/itchy in winter/summer). Definitely worthwhile to think about coexistent underlying endogenous AD if you find out what the cause is and they're still not cured.

2.1.2.3.2 Irritant Contact Dermatitis (ICD)

Around 80% of contact derms are not a hypersensitivity reaction, thus quicker onset than ACD, because basically an injury to skin vs. immunologic (irritants alter skin permeability, allowing them to penetrate and injure the skin faster than it can repair itself).

Can be acute (potentially a severe single exposure) or chronic (potentially a mild but repetitive/cumulative exposure).

Burning, pain > itchy (particularly early).

Susceptible people: Pre-existing skin conditions (AD, etc.), occupational/ environmental exposures (usually soaps, hand sanitizers, detergents, acids, sweating, tooth whitener gel/cinnamon products). Contributory things can be subtle (baby wipes, lotions applying on their child, and so on).

- Meds can also cause ICD (tretinoin, BPO). Consider possibility of developing ICD after trying OTC stuff for a separate rash.

- Less likely to spread than ACD.

- Can't test for irritants (only true allergens). But patch testing can obviously help distinguish from ACD (which tends to stay around vs. ICD, which usually resolves quickly—although they can obviously coexist).

- Consider KOH to rule out tinea.

MANAGEMENT

Trial avoidance (clean up personal care regimen—see Section 2.3 on sensitive skin and skin care). Wear cotton gloves (can sleep with them; will help with friction).

Site-appropriate TCSs and emollients (TCSs after showering and before emollient).

TCS taper example: QD for 1–2 weeks, then QoD for 1–2 weeks, then QW for 1–2 weeks, then off.

Could also do TCIs, but will probably sting.

Eucerin Advanced Repair (despite the name) can also burn and sting (Eucerin Eczema Relief seems to be better).

Consider short course of doxycycline if patient has prominent fissuring.

2.1.2.4 Seborrheic Dermatitis

Allergy to *Pityrosporum* yeast that lives in oil glands.

Chronic without cure, so prevent and treat flares. Usually a lifelong tendency; worse with puberty due to hormones/genetics.

If they're old enough to have acne, they're old enough for seb derm. Be suspicious if from 3 months to puberty; oil glands likely not big enough (consider scalp AD if itchy).

If the seb derm scale is markedly impressive, make conscious effort to rule out psoriasis.

Sometimes patients can be concerned because it can resemble lupus rash if it affects malar cheek area (can ddx because DLE almost always has scarring after and is much less responsive to treatment than seb derm).

Acknowledge that ketoconazole is a lousy shampoo for hair; must put on scalp/face (tell patients when getting into shower, apply first, then let sit, do rest of shower, then wash out at end and use shampoo as they normally do). We only use the shampoo because the foam costs $900. Hopefully, Zoryve will be accessible by time you read this.

Ketoconazole is only prophylaxis—it kills yeast which drives reaction; need TCSs once reaction breaks out (for example, Derma-Smoothe oil 3–4× weekly for scalp, clobetasol or Lidex solution 3–4× weekly if severe; betamethasone lotion less stingy than Lidex solution).

Can do ILK if very itchy.

When local treatment inadequate, low-dose MTX for 6 months + Derma-Smoothe oil 3–4× weekly (to lift scale); can also try zinc-containing shampoo.

Additional skin-of-color considerations (see more in the Hair section):

Ketoconazole shampoo more than 2× weekly will break hair—especially in Black females. If the condition is mild and skin of color, can recommend OTC KeraCare Dry & Itchy or Head & Shoulders for textured hair.

Sometimes patients on topical minoxidil have dried-up residue that resembles seb derm scale; you can switch to PO minoxidil (no significant difference between topical + PO vs. PO alone).

Occasionally can pulse fluconazole, but for seb derm, patients benefit from QW washing, especially if mod to severe.

2.1.2.5 *Intertrigo*

Friction (thus predilection for body folds) -> eczematous eruption -> more perspiration -> more yeast. Thus, need to kill yeast on top of rash and address inflammation from friction.

Psoriasis and intertrigo harder to treat when the other exists (remember, Koebnerization is not just scratching).

TAC:SSD is a good regimen (SSD kills everything and has activity against yeast and bacteria which inevitably colonize the folds). Some pharmacies compound TAC:SSD, but if they don't, you can do TAC 0.025% cream QD PRN when inflamed and SSD up to QD.

Ddx inverse psoriasis (if no response to TAC:SSD, consider biologic), axillary granular parakeratosis (can give glycopyrrolate 2 mg BID on days expecting to sweat).

OTC options:

- Interdry AG (silver fabric, addresses moisture, friction, bacteria, fungus)— apply daily, hang, and let dry at night and wash.
- Zeasorb Antifungal Treatment Powder.

2.1.2.6 *Dyshidrotic*

One of the ~9 types of hand eczema.

Often also referred to as pompholyx (though some people separate dyshidrosis and pompholyx since can see dyshidrosis as part of ACD or hand AD, whereas actual pompholyx [larger bullous lesions that last 7–10 days then go away] is quite rare).

When hand barrier is broken, need to achieve perfect and maintain perfect for 3 months (because hands are in stuff every day, and the stuff that enhances penetration [propylene glycol—often used for thick acral surfaces] also impedes barrier repair [competing issues]).

2.1.2.7 *Periorificial*

Not just around the mouth (second most commonly around the eyes).

Sometimes had some rash slightly before and then put whatever they had at home on and get this.

Sometimes peds patients with inhalers get this (from steroid mist).

Hard to treat, and if you incompletely treat, it will come back (so need to treat persistently). Behavior and management approach reminiscent of rosaceas.
If age <7 years, PO erythromycin 225 mg BID for 3 months.
If age >7 years, PO doxycycline 100 mg BID for 3 months (some people's cutoff is 11 years).
Discontinue/taper TCSs if were on them.
Metrogel fine.

2.1.2.8 Eyelid/Orbital

Should apply TCSs + SSD for orbital eczema because easily colonized with staph (can get styes).
Patients may fear putting TCSs on eyelids, but there's never been a report of increased intraocular pressure from TCSs on eyelids (reassure patients that ophtho uses drops 1000× stronger [which go directly onto the eye] for corneal transplants).
Advise patients to wash only with fingertips with gentle wash (for example, Vanicream facial cleanser or Cetaphil liquid cleanser). Splash to rinse and pat dry.
Apply moisturizing cream (CeraVe or Vanicream) or ointment like Vaseline (especially at night). Apply thin layer of TCSs QD–BID after moisturizing.
Avoid touching face during day.
Do not scrub/pick/peel dry skin. Will prevent healing + worsen rash.

2.1.2.9 Ear

- Inside conchal bowl crusty stuff: fluocinolone oil QoD.

- If no response, can consider MTX or dupilumab.

2.1.2.10 Areolar

- Can be challenging to treat, especially when severe.

- Be careful with TCSs; use weaker TCSs or alternate with Vaselines. Avoid stuff like AmLactin.

- Apply TCSs only to red area and taper; something like BID for 2 weeks, then QoD for 1 week, then stop.

- When tapering, add in a substitute (for example, Cetaphil cream [not lotion]).

- Avoid lacy bras with seams (smooth bras are better); avoid scratching/ rubbing/scrubbing.

2.1.2.11 Asteatotic (Eczema Craquelé)

- Usually on older patients' legs (oil glands decrease over time so tend to have dryer skin). Can occur with PO retinoids, too.

- Superficially fissured "cracks."

- Prefer ointments; probably doesn't need super high-potent TCS if patient moisturizes aggressively (emphasize moisturization over TCS strength).

2.1.2.12 Stasis Dermatitis

Compression hose 15–20 mmHg are fine if higher mmHg are too hard to get on (consistency is key, and adherence is an issue with compression stockings too). *FYI*: Compression hoses are most important to wear during the day (when standing, etc.).

FYI: Unna boots are roughly 35 mmHg, so you need to be careful about those if ABI is low. However, ABI is somewhat of an irrational reference (could have a brachial artery pressure of 180 and an ankle pressure of 90 [in other words, ABI is 0.5], but with an ankle pressure of 90, there's no way you're going to collapse their arterial perfusion with 40 mmHg compression garments). Nonetheless, the ABIs are what the guidelines reference. Some people think high-compression hose improves arterial flow no matter what their pressures are because they pinch off feeder vessels, but in general should still be at least cognizant of these things (obviously, don't use high-compression stuff in someone with critical limb ischemia or something). Probably should leave at least 20–30 mmHg difference between compression strength and arterial pressures. Technically supposed to palpate a pulse (to ensure adequate flow) and do ultrasound to rule out clots before using.

TAC 0.1% cream QD PRN when itchy.

2.1.2.13 Lichen Simplex Chronicus (LSC) and Prurigo Nodularis (PN)

Taught by many as related to neurodermatitis (making an eczematous eruption by scratching or picking), which isn't really true; it's just a sign they itch.

Most appropriately framed as PN in the setting of a particular underlying condition, not just primary prurigo nodules.

Ultimate job = find out why itchy (see Section 2.1.11 on undifferentiated pruritus).

If in context of AD, treat AD (not just the lichenification of the PN).

- *Other causes*: lymphoma, renal failure, thyroid disease, L4/L5 L5/S1 neurogenic itch (positional, worse at night, has pins/needles), red bag syndrome (red itchy testicles 2/2 caudal neuropathy), Morgellons (a low-grade delusional state), and so on.

Even though dupilumab is FDA-approved for PN, it likely doesn't make sense if the PN is in setting of some of the non-AD causes earlier.

FYI: Sometimes insurance wants you to count number of nodules and document an itch score (can say TNTC or 20+ nodules or something).

If itch is idiopathic and can't target therapy at a specific underlying cause:

1. Phototherapy is usually a good option—but it costs a couple hundred dollars yearly; may take ~20 treatments to know whether they're working (usually TIW).

2. Thalidomide also a great option.

3. Some patients like Dermeleve (non-steroidal OTC topical option).

Ddx EMPD (usually itchy, can resemble LSC)—can treat EMPD with 5-FU 3–4× weekly for 6 months; ~60% clear, but even Mohs is only ~80%.

2.1.3 Vesiculobullous

Knowing the layers/antigens is mostly good for exams, but they can help you understand the diseases too. A notable layer is the lamina densa (last frontier of epidermis)—if go below, this will have scarring disease; however, if BP (lamina lucida) gets scratched at and/or infected, it can leave milia/scars too (in other words, seeing that stuff doesn't necessarily make it EBA).

For blistering disorders, ask about ENT/eye symptoms. Look in mouth and at conjunctiva.

I don't cover paraneoplastic pemphigus, but if you encounter clinical-pathologic discrepancy (such as if clinically looks like BP and path suggestive of pemphigus or something), think about paraneoplastic pemphigus (has several morphologic subtypes).

2.1.3.1 *Bullous Pemphigoid (BP)*

Prototypical type 2 hypersensitivity reaction (antibody-mediated process, linear deposits).

Almost invariably itchy (sometimes it's only pruritus, though characteristically has prodromal urticarial plaques).

Urticarial stage usually lasts weeks to months (so if receive a referral for 5-year-long urticarial BP, suspect a different diagnosis).

DIAGNOSIS

■ The main tests to know are DIF, IIF, and ELISA.

■ Usually want to use DIF. Can use IIF to improve detection of DIF negative non-bullous BP.

■ ELISA (looking specifically for NC16A domain of BP180 [which not all patients target]) doesn't help diagnose but can help with disease monitoring (though don't have to use it to monitor disease—usually doesn't impact management decisions).

■ So basically DIF or IIF is typically better than ELISA for diagnosing BP. ELISA is less sensitive, and patients can target other domains. Patients who target BP230 can be negative for DIF, be positive for IIF and ELISA BP230, and have a tendency to form non-bullous lesions.

■ DIFs should be obtained from lesional skin if no bullae; if there are blisters, then get DIF on perilesional erythema (avoid the blister for DIF; proteases in serum degrade the immunoreactants).

Always remember that false-positives are still possible with DIFs. A patient with stasis bullae could have some discontinuous C3 and fibrin at DEJ, and outside path report might say (+) DIF for instance. Thus, if a patient presents with anasarca, it gets worse with prednisone (edema), then be suspicious of stasis bullae even if has a "(+) DIF."

MANAGEMENT

For mild/localized disease (<30 blisters, <30% BSA, or BPDAI score):

■ Potent TCSs, doxycycline, RTC 6 weeks.

■ Doxycycline takes 6 weeks to work, but even if it does work, they have to stay on it (doesn't impact antibody production—only inflammatory mediators).

■ No high-quality evidence for niacinamide; could use if patient is in nursing home, bedbound, and can't sit up to take doxycycline.

If refractory and/or mod to severe:

■ Prednisone 0.5 mg/kg/day for moderate (1 mg/kg/day for severe BP) + steroid-sparing agent (MTX > MMF >>> AZA).

■ Even though you may be tempted to just give everyone 1 mg/kg/day, the difference is relevant for side effects, so try to use minimum effective dose (as always).

■ Use BPDAI scoring if not sure (usually if on fence between mod and severe).

Goal taper for prednisone is <10 mg/kg/day within 3–6 months; continue that low dose for another 3–6 months (total time on steroids 6–12 months).

So will want them to RTC Q 1 month; taper by ~10 mg/kg each month, then once below 10 mg/kg/day, have them stay on that and RTC in 3 months; if well controlled, then can stop the prednisone (continue the steroid-sparing agent).

MTX works pretty fast in BP—about 4 weeks (vs. 8–12 weeks for papulo-squamous disorders); safe in elderly unless has poor (or fluctuating/unreliably measured) kidney function, then can do MMF (which is less-effective than MTX). AZA is worst (least effective, most side effects).

For refractory disease, you should consider what patient's priority is:

- *Rituximab*: best if want complete remission; expensive (but so are a lot of office visits, morbidity from long-term pred, etc.)
  - Slowest, takes 3–6 months to see full effect.
- *Dupilumab*: safe and quick (improves within a few weeks), helps with itch, probably won't clear.
  - Suppresses inflammation and antibody production too; can yield quicker steroid tapers and result in lower relapse rates (than SCSs alone).
  - Makes sense if you have an older patient (with short life expectancy) with persistent non-bullous disease who has failed pred, MTX, MMF, and whose main goal is to not be itchy.
- *Omalizumab*: worst relapse rates; not very convenient for patient: 300 mg Q 1 month for 6 months but needs in-office monitoring after taking; would only use if can't get either of the aforementioned (though usually harder to get prior auth for this than rituximab or dupilumab).

Look at med list for strongly associated drugs (*FYI*: Different from boards answers):

- *If started within past 6 months*: aldosterone antagonists, anticholinergics, or dopaminergic drugs.
- *If within last 1 year*: DPP-4 inhibitors (-gliptins), PD-1, and PDL-1 (long latency; can develop BP even after stopping an immune checkpoint inhibitor).
- *Less strongly associated*: thiazides, statins, beta-blockers, ACEis, ARBs; unclear if loop diuretics are (in other words, worthwhile to consider trialing a holiday from Lasix to see if it works, but the other ones probably fine to continue).

The meds might act as a hapten to modify BP180, leading to exposure of an antigenic site.

DPP-4-induced BP has good prognosis if discontinuing the med (doesn't usually require long-term treatment and oftentimes is localized so can usually just use TCSs + doxycycline).

Important to let patients with immune checkpoint inhibitor–induced BP know that it's actually a good sign (better anti-tumor response). Same with having a lichenoid drug reaction or developing vitiligo from immune checkpoint inhibitors.

Usually pretty severe, so do short course (<1 month) of prednisone, then switch to biologic long-term (can give rituximab Q 6 months if need to); OK to continue the immune checkpoint inhibitor throughout.

- Reason for only a short course of steroids is because they attenuate the anti-tumor response and of course have more long-term side effects (so essentially want to transition because biologically safer).

2.1.3.2 Pemphigus Vulgaris

Usually don't see active blisters because they're so soft (often pop and all you see are erosions).

Can be bad if caught late; used to have a 2% 5-year survival before prednisone!

DIAGNOSIS

Ideally, punch biopsy uninvolved (normal-looking) buccal mucosa for DIF.

ELISA is preferred diagnostic for PV and PF (different from BP). Highly sensitive.

Both Dsg1 and Dsg3 are excellent for diagnosis.

Dsg1 much better for monitoring disease than Dsg3.

People draw ELISA for Dsg1 at baseline, then 3 months after a rituximab cycle (the idea being to try to predict relapse).

Issue with using ELISA against Dsg3 for monitoring is it detects both pathogenic and non-pathogenic antibodies. Can use a more expensive specialized test, but really no need, because a positive test indicates higher risk of relapse and majority of pemphigus patients relapse at some point, anyway.

So if they're clinically remitted and have positive Dsg3, just tell the patient that the baseline expectation is relapse (and they're at increased risk for that) and there's no indication to restart treatment based on a positive lab test in an absence of symptoms/lesions. Of course, tell them to reach out if they flare. Relapses are usually more mild (destroying more of the B-cells that produce the problematic autoantibodies).

Women with longstanding disease tend to get mildly symptomatic gingival erosions (somewhat nonspecific) after finishing treatment, and ELISA can be undetectable (no antibodies circulating). Despite being mild in terms of symptoms, it is hard to treat. The reason is that they don't have CD20+ circulating B-cell clones anymore (can't eliminate with more rituximab); it's actually tissue-based memory B-cells that lead to coordinated production of the autoantibodies. Could technically use intralesional rituximab, but not really practical. Would discuss with patient if they want to treat (symptoms might be so mild they don't care enough to want to restart medicines).

Rituximab (FDA-approved for PV—and thankfully becoming more cost-efficient) up front allows for lower dose and shorter duration of SCSs. Important because some people perceive rituximab as something that's only reserved for refractory cases, etc., like other diseases such as BP. But it's actually the first thing you should reach for in PV.

- *Can use a scale to categorize severity of disease*: PDAI (uses different names, though; moderate, significant, and extensive [vs. mild, mod, severe]).

- *Systemic corticosteroid dosing*: 0.5 mg/kg/day for moderate and significant; 1 mg/kg/day for extensive.

  FYI: Supposed to use ideal body weight for dosing (not actual body weight). Should taper over 3–6 months.

  Rituximab 1 g at day 0 and 14, then two maintenance doses of 500 mg at months 6 and 12 (or at months 12 and 18) (reduces relapse risk by 40%). No evidence to continue maintenance dosing if asymptomatic.

The rationale for rituximab can be leveraged for basically any autoantibody mediated condition (it targets CD20 on memory B-cells that differentiate to plasma cells [which are CD20-] that make IgG); so dosing based on number of cells needed to impact—less in autoimmune disease (RA dosing) than lymphoma (lymphoma dosing). CD20 cells are depleted quickly, but don't clinically see responses until later, because antibody-secreting cells still have a half-life, and IgG itself has a half-life. This is why don't have to be super worried about depleting all antibodies and getting infections (because anti-body-secreting cells causing the disease have a much shorter half-life than the plasma cells that protect us against infections). Rituximab does its job in a few days, get results in a few weeks, and hopefully get remission in a few months.

Time to treat with rituximab—important for relapse risk (2% higher for every month delayed).

Rituximab > MMF >> AZA. MTX not great for PV.

So basically don't just use TCSs.

Moderate and extensive: prednisone + rituximab; taper prednisone over 3 months (dose depends on PDAI). If doesn't work, then do longer prednisone taper + MMF.

- *Remission*: three or fewer blisters that heal spontaneously in <1 month.

- *Relapse*: do another cycle of rituximab.

At increased risk for community-acquired pneumonia and higher risk for severe outcome with COVID, so should get vaccines. Rituximab has caveats to vaccines.

Shouldn't get live vaccines on rituximab (but probably won't be recommending any live vaccines in derm). Rituximab increases risk of HBV reactivation, so check for HBV infection before starting.

Should try to get vaccines 2 weeks before starting rituximab. Important to tell patients it's not because it's dangerous to get them; it's because you want the vaccines to work (don't want to deplete their naive B-cells before getting the vaccine; otherwise, they won't make the memory B-cells you want).

So optimally you would start the prednisone, give them a list of vaccines (single-dose ones are probably most feasible: pneumococcal [conjugate or polysaccharide or both—at baseline and boosters Q 5 years], influenza, COVID, VZV [at least the first dose]) to get that day, then tell them to RTC 2–4 weeks to start rituximab.

However, this may not be realistic. If have to, just start treatment and encourage them to get vaccines at month 5 (1 month before starting maintenance rituximab). Reason is that peripheral naive B-cells repopulate 5 months after rituximab.

Of course, some people will adamantly refuse vaccines, which is out of your control. Just make sure you at least counsel them on the preceding and document accordingly.

If they are hospitalized or something and they ask for med adjustments, can hold MMF, can switch prednisone to hydrocortisone (to keep the mineralocorticoid component, can't stop that cold turkey); rituximab can't stop because already done.

2.1.3.3 Pemphigus Foliaceus

Predominantly Dsg1 (skin lesions, typically no mucosal involvement). Thus, the antibodies in pregnancy are not as problematic, because baby skin is Dsg3-predominant (resembles mucosal skin more).

Seborrheic distribution.

Uncommonly progresses to erythroderma.

Generally a benign pemphigus.

If mild, not extensive, and not progressing, can just use TCSs. If more severe/active, can follow the pemphigus vulgaris treatment ladder. Overall treat more like lupus than DM in the sense that it's more chronic (don't give systemic steroids unless absolutely have to).

2.1.3.4 Mucous Membrane (Cicatricial) Pemphigoid (MMP)

Named MMP (vs. cicatricial) because there are more publications about it affecting mucous membranes (even though a cicatrix [scar] is the hallmark of the disease and it can, of course, involve cutaneous surfaces).

Painful.

Oral > ocular > skin (in terms of incidence).

Can affect internal mucosa (nose, larynx, pharynx, esophagus, genitals). So clearly threatens function/quality of life.

Oral:

- Bright-red erosions/ulcerations. Desquamative gingivitis.

- For DIF with oral lesions: get from perilesional mucosa (more so than uninvolved mucosa).

- Can also consider ELISA instead of DIF (dentists use swish/spit Decadron so might have better luck with ELISA).

Ocular:

- Ophtho doesn't biopsy the eyes (increased risk for scarring/progression, and DIFs are more commonly falsely negative for conjunctiva than mouth), so they clinically diagnose it. You can co-manage with them, and when they do their slit-lamp exam, they can see the actual inflammatory cells in the eyes (really helpful for determining if disease is active). They also note findings (that you should honestly know too and be able to document accurately, like trichiasis, ectropion, symblepharon, ankyloblepharon) that help them stage the disease. Just like any other scarring disease, if you allow the inflammation to fibrose structures, will lead to permanent anatomic deformity/functional impairment. So need to catch early and keep the disease quiet.

Skin:

- Usually coexists with mucosal lesions.

- If predominantly skin-scarring (vs. mucosal), then may be Brunsting–Perry variant.

- Will often heal with scarring/milia.

MANAGEMENT

Control pain.

Consider other specialties to co-manage with (ENT, GI, dentists, ophtho, urology/OB-GYN).

- *Standard treatment ladder*: TCSs for mild localized lesions, dapsone/colchicine for mild to mod disease. Could make a case to just treat everyone with the more powerful systemics to optimize chances of limiting progression. MMF and MTX are great options, rituximab as well, cyclophosphamide/ IVIG if rapidly progressing. Can do short courses of concomitant systemic steroids if flaring as well, and continue the steroid-sparing agents to maintain remissions/quiescences.

2.1.3.5 Linear IgA Bullous Dermatosis (LABD)

Young children and adults. Idiopathic and drug-induced. May also be associated with IBD, RA, malignancy (but those things are so common and LABD isn't, so unclear how meaningful/relevant those really are).

Ask about vancomycin, NSAIDs, ACEis, antibiotics, lithium, AEDs.

Usually very itchy. String of pearls is from secondary vesiculation (so basically a big single bulla becomes eroded, then forms vesicles at the periphery). Remember, LABD is a subepidermal process (intact tense bullae); if the lesions appear more superficial (erosions/pustules), consider IgA pemphigus, which is intraepidermal (and is similarly an IgA process that has lesions on the periphery).

Prompt response to dapsone (prednisone, if needed). Could be clear of blisters within a couple of weeks (still with post-inflammatory discoloration).

See more in Chapter 3—part of SJS ddx.

2.1.3.6 Bullous Arthropod Assault (Bug Bites and Stings)

Children > adults (adults become desensitized over time). Typically ankles. Breakfast/lunch/dinner pattern.

Itchy, sometimes painful/burning.

Can be from chiggers, fleas, mosquitos, mites, spiders, scabies, lice, bees, ants, etc.

Sterile blister fluid.

Patients with lymphoma more likely to get (can precede blood cancer diagnosis).

Management: Same as regular bug bites/stings. Can do TAC QD–BID for 2 weeks to lesions only (still never to face obviously). Or can use Sarna Sensitive or pramoxine spray for the itch. Better to avoid topical Benadryl/benzocaine—can cause contact derm.

2.1.3.7 Porphyria Cutanea Tarda (PCT)

Most common porphyria. Type 1 most common (sporadic, acquired; possibly from iron overload [such as hemochromatosis, including heterozygotes, which are quite common—roughly 1/50 people], EtOH, smoking, HCV, HIV).

Chronic, relapsing. Photosensitivity is delayed.

No red base because non-inflammatory bulla.

MANAGEMENT

Preventing flares is key (avoid EtOH, decrease iron-containing foods, stop smoking, etc.).

Can use HCQ 200 mg 2–3× weekly (*FYI*: It's different than other dosing for lupus). If can't tolerate, sometimes phlebotomy works. Treat HCV or HIV if present, obviously.

2.1.3.8 Dermatitis Herpetiformis

Very itchy. Chronic. Male > female, northern Europeans usually; 90% have gluten-sensitivity, but only 20% have GI symptoms. Ask about bloating/diarrhea and what they eat.

Some flare with iodides and NSAIDs.

DIAGNOSIS

Often eroded because vesicles are so thin and patients scratch them. But classically tense, taut, unilocular bulla; can affect acral surfaces.

For DIF: Go for normal-looking skin perilesionally (not perilesional erythema like for BP, etc.—because higher chance for degradation of immunoreactants closer to blisters).

Remember TTG3 deposited in skin—not a serum test.

MANAGEMENT

Gluten-free diet (decreases lymphoma risk; can lead to skin remission, but slow to do so).

Dapsone yields fast relief within days but can be a lifelong need (though gluten-free diet may decrease this need). Dapsone also doesn't impact lymphoma risk.

Don't refer to GI for small bowel biopsy unless has GI symptoms.

2.1.3.9 Hailey–Hailey

Autosomal dominant (complete penetrance, variable expressivity), intracellular calcium signaling issue.

Chronic. Waxes/wanes. Flares with heat, humidity, friction. Thus tends to affect body folds. Looks like blood-red tears in macerated tissue paper–looking skin.

No cure. Many treatments target exacerbating factors (Botox and glycopyrrolate target the hyperhidrosis/maceration), etc. Some use TCSs.

Systemic options conventionally used: MTX, MMF, acitretin; not sure if isotretinoin has been tried much but perhaps might help. Can also consider naltrexone 50 mg QD (debatable that low dose works, so probably should just use the addiction medicine doses; need to follow liver functions).

Some people also use lasers (ablation). Because follicular epithelium is rarely involved, if doing ablative therapy that destroys the entire surface epithelium (forces them to re-epithelialize from the follicles), can get sustained benefit. Wouldn't want to do something like Fraxel (which would only punch holes and leave lots of epithelium behind).

Can try topical cinacalcet (sensitizes calcium receptors).

JAKi probably not good because risks Kaposi's varicelliform eruption (AKA eczema herpeticum).

2.1.3.10 Grover's

Benign red (usually itchy) bumps on chest and back. Acquired. Usually older White males. May be related to heat/sweating, sun exposure, some meds, comorbid skin conditions, such as xerosis/AD.

Chronic. Waxes/wanes for years. Hard to treat.

Most people manage with TCSs (creams preferable to ointments because less occlusive). Can do topical vitamin D analogs on weekdays and TCSs on weekends.

MTX or systemic retinoids may be worth trying if patient non-responsive to topicals and desperate for solution. Dupilumab also reported.

2.1.4 Vascular

2.1.4.1 Urticaria

About 25% of kids get hives.

Circle a lesion; if goes away <24 hours, then it's urticaria (if > 24 hours, then it's not urticaria; clinical ddx: urticarial vasculitis, urticarial multiforme, urticarial phase of bullous pemphigoid—see those sections).

If truly urticaria and <6 weeks, then it's acute; if >6 weeks, then it's chronic.

- *Acute*: find the cause 60% of the time (40% don't because people breathe in different stuff, might eat the same foods with different ingredients, etc.).

- *Chronic*: find the cause 1% of the time (because usually autoimmune disease where you have direct activation of receptors on mast cells), and 60% of them have it on/off. Could be thyroid; consider checking TSH if have other signs/symptoms.

In both acute and chronic, should probably recommend not doing allergen tests because most likely never going to find the cause (and the results are not predictive, anyway). Only thing it does is make their insurance go up. Just tell them to keep a diary of what they did and what went into their system for the 24-hour before breakouts.

The only meds that can take red away from urticaria lesions are CsA + prednisone (which are obviously inappropriate for chronic urticaria because of their inevitable long-term side effects). Xolair (omalizumab) is useful, but not as miraculous as CsA + prednisone. Some patients also may not be destined to respond to Xolair (only a subset of chronic spontaneous urticaria patients are autoallergic; the others are autoantibody-mediated). A realistic goal is to make their lesions flat and not itch with antihistamines.

Can use combinations of antihistamines or do the French way and give four of same (Allegras, Claritins, or Zyrtecs).

Need around-the-clock suppression of H1 and H2.

Many providers use hydroxyzine (Atarax) for itch relief, but only works for 6 hours and makes sleepy. Cetirizine (Zyrtec) works 24 hours, but 18% get sleepy. Levocetirizine (Xyzal) (works 24 hours) and fexofenadine (Allegra) (works 12–24 hours) are more favorable because they don't cause sleepiness.

FYI: Benadryl isn't great because only has 6-hour half-life and is sedating for ~19 hours (makes patients groggy). Pepcid not great because blocks the feedback inhibition of a mast cell (H2 receptor); never use H2 blocker without H1 blocker.

- *Example regimen*: Allegra QAM, Xyzal QPM + 10 mg doxepin QHS (sedates for 6–8 hours—potent blocker of H1 and H2 on blood vessels [great because blocks what usually makes them dilate and leak]). Start doxepin at 10 mg QHS (at 150 mg, it is an antidepressant and can have cardiac effects. Shouldn't have those issues with derm doses [explain this to patients]; can go as high as 75 mg QHS). For context: 1 mg doxepin = 10 mg Zyrtec.

- *Avoid aspirin/NSAIDs*: will make urticaria worse because when they block cyclooxygenase, causes leukotriene shift, which exacerbates histamine reactions in 60% of patients.

While antihistamines address the inside, it is also worthwhile to recommend all free/clear, etc. (could be bedsheets, etc., and need to optimize avoidance of outside irritants).

Important to maintain consistency with meds even when clear (in other words, when lesions pop up, it's too late; emphasize antihistamines need to be IN the system when skin is irritated).

Sarna Sensitive (numbing medicine), nice because can use as much as desired, but only works for 30–45 minutes.

Other urticarias and dermatographia:

Dermatographia is a mast cell reaction to friction (scratching skin changes a protein; body is allergic to those proteins). Roughly 5% of people are dermatographic (back is most sensitive place to test for it). Dermatographia isn't a true physical urticaria unless it's symptomatic.

While symptomatic dermatographia is the most common physical urticaria, it can also be from exposures to heat, cold, sun, water, etc. These urticarias are IgE-mediated (can take blood from someone with symptomatic dermatographism and inject into a pig and inject blood from normal person into pig; scrape the pig skin and it welts up, but if you treat with anti-IgE, the ability to transfer it goes away, so presumably in physical urticaria you're allergic to a product that comes from physical stimulus).

Cholinergic urticaria (breaks out into hives without shortness of breath when gets in hot tub and starts perspiring—differentiates from exercise-induced anaphylaxis). If concerned may have exercise-induced urticaria or something, ask if they use pre-workout stimulants (some have a bunch of B vitamins that make them flush, etc.).

2.1.4.2 Vasculitis

Prototypical reactive dermatosis.

Can be limited to small vessels in skin or life-threatening organ involvement. Skin signs reflect the size of vessels affected.

See Chapter 3 for more.

2.1.4.2.1 Leukocytoclastic Vasculitis (LCV)/Cutaneous Small Vessel Vasculitis (CSVV)

"Palpable" purpura doesn't need to be papular (can just be indurated); to be honest, sometimes I don't really feel like it's that palpable but has a pretty distinct appearance.

Extracutaneous involvement is relatively uncommon in non-syndromic, idiopathic CSVV.

Skin-limited CSVV usually has 12-week lifespan: 50% never will have again, 50% get again over lifetime (possibly multiple decades later).

Significant proportion of young CSVV patients have strep-induced LCV (if [+], then prevent future strep infections with erythromycin 250 mg QD for 1 year. Same with strep-induced guttate psoriasis).

If it's viral-related, usually HCV. Don't forget about deep fungal (ask if been to Ohio River Valley for histoplasmosis). COVID and COVID vaccines can do it too.

AICTDs (usually Sjögren's, SLE, RA, juvenile DM), IBD, Behçet's, myelodysplastic malignancies, etc., can cause it as well, and vasculitis of the skin is the #1 predictor of systemic flare in SLE (because better than falling complement or rising dsDNA, you're actually seeing evidence of what could be occurring in kidney). Chemo tends to help LCV and lupus, but they do intermittent pulsing for cancer, so their LCV/lupus tends to become labile.

Lesions can become confluent and favor-dependent sites (for example, if hospitalized/bedbound, may be on their butt).

■ *Reason*: Your body's goal in a type 3 hypersensitivity reaction (where you have an antibody against a protein/antigen) is to get to a lymph node and destroy it.

Legs and dependent sites have gaps in post-capillary venules (endogenous histamine, etc.; other mediators are prevalent in dependent sites).

Circulating antibody-antigen complexes get stuck in those post-capillary venular gaps and do what they do (activate complement), which is very chemoattractive for neutrophils, which do what they do (release lysosomal enzymes), and the vessel wall is the innocent bystander.

Work-up (don't need all of it for all patients):

- Biopsy prove w/DIF (especially in kids to rule out HSP)
- Eval GI + GU: UA/stool guiac
- Eval for infection: anti-HCV, anti-DNAse B
- CBC, CMP
- RF/CCP, SSA/SSB, SPEP, ANA, c-ANCA

Ask about nervous system symptoms, pleura/pericardium (perhaps do EKG), joint symptoms (**FYI**: not an erosive arthritis when immune complexes deposit in joints).

Number of LCV spots is not always correlated with what is going on internally (so even if skin appears mild or moderate, usually worthwhile to do some work-up to make sure no residual systemic consequences).

While should ask about systemic signs/symptoms (and potentially do work-ups) every time the patient flares, should only do etiology tests ONCE (in other words, if you have patient with vasculitis who has four episodes a year, don't get four ANAs or HCVs); must separate tests you do for the extent of disease vs. tests for etiology.

Should biopsy lesions that are just starting to get purpuric for H&E; for DIF has to be earlier lesions because the LCV destroys the immune reactant; same with autoimmune bullous diseases because once have the full-blown histology, the immune reactants have already disappeared; that's why they say get the edge—see more in Pemphigoid section.

MANAGEMENT

TCSs typically aren't super helpful unless it's one or a few localized lesions and you don't want to escalate their systemics.

If it's just skin spots, you can probably do gradient support hose only; **FYI**: Pressure from socks doesn't induce lesions because the stockings, even if tight, are 30–40 mmHg (compared to normal BP 120/80); blood gets through to the heart fantastically (pressure on post-capillary venule is determined by how hard it is to push blood up to the heart, so if pushing it up with stockings, you actually are decompressing the leg). Additionally, CSVV causes lymphedema for some reason, so essentially all patients will do better with gradient hose.

If bothersome or joint pains can consider dapsone/colchicine; maybe MTX and slow taper prednisone for ulcerative spots; if renal disease perhaps IV methylprednisolone, pulsed cyclophosphamide, and so on.

Reminder about being careful about prednisone taper duration: can't be a 2-week taper (risk rebound—for instance, could go from small vessel to large vessel, non-ulcerating to ulcerating, no systemic to systemic, etc.); should be 8–12 weeks taper at least—come down slowly (for example, if lowest to achieve perfect is 30 mg QD, then start there and decrease by 5 mg per week until 20 mg QD, then decrease by 2.5 mg per week until off).

Obviously stabilize their underlying disease if they have one (such as IBD, RA, etc.).

The preceding pertains to regular LCV (not otherwise specified). But *small-vessel vasculitis* is a pretty umbrella term and encompasses some of the conditions that follow. Also includes cryoglobulinemic vasculitis. (Didn't cover specifically but should appreciate that cryoglobulin can act as both an immune complex [get LCV] and as a hyperviscosity state [get vasculopathy findings, such as livedo]. These findings can be seasonal too—for instance, a patient with cryoglobulin issues could have LCV lesions in summer and purpuric legs in winter [when cryoglobulins settle in thighs from the cold].)

2.1.4.2.2 IgA Vasculitis

Tetrad: purpuric rash without low platelets/coagulopathy, arthralgias, abd pain, hematuria.

Rash tends to onset first.

Usually children (>90%), who tend to have joint pain (2/3), abdominal pain (1/3), fevers (usually self-resolves; very small fraction progress). Adults tend to have joint pain/renal issues (should be more concerned for possible fulminant course [ESRD, etc.], so have lower threshold to treat adults).

Tends to be in fall/winter (may be associated with infections).

Kids tend to self-resolve over ~6 weeks. Recurs in 1/3—recurrences usually more mild than initial episodes.

Although most common vasculitis in children, kids can have vasculitis from juvenile DM, from strep (very common), etc., so don't forget about other entities.

Rheum is sometimes already involved by time consulted if patient is admitted.

If mild, can do symptomatic control (NSAIDs if no renal/GI issues, etc.).

If systemic stuff going on, can do systemic steroids. If having rapidly progressive renal issues (rare), can consider cyclophosphamide.

Anti-neutrophil meds (colchicine, dapsone, etc.) tend to work well for IgA stuff and vasculitides, but relapse common with dapsone for IgA vasculitis.

2.1.4.2.3 Urticarial Vasculitis

Typically middle-aged women. Painful, longer-lasting episodes of urticarial lesions (>24 hours). Not as characteristically itchy (vs. true urticaria). May leave discoloration as it resolves (vs. actual urticaria completely disappearing). Ddx to consider: serum sickness, JIA.

Shows LCV on biopsy.

Immune complex–mediated reaction (type 3 hypersensitivity reaction), so activates complement and releases C3a and C5a, which degranulate mast cells (get hives, 50% get angioedema). Have to treat both the acute urticaria and the chronic vasculitis parts.

However, they can of course also get low complement (which is more commonly associated with systemic involvement than normocomplementemic), so something more profound happens to affect the serum in this (unclear why happens; hypocomplementemia doesn't occur in LCV).

At the most severe end of hypocomplementemic urticarial vasculitis, they meet criteria for SLE; thus, if have urticarial vasculitis, work them up for SLE.

Management best practices are not well-defined. Flares are common with systemic steroid tapers; can follow a similar treatment ladder/algorithm to LCV.

2.1.4.2.4 Medium and Large Vessel Vasculitides

If immune complex gets stuck in larger vessel (medium, large, largest), such as an artery (vs. postcapillary venule in LCV), get a wedge of infarct.

Will probably get asked to biopsy, but hard to biopsy-prove larger vessel vasculitides (if you biopsy end of finger, will just see dead finger [because the pathology is proximal to the infarct against the bone], and by the time surgery does biopsy the artery, the patient likely already going to be on pulsed cyclophosphamide and the pathology likely gone).

Another problem is, the clinical ddx for vascular issues is quite broad: hyperviscosity (plugs it), emboli (plugs it), vasospasm (like ergot intoxication, etc.), -itis (closes wall of muscular artery). Example for context: SLE patient—could have APLS, cryoglobulins, Libman–Sacks lesions on heart that are embolizing, etc. So need further work-up because even biopsy can be hard to differentiate vasculitis vs. vasculopathy (might see both plugging of vessel and inflammation of the vessel wall—and don't know which one came first).

Wegener's (necrotizing granulomatous inflammation): often periorificial. Hard to prove in the skin because the most common skin lesions usually don't show the histology (usually shows LCV, which may be some spillover phenomenon).

If have PG (which looks like Wegener's lesion), should check c-ANCA.

- *PAN*: best lesions to biopsy are the nodules, which are classic in cutaneous PAN (though not usually seen in systemic PAN, in which only 30% of patients have skin lesions—most commonly palpable purpura, second most commonly peripheral gangrene, third most commonly necrosing livedo).

- *MPA*: palpable purpura on skin with coexistent lung and renal involvement (alveolar hemorrhage and crescentic necrotizing glomerulonephritis). Apparently has distinctive histology.

- *Churg–Strauss*: a lot of IL4-responsive stuff + skin vasculitis. High eosinophil counts. Histologically can see features of granulomas and vasculitis (just like rheumatoid vasculitis, etc.).

2.1.4.3 Vasculopathy

Clinically can have overlap of findings with vasculitides, as alluded to earlier.

For vasculopathic issues, ask yourself if there is atrophic change (cell death from not getting enough blood to feed the skin).

For livedo reticularis (reaction pattern, not really a stand-alone entity):

The livedo changes are due to spasms pulling blood into the deeper vessels (deoxygenated blood accumulates in superficial venous plexuses, which causes the erythematous part [arterial blood is the skin colored/spared areas]).

Would emphasize differentiating blanching vs. necrotizing.

Necrosing livedo tends to be more stellate purpura. Could be seen in purpura fulminans in setting of some kind of shock, for instance. Usually in setting of something bad.

If the livedo is blanchable, usually not due to a serious underlying issue (of course can be seen in babies when they're cold, and adults with vasoactive skin). If it's blanchable in a patient with vasculitis and there's no ulceration, then it suggests the vessels aren't being destroyed (thus can actually mean the inflammation is controlled).

See more about livedo reticularis in Chapter 3 ("Concern for Vasculitis").

2.1.4.4 Capillaritis (Pigmented Purpuric Dermatoses)

Most common is Schamberg's. Sometimes itchy. Chronic, waxes/wanes. May be related to venous stasis/HTN.

1. Schamberg's

   a. Pinpoint red/brown/orange nonblanching macules (too individually small to be LCV).

b. Compression stockings.

c. Can do clobetasol QD for 2 weeks, then pulse BID only on weekends.

Many other distinct entities that are much less common.

2.1.4.5 Mastocytoses

Darier sign = stroke skin; makes urticarial lesion.
Most are skin-limited and aesthetic. But do thorough ROS.
If concern for systemic disease (more common in adults than kids), need heme-onc to manage the meds.

However, would be careful chasing systemic work-ups (because, for instance, may have a patient with telangiectasia macularis eruptiva perstans [TMEP] and fibromyalgia who ends up getting a bone marrow biopsy, etc., based off that, which is of course ridiculous).

PUVA and TCSs disperse mast cells -> useful for skin-limited mastocytosis. Avoid mast cell degranulators (NSAIDs, EtOH, narcotics).

- *Urticaria pigmentosa*—most common, self-limited in kids (usually by adolescence); usually persistent in adults.

- *TMEP*—almost only adults; chronic, stable, essentially always benign. Management directed at symptoms.

- *Mastocytomas*—more common in kids. Manage symptoms.

2.1.4.6 Urticaria Multiforme

Newer condition: looks like hives, but not hives; lasts >24 hours.
Hard to find cause (can ask them to keep diary for 24 hours before episodes).
Hard to treat; suppress when occurs.

If you know they get three episodes per year that last 1 week, can use meds that are normally too toxic to be on chronically:
Prednisone (30 to 0 over 1 week) or CsA—only PRN for flares (won't cause rebound because know duration of episodes).

Similar approach for recurrent idiopathic erythema multiforme—and can probably be translated to most episodic stuff (doesn't make sense to do continuous stuff when they only occasionally break out).

2.1.4.7 Regional Erythemas

2.1.4.7.1 Erythema Annulare Centrifugum (EAC)

Tend to not find the cause. Typically asymptomatic. Self-limited, but may get new lesions. TCSs don't seem to help.

- *Two histologic variants*: dermal and superficial type; some people think this is because if you biopsy scaly advancing rim, you'll get superficial inflammation; if you biopsy the urticarial part, you'll get deeper inflammation. But some EACs lack the trailing scale and look more infiltrated (actually look deeper clinically).

2.1.4.7.2 Erythema ab Igne

- Usually not actually erythema; usually a livedoid pigment (melanin).

- Common from heating pads, laptops, etc.

- No great treatment. Avoid culprit. Takes several months to resolve—depends on how bad it is. Can be permanent. Can offer tretinoin or laser if they want to try something.

2.1.4.7.3 Erythromelalgia

Erythematous (more violaceous in skin of color), burning pain, characteristically worse with heat, better with cooling (if just erythema with burning sensation without being worse with heat, might be vasoreactive skin—more later).
Tends to flare later in the day.
Usually feet, but also hands; less commonly head/neck, but happens.
If on legs, usually a long nerve neuropathy (not small fiber neuropathy)—should send to spine center.
If not due to nerves, most treatments don't work; thus, the following management content is actually more focused on describing thoughts regarding why certain meds (that I predict some people may consider) don't actually work (with the hope that we can skip trying these and expedite finding something that does).
Since the problem isn't a vasospasm, nitro paste will probably not work (nitro paste makes coronary vessels dilate when they're spasming); dilation isn't necessarily what you want when it's too red.
The stuff used to get the red out of rosacea (vasoconstrictors) has rebound if you use it 3 days in a row (so it'll potentially already be worse by the fourth day).
Gabapentin won't work because it's more of an autonomic type of issue.
Can try topical anesthetics like Sarna Sensitive (nice because simple, no side effects, can apply as much as they want, though obviously won't take the red away). Or maybe EMLA (but need to occlude). Pretty hard to anesthetize the skin topically, and it's obviously challenging to figure out how to orchestrate changes in localized spots with a systemic medication.
Vasoreactive skin can include stuff that presents similar to erythromelalgia (red skin that hurts and is inflamed but doesn't characteristically get worse with heat/better with cool temperatures) or non-necrotizing livedo, etc. The nerves that innervate the blood vessels are essentially screwed up (gives them a signal that they're too hot and will turn the skin bright red).
Similar to erythromelalgia, haven't seemed to find anything that works yet but wonder if capsaicin or vascular laser might work. Capsaicin depletes substance P, which mediates the triple response of Lewis (which is when stroking of skin induces an exaggerated redness [vasodilation] and urticarial swelling), so might help with the redness as well as the pain. Vascular laser may help destroy the problematic vessels (and nice because localized and superficial).

2.1.4.7.4 Flushing

Can be constant or episodic. *Possibilities*: Rosacea, emotions (blushing), menopause (hot flashes), diet, EtOH, meds (many that impact vasculature [calcium channel blockers, beta-blockers, ACEis, nitrates, etc.], niacin [more so than niacinamide, though both possible], cholinergic drugs, of course, etc.), fevers, exogenous stimuli (sun, wind). Uncommon tumors and anaphylaxis too. Do review of systems. Check med list.

■ Classically face (spares periocular), but can be hands/feet too.

■ Look for changes in redness during exam (anxiety).

■ Identify/cease culprit.

• For example, if anxiety-related: consider propranolol 20 mg QD PRN.

• Can try Rhofade (oxymetazoline) via Skin Medicinals.

• Can recommend green-tinted makeup to help conceal redness.

2.1.5 Pigmentary
2.1.5.1 Hyperpigmentation

Sunscreen obviously important for everyone, but especially important to emphasize for dyspigmentation, which is tough to get perfect.

Patients often say they want skin lightening (hydroquinone), but what they actually want is complexion blending—for which vitamin C + peels + tretinoin + sunscreen work best. Be careful with hydroquinone—more on this later.

When evaluating hyperpigmented skin on face, pull the area taut to confirm it's actually an issue within the skin. Sometimes (albeit infrequently), it's actually just an area that appears darker from a shadow cast by protruding anatomy (such as a lower lip over a concave chin), which could be addressed with filler, for instance.

2.1.5.1.1 Sunscreen in Skin of Color

Many darker-skinned individuals may have been misled to think they don't need to wear sunscreen. Although darker skin is photoprotective (melanin filters UV light to some degree), the problem is that it's not as protective as most people think.

Of course, there is UV-induced erythema, darkening, aging, carcinogenesis, but the big thing for pigmentation issues in skin of color is visible light (which we only recently realized).

To protect against visible light, need tinted sunscreen with iron oxide (if just using regular broad-spectrum sunscreen, won't be protected against visible light).

■ *An example*: Neutrogena tinted mineral sunscreen ($17 roughly).

FYI: The brand Black Girl sunscreen is a chemical sunscreen.

Should also know the difference between mineral (physical blockers, deflects light) and chemical (absorbs the photons) sunscreens.

■ Mineral: usually zinc oxide + titanium dioxide (inorganic filters); low systemic absorption; also referred to as inorganic or physical block sunscreens.

■ Should know why this is relevant for photosensitive disorders (lupus, DM, PMLE, solar urticaria, melasma, PIH, etc.) and patients on photosensitive meds (retinoids, tetracyclines, etc.).

• Chemical sunscreens may make worse because it doesn't block the UV light like mineral sunscreens do (they allow absorption, which probably isn't helpful).

• Some lupus patients can get prescriptions for tinted windows.

• Should think about people who work indoors—may be getting UV exposures from fluorescent light bulbs.

■ Vitamins C + E + B3 (niacinamide) can also help with dyschromia via tampering down reactive oxygen species.

■ Peels (*FYI*: A topical med treatment, not actually a peel) can also even complexion.

Other photoprotection things:

■ Recommend wide-brimmed hats (which are SPF7, *FYI*: Diameter needs to be 7.5, with tightly woven brim—can't just be a cap), protective clothing, sunglasses, walking in shade.

- When patients voice concerns about vitamin D: can only make so much vitamin D from sun (particularly true for darker skin) and have to take from other sources (food, etc.). Additionally, vitamin D reference ranges aren't a mean (they're just estimates of what people think they should be [so many people are, by definition, "deficient"]—which, aside from cholesterol [which is also just what people think the levels should be], is pretty unique).

2.1.5.1.2 Melasma

Chronic, thus, essentially requires continuous treatment (and constant hydroquinone is not an option—can cause paradoxical hyperpigmentation).

Usually on face, second most common area is bilateral forearms.

MANAGEMENT

Possible to treat melasma (takes 3 months to see initial improvements), but once treated, emphasize patients need to do everything they can to keep it away (5 minutes in the sun will un-do everything; and if they have sun-related hyperpigmentation at baseline [which is harder to treat than melasma] then warn them they may not get a "complete" response).

The basis of their regimen is tinted mineral sunscreen (emphasized above).

For patients who want "natural" adjuncts: OTC L'Oreal vitamin C serum (gentle), Cysteamine (put on like mask for 15 minutes, then wash off).

Topicals:

- Tri-Luma (retinoid, steroid, bleach); apply BID.
- Much better than hydroquinone 4% monotherapy and tretinoin.

Hydroquinone (doesn't literally bleach, just blocks the process that lays down pigment).

- Must wean eventually (usually only give two refills max).
- For weans from Tri-Luma/hydroquinone, can alternate with plain tretinoin QoD.
- *FYI*: OTC hydroquinone is 2%; standard prescription is 4% (some people compound it at 6% or even higher—but probably better not to, because patients will get addicted).
- If patients use 4% and take adequate breaks, you can feel confident they won't get ochronosis.
- If they do get ochronosis, can offer laser.
- The areas of lighter skin from hydroquinone eventually even out over time.

Orals:

PO tranexamic acid (TXA) (patients love the results but absolutely must not have a history of clots and cannot be on long-term).

- TXA 325 mg BID for 3 months, then must come off (absolute maximum 6 months).
  - Typically taper BID to QD to QoD.
- Topical TXA doesn't seem to work well.

Peels:

- Work too, but they are $1k–2k, and creams work just as well.

- *At home option*: St. Ives salicylic acid wash; make paste, leave for 3 minutes max on face.

2.1.5.1.3 Post-Inflammatory Hyperpigmentation (PIH)

Common complaint in eczema/acne patients (sign that they're not well controlled even if don't have active lesions).

Can of course be problematic after any inflammatory insult (can be quite bold/persistent after lichenoid rashes, less so for stuff like EACs, etc.).

No miraculous treatment. All about controlling the culprit (acne, eczema, etc.) + wearing tinted mineral sunscreen + time (takes ~1 year; thus, encourage them to judge their progress month by month, not day by day, or even week by week).

Patients might ask about lightening creams, which are probably best to avoid.

- PIH color falls deep into skin (inside melanophages), and bleaching creams mostly bleach the top of skin (so can almost make it look worse—makes the lighter surface lighter, and darker, deep pigment stays same).

  - *Can say*, "The body will heal it better than any bleaching cream, and the best lightening cream is Tri-Luma, which is $200 [insurance won't cover]."

- *Some adjuncts to consider if you get the sense they're fixated on trying something*:

  - Tretinoin.

  - Thiamidol (Eucerin has a product—have to order online).

  - OTC L'Oreal vitamin C serum.

  - Chemical peels or dermabrasion (would stop tretinoin 1 week prior to either).

  - If on legs: compression hose may help (10–15 mmHg fine [20–30 mmHg can be hard to put on]).

  - Pigment corrector products from Neostrata + SkinCeuticals.

2.1.5.1.4 Maturational

- Overlap of melasma and acanthosis nigricans; occurs with age.

- Hard to treat.

- Similar management to other pigmentary issues.

- Can try hydroquinone QHS for 3 months

  - If no response, then change treatment (perhaps Tri-Luma).

  - If better, then decrease to QoHS for 3 months, then off.

  - Can use concomitant tretinoin, though may be irritating.

2.1.5.1.5 Confluent and Reticulated Papillomatosis (CARP)

- Thick skin that lotions can't address. Looks like acanthosis nigricans and tinea versicolor combined. Do KOH to rule out fungus.

- Macrolides don't seem to work.
- Responsive to minocycline 100 mg BID for 6 weeks (give them the exact number of pills—in view of hyperpigmentation with long-term use).
- Commonly recurs. Might improve with weight loss if obese.

2.1.5.1.6 Macular Amyloid

- Darker pigment from scratching/friction (often itchy); goes away slowly.
- Usually upper back, sometimes extremities.
- Can use TCSs or phototherapy.

2.1.5.1.7 Lichen Planus Pigmentosus

- Asymptomatic (or mildly itchy) brown or gray patches. Sun-exposed areas. Usually darker-skinned patients, age 30s–50s.
- Chronic, waxes/wanes.
- Can coexist with other LPs (such as FFA/LPP, oral LP, skin LP) but usually doesn't.

MANAGEMENT

Can start with SCSs, then isotretinoin 20 mg QD for 6 months, then QoD + TCSs + lightening cream.
Tinted mineral sunscreen.
Avoid oils/dyes/henna if using.

2.1.5.1.8 Drug-Induced Pigmentation Issues

Not super common but should always check med list (notorious culprits: chemo, anti-malarials, minocycline, amiodarone, anti-epileptic drugs, HAART, can also be NSAIDs).

Usually appear weeks to months after starting drug. Take at least as long to resolve (sometimes can be years).

Usually brown but can have variable colors/patterns based on drug (look them up).

Increased melanin production or deposition of drug metabolites in dermis/epidermis.

Can also be PIH after inflammatory rashes or FDEs.

Time is the best medicine.

2.1.5.2 Hypo- or Depigmentation

2.1.5.2.1 Vitiligo

About 1% of population; 50% get before age 20.

Starts tiny macules of depigmentation; likes orifices (eyes, mouth, nose, umbilicus, genitals, areolae).

Easy to find with Wood's lamp; if you're not sure, it's probably not vitiligo (see clinical mimics/ddx).

Likes to Koebnerize, similar to LP/psoriasis (falling off bike and scraping knees—common reason).

Halo nevi—higher risk of developing vitiligo.

If vitiligo only in genital area, make sure not actually lichen sclerosus; some patients have both (which can be confusing and often requires biopsy). Want to be aggressively treating LSA (vs. treating vitiligo up to patient).

Probably better to think as segmental vs. non-segmental, though patients can have mixed segmental and non-segmental, which can be confusing.

Segmental—harder to treat, spreads quickly, but after 6 months, stops spreading forever; causes poliosis (white streak of hair).

Blaschkoid pattern indicates keratinocyte problem (keratinocytes grow in a blaschkoid pattern); segmental Darier's, linear psoriasis, etc.—all blaschkoid, because they're keratinocyte problems. So if hypopigmentation in a blaschkoid distribution problem might be keratinocytes, can't take up melanin (and the melanocytes might be normal—which grow in a segmental pattern).

Good prognostic sign in patients undergoing immune checkpoint inhibitor treatment for melanoma.

Also protective against NMSC + melanoma in regular population (probably indicative that your immune system is highly capable [perhaps too capable] of identifying and destroying problematic melanocytic/keratinocytic processes at baseline).

Although conventional wisdom is that vitiligo lesional skin is at higher risk for skin cancer, it is actually incorrect (there's no evidence to support it, and in the rare instances when vitiligo patients develop skin cancer, they seem to get it on non-lesional skin).

Do ROS for T1DM, thyroid disease; if symptomatic, can draw TSH.

Can have symptoms in brain/eye where melanocytes live -> can go blind if not addressed (usually patients have such strong eye symptoms that they go to ophtho first; but if you have vitiligo patient with weird neuro symptoms and have struggled to find a diagnosis, worthwhile to think about).

Clinical ddx:

- DLE (erythema, scale, alopecia)

- Hypopigmented MF (responds to UVB)

- Hypopigmented/depigmented sarcoid

- Lichen sclerosus (involvement of labia minora; looks atrophic/fissured, can have tight sclerosed clitoral hood; symmetric, but in figure-of-eight pattern around introitus and anus; easy to differentiate even though both cause symmetric depigmentation; the distribution is different)

- Scleroderma (salt + pepper more perifollicular sparing rather than perifollicular repigmentation)

- Ash-leaf macule

- Pityriasis alba, pityriasis versicolor

- Progressive macular hypomelanosis (treat with UVB)

- Tuberculoid leprosy (hypopigmented, anesthetic—thus might not feel the anesthetic during biopsy)

- Pinta (probably has disappeared; no one has seen it, so possibly doesn't exist anymore; let me know if anyone you know has seen it)

- Iatrogenic hypopigmentation (from ILK, for instance)

- Piebaldism (present at birth; AD, some patients think it's vitiligo passed down; islands of sparing more characteristic of piebaldism, only ventral, doesn't affect back)

■ Wardenburg (present at birth; depigmented hair, hearing difficulty, some islands of pigment)

MANAGEMENT

Good news: Often spares hair follicles (due to immune privilege [keeps immune cells out of follicle]—important, because if hair follicle remains protected, then the stem cells can regenerate melanocytes and repigment the skin).

Perifollicular repigmentation = workhorse of repigmentation—this is what you need to get significant benefit.

Can also get marginal repigmentation = repigments from the edge, weak and only a couple millimeters.

Must know whether stable vs. unstable (when unstable, use systemic immunosuppression to stop spread while getting them on phototherapy).

Signs of unstable:

1. New spot in the last few weeks or expansion >1% BSA in past 2–3 months.

2. Confetti vitiligo.

3. Trichrome vitiligo (depigmented, normal skin, hypopigmented in between).

   a. Some people look at hypopigmentation without depigmentation and wonder if early vitiligo, but NEEDS depigmentation to be vitiligo somewhere.

4. Inflammatory vitiligo—quite rare; pink erythema around edge, sometimes scaly; often very itchy.

5. Koebnerizing.

6. If see any of these, can triple the BSA within 3 months, so urgent to get treated; Koebnerized lesions usually reverse first, maybe because they're smaller, thinner lesions.

Stable = not spreading (though can still repigment—not really burnt out; it's like a constant tug-of-war, where melanocytes are regrowing but the immune system is attacking [so treating weakens the immune system pulling]).

Can flare at any time, possibly after decades of stability; waxes/wanes unpredictably.

If unstable:

PO steroid (dexamethasone 4 mg on Saturdays and Sundays only for 2–3 months [usually doesn't repigment but stops it from spreading and at least holds them in place until getting them on something that repigments]).

■ If really focal, then can try topicals (ruxolitinib best).

■ If active, then low threshold for NBUVB (2–3× weekly, starting at 200 MJ—half the minimal erythema dose [MED] for type 1 skin; go up 50 MJ each visit; try to get at least 800 MJ); no max for how long you give NBUVB (some books state 1 year).

■ Antioxidants (alpha-lipoic acid + vitamin C + vitamin E) for vitiligo appear to help respond faster, especially when combined with NBUVB.

If stable, can take it slowly:

■ If more than a couple of spots: NBUVB 2–3× weekly + topicals.

■ If >> a couple of spots: topicals (clobetasol for 1 week, then Protopic for 1 week; alternate) or straight to topical ruxolitinib, which works better and doesn't need to alternate. Can use anywhere but can only use it on a max of 10% BSA (at the time of writing, anyhow).

 • Some also pulse clobetasol (only on weekends—since the skin isn't thickened, high risk to thin the skin).

 • Protopic is a big molecule; questionable whether gets good penetration (so can consider urea cream QAM [to alter the stratum corneum] and Protopic QPM).

■ Consider excimer laser or surgery (transplant melanocytes) for segmental vitiligo.

FYI: NBUVB is safe, doesn't increase risk of skin cancer at all, plus vitiligo has 3× lower risk of skin cancer, and NBUVB doesn't impact that; so OK long-term. Face repigments in 6 months; hands/feet probably will never repigment. Rest of body is between 6 months and never (sometimes they repigment after few years); also decreases risk of heart disease/stroke in long term (maybe because increases nitric oxide in skin/arteries, but not confirmed).

Conventional therapies—relapse 40% within first year of stopping; can decrease that by treating with Protopic BIW (not BID) to <10% within first year. JAKi relapse rate is about same.

Reason it relapses is that resident memory T-cells form in skin. (T-cells go into skin, kill melanocytes, become memory [stay there forever]; if you treat with anything, it turns them off and you repigment, but if you stop treatment, they wake back up and start the process again. If you block IL15, the memory cells disappear [memory is erased] and you maintain repigmentation. IL15 induces IFN-γ, so blocking IL15 may do the same thing as a JAKi. John Harris has made an antibody that has started clinical trials—hoping it's a biologic that induces long-term durable responses without relapse.)

■ *An aside related to its applications in AA*: IL15 seems to prevent AA but doesn't reverse it; memory T-cells probably do form in hair follicle in AA, but hair follicle different than interfollicular epidermis, so the cytokines that keep those memory cells happy may be IL15 and IL7, and the interfollicular epidermis is just IL15. So may have to block both in AA.

Melanocyte transplants can jump-start return of melanocytes (they are neural crest–derived and move slowly). Works best on localized patches on face + hands (not tips of fingers). Melanocyte transplants for vitiligo:

■ If have segmental (immunologically more stable), the VASI is 90 (very much improved repigmentation).

■ If generalized, 52%, but wide standard deviation (probably because immunology not totally managed; if stable, it's a great option).

Only other ways to advance melanocytes into damaged areas (other than melanocyte transplant) are alpha-MSH and phototherapy.

2.1.5.2.2 Nevus Anemicus

- Erythema blanches on diascopy (pressing glass slide to the area).

- Interestingly, it's the actual vessel that's hypersensitive to catecholamines (not the person—in other words, if you punch biopsy the hamartoma and transfer it to another person, it'll do the same thing).

2.1.5.2.3 Nevus Depigmentosus

Present at birth or shortly after; no scale, almost always hypopigmented (misnomer).

Edges usually jagged, like torn piece of paper. Vitiligo never really looks like this; vitiligo is a round patch with smooth border.

Case reports of patients born with segmental vitiligo are probably actually depigmented nevus depigmentosus. (If you biopsy, would have normal number of melanocytes [thus not vitiligo]; they also have negative Fontana Masson, though, like Chédiak–Higashi, Griscelli [can't transfer melanin], and albinism [can't make melanin], so may just be segmental albinism—an AR inherited disease [all you need is a heterozygote albinism patient to develop a post-zygotic in other gene which will prevent melanocytes from creating melanin, so possibly a mosaic mutation in heterozygotes].)

2.1.5.2.4 Idiopathic Guttate Hypomelanosis

- White spots from sun.

- Can actually be depigmented, but only on sun-damaged skin (vs. vitiligo).

- Lesions are evenly distributed in IGH (vs. clustered in confetti vitiligo).

2.1.6 Infectious

2.1.6.1 Bacterial

Common clinical mistake is taking a swab culture as something that must be pursued.

Important to distinguish tissue infections vs. surface organisms.

Babies tend to have fecal organisms all over their eczematous eruptions, and even worse are leg ulcers (which can have all types of fungi and bacteria that should not be chased).

Biopsies can be useful at borders of ulcerative lesions if the organisms are deep (holds true in immunosuppressed patients too).

2.1.6.1.1 Impetigo

Will likely see a lot of impetiginized dermatoses, but probably not a lot of primary impetigo.

- *Non-bullous impetigo*: honey-colored crust (color is from the carotenoids in our serum [like egg yolks]), usually on face. Remove crusty stuff with warm water or hydrogen peroxide. Mupirocin if localized. Systemic antibiotics (for both staph and strep) if widespread (cephalexin, clindamycin). *FYI*: MRSA tends to be a folliculitis/abscess organism, not an impetigo organism.

- *Bullous impetigo (essentially localized SSSS)*: might present with just moist skin (look for peripheral collarette) because blisters can resolve so quickly; swab likely will just contain skin contaminants, so not very informative. Very contagious. Fully resolves within 2–6 weeks.

Goal of treatment is to decolonize (cover staph and strep).

If limited disease:

1. Place mupirocin on old spots (tell them to put on Q-tip to avoid contaminating tube).

2. Wash daily; alternate Hibiclens + antibacterial soap.

3. Stay out of school until lesions are crusted/coverable with Band-Aids.

4. Monitor friends/contacts; apply mupirocin at first sign of infection.

5. Don't share clothes/towels, etc.

If widespread/systemic symptoms:

■ Same antibiotics as previous, for ~7 days.

Raw + oozing areas ddx for peds: bullous impetigo, LABD, disseminated HSV, urticaria pigmentosa.

2.1.6.1.2 Syphilis

Great mimicker, good to have on any ddx (same with sarcoid, CTCL, etc.). Only thing it can't really be in an adult is vesiculobullous (could be in congenital syphilis).

Characteristically ham- to copper-colored papulosquamous lesions with adherent peripheral silvery scale/crust on hands/soles. Moth-eaten alopecia.

Chancre lasts 3–6 weeks, heals spontaneously. *Chancres* are erosions/ulcers on top of an area of intense induration and painless (vs. *chancroids*, which are soft, deep, painful, gray necrotic ulcers).

Secondary mucocutaneous lesions last 3–12 weeks, resolve spontaneously. Screen for other organs; refer to other specialties as needed.

For dark field, clean the chancre with saline, squeeze it, and get a drop of the serum on a glass slide and dark field that—not sure many people do this, but not a bad skill to have.

2.1.6.2 Fungal

For KOH, it helps to wipe lesions with EtOH pad before scraping the scaly borders so you don't have to catch the scales with the glass slide (the scales will stick better to the blade or whatever you use to scrape).

2.1.6.2.1 Tinea Corporis and Variants (Incognito, Majocchi's, Kerion)

Can be anthropophilic (from another wrestler or the mat), geophilic (from the soil), or zoophilic (from a pet or something). So ask about cats, dogs, etc. Anthropophilic (human host) tends to have less inflammation than zoophilic/geophilic.

There are many species of *Trichophyton, Microsporum, Epidermophyton*—should know for exams (and relevant for treatment selection, but fungal cultures are not uncommonly falsely negative [may depend on how good your lab is]). Speciation from cultures can take weeks.

Sometimes scratching/lichenification can obscure the classic annular appearance.

Patients may present after having gotten TCSs for suspected eczema (as steroids prescribed by many non-dermatologists when diagnosis is unclear). The patient will probably tell you they got better (less inflamed/irritated), stopped it, itch got worse, started TCSs again. Issue is inappropriate treatment with TCSs/TCIs/systemic steroids can alter the appearance (tinea incognito) and can also lend a somewhat misleading history; thus, if eczema-looking (or even acne-looking) rash is spreading despite treatment, consider fungus/yeast.

Would keep tinea in the back of your mind for all eczematous rashes in general, and do KOH if reasonably suspicious (ideally do a few days after stopping TCSs if suspect tinea incognito).

FYI: Lotrisone (clotrimazole and betamethasone) is marketed as something people can use if they don't know whether something is fungal or inflammatory, but patients tend to get too many refills from other providers and might get TCS atrophy (so usually best to avoid prescribing this, although it can be useful if you pulse it only on weekends for inverse psoriasis or something).

TCSs can also cause fungus to travel to hair follicle -> Majocchi's granuloma (granulomatous fungal folliculitis) -> will need longer treatment. Can also be caused by longstanding infection, shaving, or being immunosuppressed.

Kerions are fungal abscesses (often mistaken for bacterial abscesses). Essentially, Majocchi's fungal folliculitis, usually on scalp (with localized alopecia), but can be face/limbs. Can have fevers/LAD. Get (+) KOH out of the plucked hair out of the pustule; will be (–) if try to smear the pus itself. Surface may or may not be KOH (+), because the corneum might not have the fungus. Typically need 8 weeks' systemic treatment (or even longer). Alopecia can be permanent if was longstanding.

MANAGEMENT

Counsel on contagiousness. Thoroughly clean and don't share fomites (gloves, shoes, bedding, towels, combs, hairbrushes, etc.). Pets might need to be managed.

If localized:

- Terbinafine 1% cream BID (apply to slightly outside lesion; continue until 1–2 weeks after clearing)

- Clotrimazole 1% cream BID

Terbinafine more expensive than -*azoles*. Can also use ciclopirox if suspect bacterial superinfection.

If topical-resistant, extensive, or complicated variant (Majocchi's, etc.):

- Terbinafine 250 mg QD for 2–4 weeks (ask about EtOH, history of liver issues; check LFTs and CrCl).

  - CrCl 20–50 mL/min: 50% of the usual dose.

  - CrCl <20 mL/min: alternative agent preferred, but can do 50% of usual dose and monitor frequently for adverse effects (e.g., GI, hepatic).

- Itraconazole 100–200 mg BID for 1 week.

- Fluconazole 150–300 mg QW for 2–4 weeks.

- If suspect from pet (cat, dog—in other words, if you suspect *Microsporum canis*), would do griseofulvin ultramicrosize 250 mg BID until 1 week after clear.

Preceding treatment options can be used on the other tinea sites covered in the following.

2.1.6.2.2 Tinea Cruris

Inguinal folds. AKA "jock itch." Usually history of athlete's foot.
If immunosuppressed, might not be itchy.
Never affects scrotum, just the thigh (if affects scrotum, then it's intertrigo, not a fungus, and should be treated with TCSs).
Can extend to labia majora in women.
Lichenification can again obscure the annular configuration—thus low threshold to KOH if not sure.
If have been treating with TCSs, might have minimal scaling and no erythema, but KOH can be floridly (+).
Essentially same management as tinea corporis (usually terbinafine or -azoles [including topicals]; griseofulvin for 4–8 weeks if severe). Keep area dry after bathing.
Need to treat tinea pedis, otherwise will never go away (tinea usually starts on feet, then spreads to hands, then gonads; usually worse on the side that the lower gonad is on).

2.1.6.2.3 Tinea Capitis

White powdery stuff is suspicious.
Do KOH of hair (can remove with forceps or rub with moist gauze). Spores tend to be near hair shafts (not hyphae).
Fungal cultures not uncommonly falsely negative. Also can take several weeks for speciation.
Can try Wood's lamp to differentiate M. canis (fluoresces) vs. T. tonsurans (doesn't fluoresce).
T. tonsurans (no inflammation—black dots, dandruff-like scale, gray patches) vs. T. mentagrophytes (a lot of inflammation—vesicular/pustular on plaques; kerion/favus rare).
AD + T. tonsurans not uncommon in skin of color due to hair shaft type.
Management similar to previous; griseofulvin if suspect M. canis. Take QD for 8 weeks or more (take until area is perfect with hair regrowth).
Can consider ketoconazole shampoo 2–3× weekly adjunctively (might reduce spread).

2.1.6.2.4 Tinea Faciei

Not always itchy. Typically not symmetric.
Consider tinea faciei when thinking seb derm or sebopsoriasis, or even DLE.
TCS-modified tinea faciei can resemble rosacea.
If coexistent tinea capitis or hair follicle/shaft involvement -> PO treatment—same treatment regimen options as earlier.
Counsel patients on possibility of "id" reaction (initially worsening/eczema at distant site [which will be KOH-negative lesions, FYI]).

2.1.6.2.5 Tinea Manuum

Hands.
Usually asymmetric.
Similar organisms to feet and groin tinea.
Can have coexistent nail/feet fungus (two-foot, one-hand syndrome).
Assess common tinea areas (feet, groin, etc.).
Can get painful fissuring or even maceration (looks soggy)—particularly if between fingers.

If on palm, might have more fine powdery look (almost more dry or even lichenified-looking) because doesn't have sebaceous glands.

If dry palms not improving with emollients, consider this.

2.1.6.2.6 Tinea Pedis

"Athlete's foot."

Possibly from occlusive footwear/humidity/sweatiness or pools/baths, etc. Usually asymmetric. Typically lateral web spaces (vs. AD, usually medial). Characteristically has moccasin distribution. Can be macerated (soggy-looking) between toes. Can also be pustular/bullous.

If hyperkeratotic, can use keratolytics (salicylic acid 12% or urea 40%, etc.).

Cracking between toes increases risk for cellulitis/lymphangitis (entry portal).

Interdigital tinea can be asymptomatic (dermatophytosis simplex) or symptomatic, with secondary bacterial infection (dermatophytosis complex).

Interdigital tinea (dermatophytosis complex) is common in people who have fourth and fifth toes that are close together (web spaces are squished together, so less air circulation and chronically macerated at baseline, allowing diphtheroids to overgrow—thus more malodorous than pure tinea). Problem with diphtheroid overgrowth is, some of the products are anti-fungal, so hard to prove underlying tinea (which needs to be addressed as part of the process) with KOH/culture (thus a clinical diagnosis).

Management: Gentian violet (GV) + Castellani's + possibly permanganate (which is highly effective, but pharmacists don't like to hand this out because ingestion is fatal).

GV is better for yeast than dermatophyte. Castellani's is good for both as well as Gram-negatives and anaerobes (anaerobes, you can suspect based off the smell). Use the pink Castellani's (not the colorless or the phenol-free kind).

Can also debride the dead, macerated skin and apply vinegar (dilute [0.025%] acetic acid).

Stick cotton balls between toes to keep them dry (or the foam separators used to keep toes apart when painting toenails).

If erythrasma, add clindamycin or erythromycin.

FYI: For bullous tinea (multilocular—looks like tiny dots [suggests spongiotic or reticular degeneration vs. friction blisters/subepidermal splitting stuff, which is more unilocular]), the fungus is in the compact layer (bottom of the corneum); so unroof a portion of the bulla, flip it over, and scrape the wet undersurface of the bulla roof with an 11 or 15 blade for the culture (the tinea doesn't live on the top of corneum [that's just keratin]).

2.1.6.2.7 Onychomycosis

Tinea usually starts on feet, goes to groin, then hands, then fingernails (essentially never on fingernails only).

Although 50% of men over 50 have an immune blind spot that predisposes them to onychomycosis (which is permanent, thus recurrence common), many patients who think they have onychomycosis don't (often have poor-fitting footwear).

Fungus causes distal tunneling dystrophy (fungus crawls up and, with trauma, makes tunnel from the end inwards [not from proximal to distal]). If fungus in matrix -> subungual debris; if affecting nail plate -> white chalky appearance.

If it doesn't have those things, then probably not onychomycosis.

TREATMENT

Variable response rates in literature; for simplicity, can explain to patients 50% chance PO meds work, 10% chance topical meds work. High recurrence rate regardless.

Counsel on response timeline: need to clear fungus, then grow a new nail.

PO terbinafine 250 mg QD for 6 weeks (12 weeks for toenails).

■ Conventionally a 6-week course (12 weeks for toenails), but this usually fails (works best if you stay on treatment until nail is completely clear— and growing new fingernails/toenails can take ~12–18 months); consider sending 90-day supplies with a couple of refills (so they know each fill equates to one "course").

■ Discuss side effects + importance of avoiding alcohol.

■ If CrCl 20–50 mL/min: 50% of the usual dose.

■ If CrCl <20 mL/min: consider alternative agent or do 50% of usual dose and monitor frequently.

■ Some people check LFTs if on statin; perhaps more issues with lupus rash + psoriasis than liver toxicity, though. Some don't give if on high-intensity statin.

Topical meds don't work well for most (arguably not even worth trying), but some options:

■ Can soak in yellow Listerine (has thymol, which kills yeast + bacteria).

■ Topical tavaborole 5% QD for 48 weeks.

■ Topical terbinafine around nail, under nail, and in between toes/fingers.

■ Can also try the newer -azoles and ciclopirox.

■ When trimming nails, clean with alcohol pad before trimming new nail.

■ If has concomitant leg eczema, can't treat with TCSs alone, because fungus will thrive and march up the leg; spray toes with terbinafine, apply clobetasol ointment on thick active areas on legs, and alternate with SSD (different time).

2.1.6.2.8 Candida

■ Usually a secondary phenomenon.

■ Granulomatous candidiasis is analogous to Majocchi's granuloma; use fluconazole (or voriconazole) when inside, bleach baths when outside.

2.1.6.2.8.1 Candidal Paronychia

Look at cuticles. If has eczema -> destroys cuticles -> makes cave which, when gets wet, is a magnet for yeast -> creates chronic candidal paronychia (nail comes out with a ridge). Staph germs can also get on the yeast.

Nails can sometimes almost look hyperpigmented.

Can culture candida, but usually never the actual primary issue—may have to address it to get them to heal, but need to address the primary issue (this is why TCSs work better than anti-candidal agents—because the dermatitis is primary and the candida is secondary colonization).

MANAGEMENT

Treat the hand eczema and cuticle will grow back.

Gold Listerine (on Q-tip, go around each nail)—has thymol in it, which dissects under the cuticle and sterilizes it (in past, people used 4% thymol, 95% ethanol, but now they charge $250 for this).

If they don't respond, can consider clotrimazole/betamethasone (Lotrisone) QD + fluconazole QW for a few months.

Remind them to limit contact with water (especially if seen in patients who wash dishes or something).

2.1.6.2.8.2 Median Rhomboid Glossitis

Usually chronic candida (typically months). Can be from minor trauma/irritation or, of course, immunosuppressed patients (though can affect immunocompetent patients too).

The median rhomboid is an embryologic fusion point. There's something about that part of tongue—would think about this if you see any lesion on that part of the tongue (I've seen it present bright pink/purple—almost looked like they sucked on a piece of candy).

Can spontaneously resolve, but anti-fungal treatment not reasonable.

Can do clotrimazole troches (10 mg dissolved 5× every 24 hours for 10 days) or fluconazole (much more convenient/realistic for patient to adhere to—two 100 mg tablets on day 1, then 1 tablet QD for 6 days).

OTC remedies: Take hydrogen peroxide and brush with soft brush. Can also put some Activia yogurt on the tongue for a minute to repopulate the healthy bacteria after rinsing out the peroxide.

2.1.6.3 Viral

2.1.6.3.1 Varicella Zoster Virus (VZV)

Lots of older folks will tell you they have recurrent zoster, but they actually have recurrent HSV.

HSV is gentle; VZV is nuclear.

VZV is usually onetime deal (generate so much immunity you only get it once), tends to affect trunk in middle-aged females, ravages skin, and causes post-herpetic neuralgia (pain from virus scarring the nerve), which has average duration of pain of 180 days; might shorten that with valacyclovir (Valtrex) if caught early.

While HSV doesn't scar, VZV usually scars (even though infects the epidermis, because gets secondarily infected and scratched).

Can apply SSD to prevent shingles scars.

If they've had it for a week, then still give Valtrex (data states give within 48 hours, but possibly because they wanted to give themselves best chance for FDA approval; neurologists give Valtrex for Bell's palsy for 6 months or even a year after despite probably not being caused by herpes virus).

Encourage everyone to get vaccine (unless on active chemo or lympho/neutropenic), otherwise will be upset if they get disease.

2.1.6.3.2 Herpes Simplex Virus (HSV)

If recurrent and only have pain for 1 week or something, then think HSV 1/2 (vs. VZV; see earlier).

About 65% of older people have antibodies to it; very common condition—don't feel stigmatized.

Might have just had eczema as kid (poor skin barrier) and got kissed on cheeks by someone who had it (sun -> local immune suppression -> triggers reactivation).

Chemo/cancer and bone marrow transplant (BMT) patients at increased risk (new exposures + reactivations); should do HSV PCR for erosive lesions (turnaround time usually < 24 hours) or Tzanck smear if have vesicle.

FYI: Babies and immunosuppressed patients with dermatomal lesions are typically HSV and not VZV (should still cover with VZV doses [unless in renal failure, because can cover with lower doses, anyway]).

Management of HSV in patients with normal immune status:

1. Valtrex 1 g ×2 when tingles start, then 1g ×2 12 hours later.

2. SSD to affected area.

3. Can try OTC Abreva (1-Docosanol) for cold sores (but only reduces length of flare by ~0.5 days).

4. Remember, antibodies stick around forever, so if they're negative, then no valacyclovir prophylaxis.

Herpetic whitlow: when fever comes, blister comes; fever blisters on fingertips. Suspect if recurs in same place on fingers.

Lifespan 2 weeks; clears after that (so don't be fooled if another provider prescribed antibiotics and it "cleared" after 10-day cephalexin).

If has a nearly constant presence or flares multiple times per month, can consider suppressive dosing of Valtrex (500 mg QD).

Granulomatous HSV lesions can almost look like genital PG lesions. So if not responding to treatment, consider biopsy (particularly in immunosuppressed hosts, because herpetic lesions don't look classic and last for a very long time).

2.1.6.3.3 Human Papillomavirus (HPV) Warts

Around 25% of adolescents have warts.

There are 200 different types of warts; basically an immune blind spot, the virus is ubiquitous, just like toenail fungus. Possible to have virus and not develop papilloma.

There is a vaccine for HPV (but of course doesn't work if already have the infection).

Genital warts are way different than warts elsewhere. If see genital warts in kid:

1. If <2 years old, then mother had HPV.

2. If >2 years old, consider abuse, especially if anal region compromised or vaginal region is swollen.

Management directed at destruction/debulking (LN2, cantharidin, etc.) and/or immune stimulation (imiquimod, candida antigen, MMR vaccine, etc.).

Make sure to ask about lifestyle things that might be blunting their immune system (such as inadequate sleep, drinking caffeine [which is a phosphodiesterase inhibitor so technically suppresses the immune system], etc.).

Cantharidin is a blister beetle extract that causes scarring (*FYI*: Can get an OTC solution called Ycanth); may want to try one lesion first to see if they like it. LN2 + cantharidin sometimes need 10× treatments and still not gone, so sometimes better to do 12 weeks slow treatment with imiquimod (can poke holes in wart before applying). Use wart Band-Aid, reusing until doesn't stick. Wear at night.

Can compound topical cidofovir, pricey at $100–120, but pretty effective (especially if do LN2 first, or if no LN2 debulking, then maybe salicylic acid to soften it up).

Arguably not unreasonable to not treat (since often will resolve eventually), except in transplant patients—would be more careful and err more towards treating (because risk transformation to SCC). Most patients/parents often come in because they want them gone, though, anyway.

If you do MMR, make sure patients have been vaccinated before or they may not mount a response. And make sure not immunosuppressed, or may get viral symptoms.

Other site considerations:

- *Genital warts*: can try imiquimod 3 days per week for 16 weeks max (leave on for 6–10 hours each application).

- *Periungual warts*: can damage nail matrix, so do keratolytic and imiquimod for 3 months.

- *Palmoplantar*: tough to treat; Dr. Scholl's Callus Removers pads (not cushions) are the strongest OTC salicylic acid. May have to file down calluses over top warts, then LN2 to warts, then use these OTC topicals.

2.1.6.3.4 Molluscum Contagiosum

Around 25% of kids get molluscum. Loves to spread in kids with AD; probably had microscopic irritation and got from other kids, etc.

Essentially same management as warts. Can self-resolve in several months to few years.

If really young, skin of color (in other words, if LN2, cantharidin, etc. are not good options), can try tretinoin for a few months. Basically induces low-grade irritant response to draw inflammation to the area. Reasonable choice for children with lesions on the face (where can't do cantharidin, though could do LN2 on a Q-tip).

2.1.6.3.5 HIV Dermatoses/Considerations

Don't really see AIDS-defining dermatoses as much anymore since HIV medicine is better. Very testable content, though.

Several considerations to be aware of, especially if HIV poorly controlled (much of which has to do with their immune dysregulation):

- Bacterial folliculitis more severe/refractory.

- Although staph infections are common in HIV patients, they rarely get toxic shock syndrome (TSS) because of their immune incompetence (can't mount the exaggerated T-cell activation in response to the superantigens as well as an immunocompetent person can). If they do get TSS, however, may be recurrent and prolonged.

  - *Syphilis*: chancre lasts longer (can see primary and secondary manifestations concurrently), can have multiple chancres, more quick to progress to tertiary disease (meningovascular), more severe organ involvement (liver, kidneys, vasculature), can be more recalcitrant, higher relapse rates.

- *Tinea*: more severe/extensive/chronic/recurrent in HIV.
- *Tinea versicolor*: more recalcitrant/recurrent.
- *Candida*: oral most common fungal disease in HIV patients, and should wonder about HIV if doesn't have known risk factors.

■ Don't forget about deep fungal infections.

- *HSV*: atypically shallow ulcers/linear erosions. If persist 1+ months, suspicious for HIV.
- *VZV*: higher risk for shingles when <50 years old, higher risk for dissemination (for example, encephalitis, pneumonitis, hepatitis), higher risk for atypical hemorrhagic/necrotic lesions.
- *Molluscum*: more numerous, more verrucous/larger (giant molluscum characteristic of late-stage HIV).
- *Scabies*: see following.
- *Psoriasis*: HIV can unveil (immune alteration), joint involvement more common; HAART improves the skin psoriasis.
- *Seb derm*: more severe/extensive/refractory; if erythrodermic, consider HIV. Can treat with PO fluconazole.

■ **Drug reactions:** higher rates overall than gen pop (even comparing same drugs, though obviously, of course, on HAART meds and more treatment in general).

■ **Pruritic papular eruption of HIV:**

- About 15–45% HIV patients; can be presenting sign and help with early diagnosis.
- Need lesions >1 month in absence of identifiable cause (is a diagnosis of exclusion—thus rule out eosinophilic folliculitis, etc.).

■ **Management:** HAART, typically unresponsive to most traditional anti-pruritic efforts; can try phototherapy.

2.1.6.4 Infestations
2.1.6.4.1 Scabies

Parasite. Usually from other people > fomites. Contagious (but still need pretty good skin-to-skin contact for ~20 minutes, so it's not THAT easy to get it).

Mites burrow just below the stratum corneum, which leads to a hypersensitivity reaction and the development of symptoms roughly 2–6 weeks later (intense pruritus).

In other words, if you're nervous you have contracted scabies after briefly interviewing a patient and start to feel itchy, you probably don't actually have it (body hasn't mounted an immune response yet, and it was probably too brief a contact anyway). That said, symptoms will come back on a faster timeline if it is a reinfection (just like a type 4 hypersensitivity reaction).

Usually on flexor wrists, between fingers, axillae, areolae, buttocks, genitals (not usually head/neck).

Would try to entertain the possibility of scabies in any patient who is profoundly itchy and any patient with itchy bumps on genitals (men) or areolae (women). Can sometimes look a lot like eczema, and the pathognomonic burrows may not always be there. Obviously ask about family members.

To confirm a diagnosis of scabies, need to see mites, eggs, or feces.

If you don't see these things, you can clinically diagnose scabies if you see burrows.

When trying to find burrows, look for black triangles at the ends of the scale (the black part is the headpiece of the mite). The ink test might also help highlight burrows (paint ink on the skin, then wipe it off with alcohol [ink will stay in the burrow, making it easier to see]).

Burrows are most often found on the hands, wrists, forearms, abdomen and between thighs (not really the back of the legs or the face). Babies usually have them on the hands/feet. So if you're going to do a scraping, would do it from there.

For scabies prep, apply mineral oil on skin if have it, use blade to remove end of burrow (ideally where you see black speck), place on glass slide, and look for mites or scybala (fecal pellets). If crusted, use KOH to dissolve the keratin.

Negative scabies prep doesn't rule out a diagnosis, and if you see pathognomonic findings (mites, eggs, feces) on dermoscopy, then that's actually enough to confirm the diagnosis (so you wouldn't have to do a scraping in that case).

MANAGEMENT

Family members and close contacts (such as co-workers, sexual partners, etc.) need pharmacologically treated, too, even if not symptomatic.

PHARMACOLOGIC

- Treat with 5% permethrin cream after shower (leave on for 12 hours), repeat 7 days later.
  - Can do same with ivermectin 1% lotion (but more expensive and not as safe in pregnancy/breastfeeding as permethrin) or malathion 0.5% lotion or crotamiton 10% cream.
    - If a patient fails permethrin, it's usually due to application error (not resistance—*FYI*: This is in contrast to lice, which is actually more often resistant to permethrin).
    - So make sure patients know they must apply to every square inch of the body (from the neck down in healthy people or everywhere except the eyelids in older, immunosuppressed patients, babies, etc.)—including in the belly button, their back (where they likely cannot reach themselves), between toes, under nails (especially since they have likely been scratching and may have mites there; trimming nails can help get better cleaning), etc.
    - Usually will require someone to help accomplish this, especially in older, debilitated patients.
    - Must also reapply after doing things like washing their hands.

- An additional option is PO ivermectin (200 μg/kg) ×1 and repeat in 1–2 weeks (important to not miss the second dose, because it's not good at killing the eggs), though usually will still want to do permethrin regimen as surface treatment if possible.

  - If the patient lives in a huge household, somewhat hard to prescribe 10 tubes; can write a script for the patient only, and in the "notes to pharmacy" section, ask them to call you and you can write the script for the rest of the family through that.

    - Kids can go back to school 1 day after starting treatment per the CDC.

  - Probably wouldn't use lindane; can cause neuro/cardiotoxicity, etc.—definitely don't use in kids or if skin extensively involved/denuded. If absolutely have to use, don't apply right after shower.

ENVIRONMENTAL MEASURES

- Wash everything (clothing, linens, etc.) in hot water (at least 120°F), and dry on high heat.

  - If not washable, then place in sealed bag for 3–7 days.

  - Can also dry-clean the items.

- Vacuum carpets and furniture (don't have to extensively disinfect everything); throw out bags/canisters collected in.

- Previous needs to be at the same time as the permethrin for the entire household.

- *FYI*: Dogs don't tend to share the same scabies species (so if they ask about their dogs having it, probably not the case [can give/get scabies from dogs, but the mites won't be able to reproduce, so would only be temporary irritation]).

  - Nonetheless, if their rash persists despite treatment, still good to advise them to take their dog to the vet.

Lesions can take 2+ weeks to clear (immune reaction continues after killing the mite).

Nodules can take multiple weeks to months; TCSs or ILK can expedite resolution.

Itch may last 4 weeks after treatment—can use TCSs and antihistamines.

Post-scabetic itch months after treatment could be due to ACD or ICD from the topical treatments (permethrin).

Eval for secondary staph/strep infection (crusting, oozing, etc.). Could even potentially get post-streptococcal glomerulonephritis. Id reactions also possible.

Manage HIV same as non-HIV, unless have crusted scabies.

2.1.6.4.2 Crusted Scabies

More contagious (higher mite burden) and harder to treat. But usually not very itchy (because usually in patients who are immunosuppressed, so can't mount the same response). Tends to be more Th2-polarized than regular scabies (somewhat analogous to leprosy, where tuberculoid leprosy is characteristically polarized to Th1 and lepromatous leprosy to Th2).

Burrows may be absent. Impressive caked-on plaques somewhat reminiscent of psoriasis or Darier's. Fissures risk sepsis (entry portal for pathogens). Use PO + topical anti-scabies treatment concomitantly.

Pharmacologic

- Topical benzyl benzoate 5% or topical permethrin (day 0, day 7, then BIW until discharge or cured).

- PO ivermectin 200 µg/kg days 1, 2, 8, 9, 15 (maybe 22 and 29 as well if severe [if still rashy/itchy at that time]).

- Keratolytics can help break the thick crusted parts (soak in water first to soften them/improve penetration)—can apply at different time from topical anti-scabies med.
  - *Options*: lactic acid, urea, 3% salicylic acid, and Vaseline
    - Mindful of applying salicylic acid on large BSA, though (systemic absorption)

Environmental Measures

Patient needs to be isolated. Need contact precautions (gown, gloves, shoe covers). Avoid skin-to-skin contact, and treat those who had contact with the patient, the patient's bedding, etc.

2.1.6.4.3 *Other Diagnostic Considerations in Scabies*

- Bullous scabies is rare but can somewhat resemble bullous pemphigoid clinically, histologically, and immunologically (can have positive DIF with IgG and complement deposition along the BMZ).

- Scabies can also masquerade as Langerhans cell histiocytosis because it can massively recruit CD30 cells, Langerhans cells, etc.

2.1.7 Dermal
2.1.7.1 *Granulomatous*

- Body forms granulomas when immune system can't eat the problem.

- Granulomas are slow to form and slow to resolve—pertinent for management, counseling on treatment response timeline expectations, etc.

- Granulomatous processes tend to be pink and indurated without surface scale.

2.1.7.1.1 *Granuloma Annulare (GA)*

Palisading granulomas surrounding altered collagen; unclear why collagen altered (altered mucin).

Not usually drug-induced, but there are reported associated with IL17s, TNFs, and checkpoint inhibitors (which can induce almost all reaction patterns, including granulomatous diseases).

About 90% Caucasian (must be underrecognized, underdiagnosed, or underreported in skin of color); many times non-dermatologists may be concerned for sarcoid or think it's ringworm, but GA, of course, has no scale.

Localized 70% of the time, usually back of hands or tops of feet; maybe 1–2 lesions.

Typically goes away with ILK (but avoid ILK if GA goes into fat). Spontaneously resolves in 2 years in 50% patients (40% recur).

If shallow and superficial: Can try clobetasol to outer border of rings BID for 2 weeks, then BID only on Saturdays + Sundays (pulsing prevents skin thinning and might be enough to help with erythema, which is more superficial than the granulomas).

Around 10% of peds GA is subQ GA. Tend to outgrow by adolescence.

SubQ GA looks like rheum nodules clinically and histologically, but almost all GA biopsies have mucin; helps ddx from reactive granulomatous dermatitides: PNGA, IGDA, and rheum nodules.

- *Patch GA*: almost always sun-protected areas (axillae, inguinal creases); looks almost slightly purple, and tends to be responsive to phototherapy (which is logical—if showing up where patients don't get light).

Contrast to annular elastolytic giant cell granuloma (specifically in sun-exposed areas—thus probably should avoid phototherapy and instead reach for anti-malarials, which are rational for UV-sensitive dermatoses [lupus, DM, etc.]). People tend to hone in on elastophagocytosis, but almost all granulomatous diseases can have that.

Most troublesome variant is generalized GA (AKA disseminated GA). Hard to treat.

Typically don't have to worry about internal disease, but might have slightly increased risk of DM, thyroid disease, HLD—same stuff as NLD, similar to sarcoid, but these are, of course, quite common in general population.

Small increased risk for hematologic malignancies, not really solid organ malignancies (per large database studies).

Some patients may be worth working up for internal involvement. Patients to worry about are the weird presentations/patterns (for example, almost erythrodermic, etc.), or >70 years old (most are 40s–60s), or fail to respond to treatment and behave abnormally; can start with CXR, SPEP with immuno-fixation, CBC with diff, lymph node exam.

Pathology is deep and gentle. Difficult to treat gentle inflammation, in contrast to granulomatous dermatoses with rapid inflammation, such as sarcoid, etc.

One of the big mistakes is people consider failure too fast; slow to form and resolve; takes at least 3 months to see if therapy is actually helping.

TREATMENT LADDER

1. *Anti-malarials*

   a. If works partially, can add tetracycline class antibiotics (which have anti-granulomatous properties), such as doxycycline or pentoxifylline (FDA-approved for LE ulcers, helps with RBCs, a little bit of anti-TNF properties, has been studied for pulm sarcoid, and used for skin granulomatous diseases).

2. *Phototherapy*

   a. Probably first choice for patch GA; PUVA will likely clear it.

      i. PUVA works better than UVB since stronger and penetrates deeper—good for deep infiltrates. However, much harder for patients to do; if partially respond to UVB, then PUVA might be good, but patients usually aren't very enthusiastic about it (they have to wear wraparound sunglasses, take photosensitizing medicine [psoralen] at a certain time, etc.—which is a hassle vs. stuff like HCQ that just needs annual eye exams).

3. *Dapsone—if fail to respond to anti-malarials*

   a. Might also consider adding colchicine if partially responsive (they tend to work well together for conditions like vasculitis, complex aphthosis, etc.)—not a ton of data for this, but let me know if you've tried.

4. *If previous treatments fail, can think about more traditional immunosuppressives*:

   a. MTX—of course a workhorse for other granulomatous stuff like sarcoid, Crohn's, etc.

      i. MMF/AZA not good options, poor efficacy for granulomas.

   b. TNFs + JAKis—might work, but expensive and off-label; have heard variable opinions. If TNFs don't work, can try a different TNF or a JAKi.

   c. Some say isotretinoin helps, but may make more sense if partially responding to phototherapy (intentionally make them more photosensitive to get a PUVA-like effect).

Granulomas are characterized by IFN-y and TNF-a; also appears to have Th2 profile with elevated IL4, so some data for dupilumab; but granulomas are primarily Th1, and when you use dupilumab, it can sometimes skew the immune system away from Th2 and towards Th1 (so it might actually induce or worsen GA). Thus, probably shouldn't reach for dupilumab in GA (unless have severe AD and mild coexistent GA or something).

The JAK–STAT pathway is a heavily IFN/IFN-y pathway. Topical and/or systemic JAKis may work for GA; should be aware of black box warning (particularly for older patients or patients with multisystem sarcoid involvement), risk for clots, CVD, skin cancers, chickenpox reactivation, etc.

May have leftover puckered skin (almost looks anetodermatous) as papular GA resolves.

2.1.7.1.2 Sarcoidosis

Great mimicker. Can affect the hair and nails. Lacrimal glands tend to be big (pull up their eyelid and look to the top lateral corners to check). Can check for the classic "apple jelly lesions" with diascopy (press a glass slide on a lesion to squeeze all the blood out and you'll be left with carotenoids—which is the "apple jelly" [yellow] cytoplasm of histiocytes).

Primarily Black patients, female slightly > male, 30s–50s.

Usually EN-associated sarcoid presents in White patients in setting of Lofgren.

Possible inducers of granulomatous inflammation:

- IFNs (old MS, CTCL treatments) are critical cytokines in granuloma formation.

- Checkpoint inhibitors (which can cause almost any reaction pattern).

- Also reports of paradoxical reactions to TNFs (particularly etanercept).

Arguable whether TNFs (and even IFNs) actually cause sarcoid; patients potentially just had sarcoid, discontinued systemic steroids, then got diagnosed (in other words, could be the drug that wasn't adequately treating the sarcoid [etanercept not great at breaking up granulomas]).

■ *Lupus pernio*—misnomer; nothing to do with *lupus* or *perniosis*. Basically sarcoid of nose and cheeks; usually plaques and nodules that are scaly (not just rosacea type of changes).

■ *Poor prognostic sign*—oftentimes isn't skin-limited and involves granulomas of cartilage -> notching of the alar rim; even if goes away, can have permanent nasal deformity. Thus, treat lupus pernio aggressively.

1. More likely to involve upper airway, sinus/larynx. Nasal papules strongly associated with upper respiratory tract involvement, which can be highly destructive. Some people say hoarseness is predictive of respiratory involvement (but could just have reflux); if have nasal papules, refer to ENT for laryngoscopy.

2. More likely to have chronic sarcoid, lasts decades.

3. All treatments have 30% response rate, such as SCSs + MTX, but TNFs may have higher.

Most patients with sarcoid have it in their lungs.

Most pulmonologists get high-resolution chest CTs (*FYI*: Different study from a regular chest CT, so make sure you order the right one if you choose to order it), but depends on your comfort level.

Would at least get CXR PA lateral, PFTs including DLCO (because can have interstitial involvement that doesn't pop out on CXR and have gas exchange issues).

Even if CXR normal, >90% have lung involvement.

Second most common is eyes.

Do eye exam. If looks like pink eye with inflamed blood vessels, should refer to ophtho.

Liver and lymph node involvement usually isn't critical. CNS pretty rare.

Cardiac symptoms include sudden death; thus, get screening EKG and ask if palpitations. If have abnormalities in either, then refer to cardiology, who can decide if they need MRI/PET or Halter monitor, EP study, etc.

WORK-UP

Usually get basic blood work, though bone marrow involvement (cytopenias) very rare; mainly looking for hypercalcemia (ask about kidney stones).

If you screen sarcoid patients' vitamin D level, it will read low even though their active vitamin D is very high (so don't keep giving them vitamin D supplements—can cause iatrogenic hypercalcemia).

The reason is that granulomas are accustomed to being made in effort to do something (for example, they fight mycobacteria by converting 25-vit D to 1,25-vit D, etc.); in sarcoid, you're making too many, and they are pulling vit-25 stores down (busy converting to vitamin D-1,25).

MANAGEMENT

The same drugs that don't work for Crohn's don't work for sarcoid.

TREATMENT LADDER

TCSs don't work for most lesions but can make them softer, lighter, and certainly less scaly (which is what most patients want).

ILK (usually 10 mg/mL, sometimes 20 mg/mL, rarely 40 mg/mL). Trial anti-malarials and tetracycline class antibiotics. Declare response vs. failure at 3 months (at earliest); if fail, can add to that MTX + TCSs + ILK (OK to do all at once). Thalidomide an option, but toxic; requires monthly visits. Adalimumab or infliximab also options—higher doses than for psoriasis; 40 mg QW or 5 mg/kg Q 6 weeks up to 7.5–10 mg/kg as frequently as Q 4 weeks. Most lupus pernio needs a TNF to clear.

Can also stack on pentoxifylline, maybe even apremilast in some cases (but usually not). Although psoriasis response to MTX is 6–8 weeks, in sarcoid it's 6–8 months.

Worry about body making neutralizing antibodies that make biologics lose efficacy. Doesn't tend to happen in sarcoid as much because naturally more anergic in general, so if you find an effective TNF, they usually can stay on for some time, which is good, because many patients may tend to flare if try coming off of it (plan for long haul). Topical JAKis doesn't seem to work well.

Prednisone is basically cheating for granulomas, usually will come back in same spot, but if someone has terrible, ulcerating, disfiguring disease and has an upcoming wedding or something and want to use steroids while the other things are kicking in, then probably fine.

Just be careful of prednisone tapers for skin sarcoid and rebounding systemic sarcoid.

2.1.7.1.3 Necrobiosis Lipoidica (NL)

Slightly more well understood than GA because NL correlates with vascular disease (such as retinal toxicity, renal toxicity, HTN), so must be that blood vessels are choking off collagen, resulting in deposits of fat in altered collagen.

About 98% of cases on shins, and the 2% that are ectopic (lesions not on shins) almost always also have NL on shins; pretty consistent clinical presentation (which is seemingly quite rare in derm).

Around 10–30% ulcerate, and has a lot of overlap with ulcerative sarcoid—clinically and histologically.

A lot of people have diabetes, and not many have NL; some wonder whether controlling their diabetes will actually improve their NL (moot point, because should try to control the diabetes regardless).

If they have NL and don't have diabetes, should probably screen them. Also associated with HLD, thyroid disease—similar to GA.

MANAGEMENT

Prognosis depends on how bad it is.

If superficial and not sclerotic/atrophic, can achieve normal skin eventually (PIH takes long to resolve).

If an ulcer, will always scar and usually hypopigmented, thin, telangiectatic.

Mainstay: TCSs under occlusion, phototherapy (PUVA >> UVB—since infiltrate is so deep, but some patients might respond to UVB).

■ High-potency TCSs to entire lesion (consider risks/benefits if tendon exposed, as TCSs prevent wound healing and increase risk for infection).

• Managing inflammatory ulcers/wounds is a balance between inflammation and preventing infection (usually wound care used to prevent infection and systemic treatment used to stop inflammation). All wounds have bacterial biofilms and colonization.

- If patient has ulcers with muscle/bone showing, then may not want to apply TCSs (probably not worth it) and probably need systemic antibiotics due to easiness of developing osteomyelitis, etc.

- Other parts of treatment ladder mostly adapted from other granulomatous diseases; some patients do well with PTX, reasonable to try.

- Topical JAKis might work because so thin and atrophic that might penetrate better than for other granulomatous diseases.

2.1.7.1.4 Crohn's

Many patients with IBD will have some sort of skin manifestation.

Can have IBD-specific lesions (Crohn's directly extending from anus, etc.) and secondary complications (disease associations, such as HS/psoriasis, reactive dermatoses such as PG/EN, or therapy-related, like TNF-induced psoriasis).

For IBD-specific lesions, can see contiguous or non-contiguous spread of IBD to skin in genital, orofacial, or peristomal areas. Gut goes from mouth to anus, so oral aphthae can be part of the inflammation. Can also have gingival infiltration, which can be seen in leukemia cutis, granulomatosis with polyangiitis, side effects of anti-epileptic drugs, CsA, etc., as well.

Then, ~30% of intestinal Crohn's patients have genital involvement (and some patients have genital Crohn's but never get luminal Crohn's).

Genital Crohn's can present variably—usually vulvar or scrotal swelling.

If you see persistent vulvar dermatitis (can look like contact derm, AD, or inverse psoriasis), sometimes it's actually Crohn's (blocked lymphatics with fissuring [inflammation in and around vessels, including in the lymphatics -> plugging of lymphatics -> lymphangiomas, lymphangectasias, swelling]).

Peds often present with scrotal or labial swelling; can get skin tags too, perhaps because of pooling of lymphatic fluid.

Can get small ulcers that resemble PG, but Crohn's often shows up with linear fissures in skin folds (knife-cut ulcers almost pathognomonic). Sometimes, ulceration can be so severe that muscle/tendon exposed.

You will probably see Crohn's flares on consults and will likely discover that GI doesn't like to do inpatient scopes. However, sometimes abnormal blood tests, etc., can help push them to do them.

Non-invasive imaging (MR enterography), fecal leukocytes, fecal calprotectin, anti–*Saccharomyces cerevisiae* antibodies, HACA (human anti-chimeric antibodies [such as anti-infliximab]) if not responding to infliximab, or check dosing (might need 10 mg/kg for Q 4 weeks for severe).

Infliximab is probably the best and strongest treatment because can be weight-based and dose-adjusted; would be surprising if doesn't respond, so if recalcitrant to that, would also check for co-infection.

2.1.7.1.5 Orofacial Granulomatosis

Granulomatous cheilitis. Should assume IBD until proven otherwise.

Eval for contact dermatitis; tell them to go on a cinnamate- and benzoate-free diet.

Eval for other things that cause granulomas (sarcoid, GPA, etc.); most get evaluated for Crohn's, and it often heralds a diagnosis of Crohn's (sometimes years later).

Can have infiltration of philtrum and outpouching of upper lip. Treat or will be swollen forever.

Can use ILK (may need nerve block); HCQ helpful for some, antibiotics like metronidazole (which is used for luminal Crohn's and might be helpful for some other granulomatous skin conditions).

Melkersson–Rosenthal syndrome—stereotypical derm thing—a triad that never presents with the full triad, rarely actually seen. Good to know for exams.

2.1.7.2 Neutrophilic

These are really like neutrophilic vascular reactions, because they are mostly reactive to things like IBD, RA, myelodysplastic syndrome, etc. If we were talking about all neutrophilic dermatoses, that would include epidermally focused processes, like pustular psoriasis.

For these reactive dermatoses, the skin is talking to you—telling you their disease is not well controlled (in other words, disease is fluctuating and immune complexes are spilling out of joints, getting through subtle cracks in bowel, or coming from bone marrow).

One issue is, we try to make a treatment ladder for all causes, but management is really about combatting the underlying disease (in other words, some of the things reported to work well are because they were good at treating underlying diseases associated with these dermatoses). For example, thalidomide good for myelodysplastic patients. Getting to a more stable biologic is the way to go for IBD/RA (for instance, a patient on infliximab for multiple years without MTX and now has anti-biologic antibodies [might manifest as a few lesions right before last infusion, now have lesions all over place before their next infusion—means the disease is becoming labile]). If idiopathic, then can just do the derm treatment ladder.

2.1.7.2.1 Sweet Syndrome

Juicy lesions (correlates histologically). Typically tender/painful.

Usually due to mucosal tract infection (ask about URI symptoms, GI symptoms, etc.), though despite name (acute febrile neutrophilic dermatosis), don't need a fever to diagnose.

Can also be 2/2 IBD, myelodysplastic problems, MGUS (roughly 15% are malignancy-associated—usually hematologic), pregnancy.

Usually red, hot, juicy, but when associated with hematopoietic disease, can be more dusky.

Look inside mouth; if they have canker sores, usually have underlying IBD.

Although drugs clearly cause things, their associations are probably overstated (for example, drugs that are used to treat neutrophilic dermatoses are blamed on causing—thus should always ask what was stopped when the suspected culprit drug was started and how long it takes the new drug to work). Most common drug inducer of Sweet's is G-CSF (makes sense, because it is a neutrophil stimulator).

Characteristically rapidly responsive to systemic corticosteroids (look up major and minor diagnostic criteria). Dapsone/colchicine/SSKI are fine but are obviously slower-onset. May help suppress recurrences (which are common).

Thalidomide works well for myelodysplasia-associated Sweet's. Sometimes onc is OK with MTX or SSKI as well.

See more in Chapter 3.

2.1.7.2.2 Pyoderma Gangrenosum (PG)

Initial onset is usually a suppurative folliculitis that turns into a pit that oozes pus, becomes chronic, and the pits merge into a cribriform pattern (thus heals with cribriform scarring). If from needlestick, can be more of a pustular vasculitis.

Histologically, a diagnosis of exclusion (in other words, if you biopsy, you're not technically doing it to "confirm PG"; you're biopsying to rule out the ddx of things [infection, malignancy, vascular issues, etc.] that can look like PG— for example, iododerma, bromoderma, AFB fungi-like sporotrichosis, routine bacterial infections, SCCs, Wegener's).

- Include the wound edge (characteristically undermined).

  - Peripheral biopsies (H&E) will help rule out lymphomas.

- Don't biopsy the middle of the ulcer, or it will just show an ulcer.

  - If the lesion is still early (the middle isn't pure ulcer), can biopsy more centrally to rule out infections (get H&E + tissue culture).

- Old lesions are lymphocytic; early lesions look like Behçet's/BADAS (and are associated with same stuff as them).

- Don't debride (pathergy).

  - Though, **FYI**: Pathergy is only relevant on viable normal skin (so debriding necrotic stuff is not necessarily an issue but could get from needlestick sites from injecting anesthetic).

    - Patients are actually less likely to get pathergy from abdominal surgery than from where they draw blood for a CBC (thought to be a histamine trap phenomenon, where immune complexes form, resulting in a pustule that subsequently expands).

    - Can test for pathergy by poking small holes with a 30G needle, and if develops pustules 24 hours later, then there's pathergy.

    - As an aside, *pathergy* is an acute suppurative inflammation at a site of minor or greater trauma.

    - Contrast to *Koebnerization*, which is injury that a dermatosis localizes to (like getting psoriasis in a scar from abdominal surgery, or overdo phototherapy and psoriasis get worse rather than better).

    - Contrast to Wolf's isotopic response, which is when you have an inflammatory something and a second inflammatory something localizes to that area because of vasodilatation, etc. (EM localizing around surgical sites, bullous disease and, later, LP showing up in that area, etc.).

When evaluating, the main question is whether inflammatory or non-inflammatory (because there's the inflammatory component and a wound healing component). Critical to distinguish.

- When active = has undermined borders, needs anti-inflammatory meds.

■ Gulliver sign = threads of epithelium crossing border to bed of ulcer (making a pterygium across border to bed of ulcer)—correlates with a lack of inflammation.

• If see this, can start to taper treatment (and if see this in absence of treatment, then probably not PG).

– However, also consider the underlying condition:

– If have PG from IBD or RA, must realize if you only focus on skin disease, they will flare their internal disease when you taper MTX/prednisone too far.

– The dream treatment for PG/Sweet's is treatment for the underlying disease (problem is, many get put on treatment before having their colonoscopy, etc., and then they can't get the biologics they need [or at least can't get the IBD dosing they need]).

– Tacrolimus topically seems to help PG heal better; can consider soaks—see DIY section.

– ILK is fine (don't really get pathergy since instilling steroids right at the site where there'd potentially be problems with pathergy).

– Dapsone and colchicine are more for indolent disease.

– Prednisone, CsA, infliximab are the fast-acting options.

– CsA has some anti-fungal properties, so may be reasonable for PG if think might have infectious stuff on ddx.

– If highly recalcitrant, consider SSKI, thalidomide (see Systemic Treatment section).

– If continuing to get more lesions, biopsy again (the prednisone might be like fertilizer to sporotrichosis or atypical AFBs or something; always think about infectious granulomas).

– Also remain vigilant for SCCs; sometimes patients can have classic PG and, in the middle of their ulcers, have an SCC that looks like a PG lesion.

– *FYI*: Some labs are not good at detecting AFB, which makes the conversation with ID difficult (they're not as inclined to help if cultures are negative).

– If tendon is exposed, will need graft because can't grow epithelium over it if it's always moving (derm job is to control the inflammation; if controlled, then surgery is OK—if controlled and border not raised, then pathergy is not an issue).

– Patients want to shrink, but shrinkage of lesions occurs last; first things noticeable to improve are redness, drainage, and pain. Need protein intake. Don't want dressings to stick. See wound healing.

2.1.7.2.3 Behçet's

Multisystem disease.
Has non-erosive and non-axial (trivial peripheral polyarthritis) arthritis.

Only bowel lesions are canker sores (can be from nose to anus). Start as neutrophilic vascular reaction and go to lymphocytic lesions; clinically hard to distinguish genital (and potentially oral) lesions from HSV—so get a PCR.

Causes aneurysms/pseudoaneurysms due to vaso vasorum vasculitis not hypercoagulable state (the clotting is also not due to hypercoagulable state—even though this is hard to prove).

Superficial migratory thrombophlebitis can be due to vaso venorum vasculitis; leading cause of death is pulmonary artery vaso vasorum vasculitis (people bleed out), while leading morbidity is blindness.

Very prevalent from southern Europe (originally described in Turkey, through Middle East, Southeast Asia, Japan, China).

However, overdiagnosed due to criteria issues:

- Oral aphthae, genital aphthae, and pathergy—all same thing in a different place.

- Ocular abnormalities are essentially neutrophilic dermatosis of retinal vessels.

- Skin lesions are acneiform (common in patients without Behçet's).

- So if you have a conjunctivitis episode (anterior uveitis) + canker sores + acne, then you meet criteria for Behçet's.

- Having to exclude IBD and RA was a brilliant addition, but still overdiagnosed due to the earlier criteria issues.

For mouth sores, can use TCSs (clobetasol gel). Genital sores can use lower-potency TCSs.

Systemics: Typically dapsone and colchicine (combination works well). Thalidomide if recalcitrant or if cannot tolerate.

FYI: MTX doesn't work for true Behçet's; evidence likely for patients with erosive arthritis of Crohn's, not actual Behçet's.

2.1.7.2.4 Simple and Complex Aphthae

Simple aphthosis = small and resolve without treatment. Have periods of remissions.

Complex aphthosis = constant or nearly constant 3+ oral or oral and genital aphthae in the absence of Behçet's.

Punched-out appearance, more easy to separate from oral herpes, resolve in 1–3 weeks (vs. anogenital aphthae, which are hard to distinguish clinically from genital herpes).

Exaggerated response to injury in mouth. Can be from stuff like walnut pickles.

Can do ILK and then send out with clobetasol or Lidex (remind them OK to use in mouth despite what package insert says).

If no response, can consider dapsone/colchicine. Also tacrolimus swish/spit. Thalidomide if highly recalcitrant.

2.1.7.2.5 Bowel-Associated Dermatosis Arthritis Syndrome (BADAS)

Basically from a bowel procedure that creates blind loops of bowel (bowel loops that are not connected to functioning part of GI tract) -> bacteria grow, create antigens -> immune complexes form, enter circulation -> serum sickness–like reaction (fever, skin lesions, non-erosive polyarthritis [immune complexes deposit in joint fluid]). IBD an important cause.

Lesions are usually not urticarial; usually black/blue marks with pus in middle (pustular vasculitis).

Skin lesions are indistinguishable from Behçet's; histology is same too.

Usually few months to multiple years post-op.

Recurrent episodic flares that spontaneously resolve.

If isn't self-limited, can do long-term antibiotics (doxycycline or metronidazole), but remember probiotics and treat for yeast.

Anti-neutrophilic meds also rational (dapsone, colchicine, thalidomide).

2.1.7.3 Lymphocytic

2.1.7.3.1 Polymorphic Light Eruption (PMLE)

Pathologic response to UV light (minutes to hours after exposure—including via windows, etc.).

Often spares face.

Generally resolves within a few days, sometimes weeks.

More UV exposure -> reduces tendency/severity of flares (called "hardening"—similar to desensitization phenomenon).

Still should recommend photoprotection.

FYI: Chemical sunscreens make worse (absorbs and creates chemical reaction in skin—in contrast to mineral sunscreen, in which light never gets into skin [good barrier, and iron oxide blocks visible light]).

Can also use TCSs, HCQ (particularly for spring months).

2.1.7.4 Depositional

Many entities can deposit materials in skin (NLD deposits lipid, rheumatoid nodule deposits fibrin [treat RA, nodules go away], GA deposits mucin [unclear why]), etc. These are a few that are most classically thought of as depositional disorders.

2.1.7.4.1 Calcinosis Cutis

Need to obsess about keeping AICTDs perfect so they don't develop this (in other words, don't leave the CK smoldering in DM; can probably be avoided with 2 years of proper tapering in EF, etc.).

Not only have palpable calcium but can also have ulcerations from transepidermal elimination of calcium. Painful.

If you see this, don't be fooled by widespread erythema (from the calcium pushing up on the skin). Can almost mimic active eosinophilic fasciitis (EF), for instance, if on bilateral legs—especially if have an EF patient who was treated late or undertreated or inappropriately treated, etc., and "isn't responding" to immunosuppressives and hasn't cleared after multiple years of treatment. Patients may say "prednisone helps"—probably because it helps keep calcium from rubbing against skin and making it hurt.

Can see easily on XR.

Has high calcium burden in soft tissue (much different than calciphylaxis, which has a low calcium burden [basically a little sprinkle of calcium in a bad location that results in widespread disaster]). Usually, plain XRs don't have enough resolution to detect calciphylaxis; if on HD, might see large vessel calcium deposition (but those aren't the small vessels of calciphylaxis, so can't go off that).

Limited treatment options for calcinosis cutis (no blood flow to pathology). Only thing that will work is procedural removal. But not really feasible if super extensive.

2.1.7.4.2 *Tumoral Calcinosis*

Usually periarticular calcification; looks like sarcoma on XR (almost like cauliflower), which is different from calcinosis cutis.

2.1.7.4.3 *Amyloidosis*

Macular, lichen, and nodular—look different clinically. Distinguishing is relevant for work-up and management.

Macular/lichen are pretty similar; both typically itchy and associated with scratching, differing in location and lesion morphology.

For instance, should definitely get an SPEP for nodular amyloid (since 7% are associated with systemic amyloid). But don't need to order SPEP for macular/lichen because they're so clearly keratin-associated. Obviously, don't need a SPEP for localized amyloid associated with a DF or BCC or something either.

If have high suspicion for systemic amyloid, should get an SPEP, UPEP, IFE (immunofixation electrophoresis), and FLC (free light chain)—getting all these will increase sensitivity/specificity (don't just get SPEP/UPEP). Supposedly, the abdominal fat pad is the best place to biopsy (telescope punch to get fat), but positive findings still very rare (and they will always say you needed more fat because it's never positive).

For SPEP, they take your blood, centrifuge it, take out your plasma, and look at the protein content in that. (Separates the proteins by size and charge via electrophoresis. UPEP basically the 24-hour urine version of that. IFE is a counterpart to SPEP/UPEP, in that it tells you the type of monoclonal [abnormal] protein in the blood/urine—in other words, tells you whether it's present or absent; doesn't tell you the amount.) FLC is a blood test where they're just looking for light chains.

Nodular amyloid does really well with thalidomide.

2.1.7.4.4 *Gout*

Can be debilitatingly painful. Usually men 40s–50s.

■ *Acute* = swollen, warm, erythematous, usually one joint (first metatarsophalangeal, ankle, foot, knee)—flares last days to weeks if untreated.

■ *Chronic* = nodules with yellowish creamy color, usually ear, sometimes distal toe, fingers, Achilles, elbow/knee bursa; can ulcerate and with chalky stuff, and if uncontrolled -> destroys joints -> deformities.

FYI: Uric acid crystals are destroyed in routine H&E processing (formalin)—so if concerned for gout, process in EtOH fixation.

MANAGEMENT

Avoid triggers (EtOH <2 drinks QD, avoid high-purine foods [anchovies, asparagus, cocoa, mushrooms, spinach]).

■ *Acute flares*: NSAIDs, colchicine

  • Ibuprofen 800 mg TID for 5 days, or naproxen 500 mg BID for 5 days, or indomethacin 50 mg QID for 5 days

  • Colchicine 0.6–1.2 mg QD (max dose 4–6 mg)

■ Prophylaxis (if 3+ flares yearly): allopurinol, febuxostat

■ Careful with dosing in renal insufficiency (which is risk factor for gout)

2.1.8 Panniculitides

Diseases on surface and in dermis are easier to classify because of so many structures.

Although can have infections/calcification/deep GA in fat, fat otherwise usually not a super helpful histologic tissue.

Possibilities for lobular panniculitides: infectious, autoimmune (lupus, DM), pancreatic (calcification + saponification); all the rest is inflammatory (associated with things like IBD, bone marrow problem [MGUS], myelodysplastic problem [someone on the way to having leukemia]), or something in fat cells that triggers an autoimmune response.

Most common panniculitis is EN (a septal panniculitis).

2.1.8.1 Erythema Nodosum (EN)

Reactive condition, but 50% idiopathic; other 50% related to drugs (OCPs in EN), infections (TB in world, strep in USA, histoplasmosis/coccidiomycosis), or IBD, sarcoid, etc.

Because EN is a septal panniculitis, cannot suppurate (can't ulcerate and have degenerated liquid fat/other material coming to surface; only inflammation of the lobule can do that).

■ So if you see stuff draining at the surface, then think infectious panniculitis or any of the other lobular panniculitides; EN would be the one thing it couldn't be.

• Important to emphasize this distinction because there's a misconception that RA/IBDs are only associated with EN, but can get reactive lobular panniculitides with them too (that actually suppurate).

■ Ask if they shaved before going to a nail spa or similar (can get atypical AFB from that).

Typically lasts 1–1.5 months. Spontaneously regresses. Can manage symptoms conservatively (rest, elevation, compression, NSAIDs). Anti-neutrophilic migration meds may help (dapsone, colchicine, SSKI).

2.1.9 Acne, Rosacea, Papillomatoses, Keratotic, and Follicular Disorders

2.1.9.1 Acne

Corneocytes ("dead skin" surface cells) stick together + increased oil production -> acne bacteria -> inflammation.

Begins at puberty, when oil glands enlarge.

Reasonable to follow teenagers (vs. having them RTC PRN) as they go through puberty, because hormones change and they may develop different types of acne.

If persists >19 years old, acne may be lifelong, so isotretinoin reasonable to consider.

Easy to be inadvertently incomplete with these patients; look at their back and shoulders (sometimes you'll be surprised!) and actually palpate their acne to see if there are deeper lesions.

Back acne more stubborn than face acne.

Face acne usually not from hair touching forehead, etc. (unless putting gel/stuff in hair).

Sun typically good for acne, but can occur in summer if put comedogenic stuff on (such as sunscreen). Ask about what they put on their skin, like cosmetic products. Or if they wear sports helmets, hats, etc.

May flare around periods.

Don't forget about med-induced acne.

Treatment considerations:

- Topicals take 2–3 months to see effect.

  - Acne takes 3–4 weeks to flare, 3–4 weeks to get better after starting or restarting medicine, so need to stay consistent regardless of how doing.

  - Prescriptions can be irritating; recommend gentle cleansers/moisturizers (CeraVe, Cetaphil).

  - Topicals don't work well for deeper lesions.

- Patients will often be concerned with the PIH, which is evidence their acne is not controlled; so explain need to be proactive with acne treatment to get rid of the PIH and the discoloration can last up to 12 months after the acne lesions resolve.

  - Red spots should fade every month up to 1 year (tell them to judge month by month vs. day by day).

General treatment ladder:

I. *Mild to moderate*

  1. Tretinoin (conventionally for "non-inflammatory" comedones, but they are still inflammatory, and most everyone would benefit from a topical retinoid).

    a. Harder to tolerate in winter; avoid where skin folds onto itself or will peel.

    b. Can tell them every other night to start with and work up to QHS as tolerated.

      i. Explicitly mention pea-sized amount for whole face.

      ii. Needs to be at night (inactivated by light); don't apply retinoids to folds or eyelids because will peel.

      iii. Moisturize.

  2. BPO (conventionally for red inflammatory papules—important to prevent these to prevent scars).

    a. BPO stains clothes (can apply QAM in shower to face/back/chest).

    b. Recommend buying cheap white hand towels to avoid ruining nice towels.

  3. Clindamycin much better (especially for back, which it was specifically made for), but more expensive.

    a. Clindamycin 1% swabs BID for back acne.

    b. Not really supposed to use as monotherapy (AAD guidelines).

  4. Clindamycin–BPO gel (Benzaclin, Neuac, Duac, Acanya, Onexton).

  5. Azelaic acid (one of few options that is OK during pregnancy).

6. Salicylic acid can help with comedonal superficial acne. Can use as DIY at-home chemical peel.

7. Clascoterone (Winlevi)—novel topical, cousin to spironolactone; helpful for adult females with hormonal acne.

8. Topical dapsone 5% or 7.5% gel (Aczone).

   a. Do NOT apply at same time as BPO (will cause orange discoloration; self-resolves 1–8 weeks), but OK to separate them QAM and QPM.

   b. Females tend to be more responsive to dapsone gel than males.

9. Sodium sulfacetamide—a topical (lotion, cleanser) option if dapsone gel too expensive (though may smell bad).

10. Topical minocycline (Amzeeq, Zilxi) 4% foam.

    a. Express a "cherry-sized" amount to fingertips and apply QD. Also available in 1.5% foam for rosacea.

    b. Insurance may not cover; can use patient coupon at www.amzeeq.com/.

II. *Moderate to severe*

1. PO antibiotics (not a forever plan [stewardship]) + preceding topicals.

   a. PO doxycycline 100 mg BID for 3 months, RTC 3 months.

   b. Non-photosensitive options include cephalexin 500 mg BID or TMP-SMX 1 double-strength tablet BID.

   c. Can try macrolides.

2. Spironolactone 100 mg QD (hormonal/PCOS/older women); range 50–200 mg daily (acne dose lower than FPHL dose).

   a. Probably don't need to monitor K+, but consider in older patients on many meds.

   b. Some get breast tenderness; of course, increased urination, possibly orthostasis, related to diuresis.

   c. May not be the best acne med but helps avoid long-term antibiotics.

   d. Not good for women with irregular periods (makes them even more unpredictable).

   e. If not better after 3 months, then consider isotretinoin.

III. *Severe*

1. Isotretinoin (Accutane, Absorica, Amnesteem, Claravis, Myorisan, Sotret, Zenatan).

   a. Essentially curative (some patients might still get a few small pimples occasionally); permanently shrinks oil glands.

   b. Target total dose is conventionally 120–150 mg/kg.

      i. About 85% clear for 2 years, and 1 in 6 get it back (according to older data; today's Accutane isn't as well absorbed so usually need to overshoot to ~200 mg/kg for best odds of complete and sustained remission).

c. Fat-soluble—better to take with fatty meal (except Absorbia, which doesn't need to be).

d. Can't take doxycycline until 1 month after finishing (and of course not concomitantly) (pseudotumor cerebri).

e. Photosensitive until 1 month (at least) after stopping isotretinoin.

f. If flare within 6 months after finishing isotretinoin, can complete another month; has 27-hour half-life, so essentially out of system in 3 days.

g. *Common side effects*: dry skin/lips/eyes, muscle/joint aches, irritability; can also cause hair loss (basically vitamin A toxicity side effects).

   i. For dry eyes: Systane preservative-free eye drops.

   ii. For dry nose/nosebleeds: AYR gel or spray (ENT commonly uses); *FYI*: Vaseline not great because can be inhaled and cause pneumonitis.

   iii. For retinoid dermatitis: hydrocortisone.

   iv. For joint pain: Tylenol PRN; usually improves over time.

   v. For chapped lips: Aquaphor or ChapStick (Burt's Bees—the moisturizing one).

   vi. Doesn't cause the three scary things it was initially thought to: depression (initially thought because some patients had such bad acne they were depressed), IBD (initially thought because certain types of acne go along with inflammation of the bowel), or liver effects (initially thought because it's a vitamin A derivative).

      – Still, of course, a hassle coming in Q monthly.

      – Still ask them to let you know if they notice anything while taking the med.

h. Can't donate blood while on it.

   i. Females must have two negative pregnancy tests 1 month apart prior to starting. Need two forms of contraception (or abstinence alone)—which must stay the same during the treatment course (can't switch from IUD to Nexplanon or something).

j. Can't share with others.

k. After stopping isotretinoin, recommend mild foaming face wash, because if recurs after finishing, might want to start topicals and don't want irritated skin at baseline.

l. For acne scars, after finishing isotretinoin, can consider dermabrasion/microneedling/peels/CO_2 laser (few months after finishing).

m. Once finishing isotretinoin, will slowly start to look better as skin heals; the oiliness will also return.

IV. *See PIH*

Can also try OCPs (decrease androgen production, increase sex hormone–binding globulin in blood [binds/makes free testosterone unavailable], reduce

5-alpha reductase activity [limits conversion to more potent DHT]). Any of the ones that have estrogen should help (not the progestin-only ones, like the implant). May also get acne flares when hormonal contraceptives inserted/ started.

OCPs are nice if also having irregular periods (will make them more regular and lighter). Would avoid spironolactone in patients with irregular periods since makes them even more unpredictable.

Four FDA-approved options for acne:

1. Ethinyl estradiol/norgestimate (Ortho Tri-Cyclen).

2. Ethinyl estradiol/norethindrone acetate/ferrous fumarate (Estrostep FE)— iron overload possible, so check if history of hemochromatosis, etc.

3. Ethinyl estradiol/drospirenone (Yaz)—higher risk of blood clots.

4. Ethinyl estradiol/drospirenone/levomefolate (Beyaz).

Works well if you tell them to start taking the Sunday after their next period (vs. just picking up the med and starting whenever). If their next period is on a Sunday, then take it on that day. If next period is on a Monday, take it the next Sunday (6 days later). This helps sync with hormones.

Possible side effects of OCPs: Blood clots, heart attack, stroke, breast and cervical cancer (primarily 35-plus-year-old smokers with HTN).

Should avoid if pregnant, history of breast cancer/clots/heart disease/ stroke, breastfeeding <6 weeks after delivery, HTN (>160/100), diabetes (with end-organ damage or 20+ years), undergoing surgery with immobilization, migraines, 35-plus-year-old heavy smoker.

Also probably best to avoid within first 2 years of starting menses or if <14 years old (possible risk of decreased bone mass, especially younger patients).

FYI: OK to add OCPs during isotretinoin if desired (for example, if their method of contraception was abstinence at the start of isotretinoin course, you can add OCPs during treatment but just have to document that their method of contraception remains abstinence).

Acute fixes (if has upcoming wedding or prom, etc.):

- If diffuse: prednisone 40 mg × 3 days (last dose am of event)

- For individual lesions:

  - Pustule: I&D

  - Papule: ILK (2.5 mg/mL max concentration, low volume, stay shallow)

    - Topicals also work: class 1 steroid on papule for 2–3 nights (apply with Q-tip, avoid surrounding skin)

    - For example, Duobri (halobetasol + tazarotene)

Acne Scars

Most are atrophic scars (80–90%), which are caused by collagen degradation during healing process (vs. hypertrophic scars = gaining of collagen).

First figure out type of acne scars (ice pick vs. rolling vs. boxcar, etc.).

- Can turn off lights and shine flashlight under their chin to help with determining depth and type.

■ Also consider skin type.

■ Set expectations to avoid disappointment (scars will be improved [less deep] by 50%, not going to be perfect).

■ Active acne needs treated before procedural stuff (shouldn't have had breakout in past 6 months, really).

- If been on isotretinoin, data states needs to be 6 months after finishing, but can probably do slightly less than that, unless doing ablative lasers (which are more aggressive than vascular lasers, hair removal lasers, RF, etc.).

■ If still red, means body is still healing—probably need PDL (to treat the redness and telangiectasias [also mildly helpful in stimulating collagen production]) more so than CO_2/subcision (which are more aggressive).

Should treat the individual scar lesions before smoothing things out via field treatment (lasers, peels, dermabrasion, microneedling, RF).

■ *Ice pick scars (most common)*—narrow, sharp, can be deep (into deep dermis or even subQ).

- If shallow, can do TCA cross (65–100%, which is way stronger than what they use for chemical peels).
  - TCA denatures the collagen (scar tissue), stimulates remodeling immediately after treatment (basically creating new collagen to raise the scar).
  - Have patients remove makeup (don't want the scars to be plugged with makeup).
  - Do lower concentration on skin of color (risk hyperpigmentation).
  - Don't need to numb; feels like small ant bites.
  - Ideally, don't get the TCA very far outside the scar (can use end of Q-tip or end of culture swab [acts more like a syringe]).
  - Will see frosting pretty quickly (just like chemical peels), then turn red, then will scab (tell them not to pick them off).
  - Need 2–4 treatments, Q 4–6 weeks.
  - Nice because quite easy to do.
- If deep, can do 2 mm punch excision and put a fast-absorbing plain gut through it.

■ *Boxcar*—rigid straight lines (looks like punch biopsy that was never stitched).

- Wider, TCA would be too aggressive.
- If shallow, can do lasers, dermabrasion, or microneedling.
- If deep, then punch them out and put tiny sutures through them.
- If bigger, can do punch and then graft (usually from retroauricular) inside the area you punch; some people use Dermabond rather than stitch, or even Steri-Strip the graft on.

■ *Rolling scars*—smooth edge in and out (looks like over-aggressive shave biopsy).

- Probably hardest to get rid of; it's when you have the fibrous tethers that pull down the dermis to the subQ, thus have to subcision (break the tether so skin can rebound upward).

- If subcising just a few, can numb them individually.

- If subcising a lot (like a whole cheek), then should tumesce.

  - Tumescent is nice because helps you find the plane because pumping so much liquid in there.

  - The needles are pretty big, but the entry points heal up much better than you might think.

    - *Needle option examples*: 27G, 23G, 18G, Nokor 18G, cannula (but cannulas have blunter ends, so they don't work as well in breaking up the tethers).

  - Pick a good area to move in for your entry point (want a lot of area to swing your hand—like a pivot point with a big arc).

  - Usually either from lateral cheek or inferior.

  - Should almost see the needle (should be right under the epidermis—and keep it shallow), move it back and forth (end of needle is basically a scalpel), and turn it sideways (can feel and hear the bands snap).

  - Can see skin rebound up essentially right after doing it.

- Warn patients about bruising.

- After treating the deeper lesions, can think about laser resurfacing, or if mild scarring at baseline, can just do ablative (Erb:YAG, fractionated CO_2, etc.).

2.1.9.2 Rosacea

Usually in 30 year olds or older (not really kids).

Ask about eye involvement (FB sensation, blurry vision, etc.). If (+), encourage ophtho follow-up + start PO doxycycline 100 mg BID. Can also recommend lid hygiene (helps when meibomian glands are inflamed or clogged up, such as in blepharitis) and preservative-free eye drops (such as Systane—the single-use ones that come in a box are better vs. the bottle; can store in fridge to make it feel better).

FYI: Restasis drops have preservatives, as do many eye drops.

There are two rosacea reds:

1. Inflammatory red (acneiform papules or centrofacial edema)

2. Stretched blood vessels that are scarred red (doesn't matter what you put on topically, won't go away)

For inflammatory red:

Usually start with Metrogel or Metrocream QHS. PO doxycycline 50 mg BID if moderate to severe.

Other topicals are options but have their issues: azelaic acid (doesn't work super well; can try for pustules) QHS, topical ivermectin (Soolantra) QD ($$$), sodium sulfacetamide (smells bad) lotion, brimonidine (rebound).

Obviously, counsel on common triggers (EtOH, sun, spicy foods, etc.) and to avoid any suspected inciting factors.

Isotretinoin if refractory.

Laser works but is not covered.

For steroid rosacea, give PO doxycycline 50 mg QD + low-potency TCSs (to replace the high-potency TCSs that caused it; otherwise, will have scale + itch).

Rhinophyma:

Patients with background tendency for rosacea can have soft tissue changes on nose—consider low-dose doxycycline and/or procedural resurfacing if symptomatic/develops noticeable rhinophymatous changes.

Isotretinoin >>> doxycycline.

Similar to sebaceous hyperplasia, will need to pulse it on/off and is more of a maintenance thing to do after getting improvements with procedural stuff.

Procedural for rhinophyma: Will need to numb and let sit for 10 minutes to get to epinephrine effect.

For large nodules:

- Should debulk with a 15 blade or shave blade (but keep the blade flat; don't curve it like done for BCCs).

- Then do loop cautery (requires a special attachment for the hyfrecator or Bovie).

  - Hit the yellow button (cut), not the blue (coag).

  - Want to get to just below the yellow sebaceous lobules (in other words, if it's barely yellow, then you're not deep enough).

    - Saves time to just get to the level you need then do the entire nose (don't repeatedly take a bunch of thin layers until you get there).

- Once bulk is gone, can do dermabrasion, CO_2, or erbium to touch it up/smooth it out.

- Post-op care:

  - Heals in 1 week; cover with Telfa and paper tape (weeps a little in beginning).

  - Keep greasy with mupirocin ointment (antibiotics rational given it's the whole nose).

- Covered by insurance if for example it's medically necessary (if they can't breathe well through their nose).

2.1.9.3 Acrochordon (Skin Tag)

Can snip off with scissors or LN2.

1. Usually don't numb (hurts more than just snipping)—unless on large stalk that think might bleed (epinephrine in the lidocaine can help with that).

   a. I prefer snipping; LN2 harder to judge whether effective and entails a longer healing process.

2.1.9.4 Acanthosis Nigricans

Darker and thicker skin. Typically body folds. Sometimes related to insulin/ diabetes (body has to make more insulin to keep sugar normal, and insulin can act as epidermal growth factor).

A papillomatosis, not a hyperkeratotic disorder; thus, keratolytics (AmLactin) don't work and aren't rational. There are no medicines for papillomatosis.

Best thing can offer is to avoid colonization/eczematization; also should address manifestation of insulin resistance.

2.1.9.5 Corn

From repeated friction (possibly ill-fitting shoes, not wearing socks, bony prominences in feet).

Soft corns (more soggy-appearing) and hard corns (tops of toes, painful, press on nerves; usually dry-appearing).

Ddx corns vs. calluses vs. warts (warts have thrombosed capillary [black dots] on dermoscopy).

Can cut it out in clinic (thin it down with 15 blade; make sure you remove the core).

Can also recommend OTC 17% salicylic acid pad (usually QD for 4–6 weeks at least).

Need better-fitting shoes, possibly insoles.

2.1.9.6 Porokeratosis

- Use marker and wipe to accentuate cornoid lamellae if can't see. Sometimes it's very subtle (in some cases arguably nonexistent).

- If opt to biopsy, try to get what you think might be the peripheral scale— histologically pathognomonic.

- When have multiple lesions (such as in DSAP), can try TCSs, TCA peels/ chemo wraps, or blue light.

2.1.9.7 Keratosis Pilaris (KP)

Arms get prickly when dry (basically the keratin pooches up around the hair follicles). Bad news is that keratin is the cement that holds the skin together, so will probably never get KP perfect because it would theoretically dissolve the skin. But usually gets better with age.

Can affect thighs.

Not as itchy as follicular eczema.

MANAGEMENT

Keratolytics (salicylic acid [CeraVe SA cream], lactic acid [AmLactin lotion— may get stingy in the winter], or urea creams).

Acitretin would probably work, given it's a disorder of keratinization, but needs to be bad to justify this.

An aside on KP atrophicans (KPA):

KP is when it's just bumps on arms/legs. When on face, it's different, because this means there's inflammation deep down in the hair follicle, which is problematic, because it will leave pits/scars if not addressed. KPA is the overall category. If involves eyebrows, then it's called ulerythema ophryogenes. If has the pitted lesions on cheeks (looks like acne but it's not), then it's called atrophoderma vermiculatum. And so on.

While it supposedly tends to become less noticeable with time (generally after puberty), important to treat to minimize the disfiguring scars. *The books essentially say nothing really works, but a regimen that may help slightly:*

- Clindamycin gel QAM (has propylene glycol and takes the clindamycin down deep into the hair follicle and makes the immune cells disperse and stops them from attacking).

- Hydrocortisone 1% or 2.5% max at lunchtime (reduces the irritation from the retinoid).

- Tretinoin QHS (helps sand it down a little).

2.1.9.8 Folliculitis

Many non-dermatologists make the mistake of perceiving pustules as a sign of infection (even though most pustules in derm are sterile—such as acne [sterile except for floral, rosacea).

So when see pustules, question if patient has history of eczema (or other itchy conditions), using TCSs (smearing back and forth or something), has been treated with prolonged antibiotics (Gram-negative folliculitis), shaving habits, other exposures to waters/oils.

Relevant because can have recurrent folliculitis from scratching scalp in setting of pruritus from seb derm, and thus, what you really need to treat (perhaps all you need to treat) is the itch (pustules can sometimes be more of a sign they itch than a sign of an infection).

However, can of course also truly be bacterial, fungal, viral, parasitic, etc. If immunocompromised, can evolve to furunculosis (*furuncles* are deep; *carbuncles* are deep sinus tracts between furuncles).

So again management is all about etiology:

- Staph most common (characteristically gold pus—hence the name *aureus*); if mild, may not even need to treat. Can use BPO or something. If extensive or not resolving within few weeks, can do topical clindamycin BID for 1 week or so. Mupirocin also fine. Cephalexin if doesn't respond, or doxycycline (or TMP-SMX) if suspecting MRSA.

- Strep less common; tends to make white pus.

- *Pseudomonas* (contaminated pools) often self-resolves.

- *Pityrosporum* (Malassezia) can do ketoconazole shampoo 3–4× weekly for 1 month (let sit for 5 minutes), or PO fluconazole 200 mg QD for 2 weeks, then 300 mg QW for 1–2 months.

  - *Pityrosporum* folliculitis is characteristically widespread; can check with Wood's lamp (center glows green vs. acne, where it glows neon pink due to the porphyrins in *P. acnes* vs. just keratin [such as KP or eruptive vellus hair cysts], which reflects the blue light as bluish white).

- Dermatophytes (tinea or Majocchi's) can do PO terbinafine 250 mg QD for 4 weeks.

- Candida can do fluconazole.

- HSV/VZV can do Valtrex 1 g TID for 7 days.

- Molluscum can do cantharidin or LN2.

FYI: Solitary lesions of folliculitis/furuncles heal just as well with or without antibiotics when you nick them (so drain anything with pus). While PO antibiotics for MRSA abscesses don't lead to faster resolution, they give a lower rate of recurrence of abscesses (and patients do better when you address all sites of carriage—so give PO antibiotic + topical toward the nose + bleach bath or chlorhexidine [or whatever you're doing for surface carriage]).

If they're using the same razor, same loofah sponge, same soap, same towels, all that stuff is carrying staph; so use liquid soap, encourage using their own towel (and launder the towel after using it, because if it's still moist, the staph will still be there the next day).

For cold-indolent abscesses, think AFB, especially if developed after procedure (routine culture tends to make you miss fungi [other than yeast; candida grows fine], anaerobes, and AFB [requires special media]). Clarithromycin has the broadest anti-mycobacterial coverage; question is whether to use as monotherapy (can do for skin-limited infections). For more serious infections, would want to do with rifampin or triple-drug therapy. When purely an abscess, drainage alone will heal a lot of AFB abscesses.

2.1.9.9 Pseudofolliculitis Barbae

Shaving bumps.

Noninfectious folliculitis from foreign-body reaction.

Usually in curly-haired individuals who need to shave (military, etc.), especially if using razors with multiple blades, plucking hairs, shaving against direction of hair growth.

Can see entrapped hairs within the papules sometimes. Usually beard. Possibly neck, cheeks, groin. Darker lesions are older. Can get keloids, scarring.

MANAGEMENT

1. Some people say shaving makes worse, but the actual problem might be how often they shave and their shaving technique.

   a. Shaving somewhat frequently is preferable (3× weekly or more), because it may prevent hair from growing long enough to cause irritation.

   b. If they shave in the shower, they should do it first (the warmth and steam from the shower will swell the skin, so the shave won't be as close and the hairs can dig back in and cause irritation).

   c. Patients should pre-treat before shaving with a gentle cleanser like Gillette or Aveeno.

   d. Can recommend Gillette Labs razors. The Art of Shaving products are also nice.

   e. Shave in direction of follicles. Don't pull skin taut, and don't shave over area twice.

   f. Don't pluck; can try to lift the end of the ingrown hairs out of the papules with tweezers.

   g. Apply OTC hydrocortisone after shaving, possibly topical clindamycin.

   h. Tretinoin QHS might help.

   i. They will often want doxycycline. Try to be a good steward. Can give short courses if flaring badly or if superinfected.

2. Need to eliminate papules/pustules/ingrown hairs to fix color problem.

a. If dark, then need laser hair reduction.

   i. Laser hair reduction is ~Q 6–8 weeks for facial hair for 8–10 treatments, then maintenance Q 1 year.

     – Have to repeat because lasers only kill the anagen hairs. Thus, tell patients when they get offered a package of "three treatments or something" seems like salesmanship but is actually worth it.

     – Tell them fine to shave a few days before, but don't wax.

   ii. Prices vary, but probably around a couple hundred per treatment.

   iii. Patients may wonder if there is such a thing as having too dark a skin for laser (isn't true; just need the right laser).

b. If dark + gray, then can get electrolysis.

   i. Electrolysis (probe individually damages the hair follicle so it can't grow) is cheaper but more painful, and more rounds of treatments compared to laser (20–30 treatments).

2.1.10 Psychiatric
2.1.10.1 Approach

1. Change your mindset to think more like a psychiatrist (part of the therapy is connecting with provider, not the prescription you write—much different than the usual medical mindset [evidence-based, objective]).

2. First, find out whether they will admit to picking.

3. If they admit, then it's easy—find out why.

a. If they say they do it because they're feeling bad, anxious, stressed, depressed; easy, because then you can just refer to psych.

b. If scratching because stressed, can try asking them to think of something that helps relax them—tell them to do that once per day every day until next appointment, and then you'll talk about it.

4. Not uncommon that they deny it ("It just came up").

a. If you encounter denial, don't be confrontational (usually, it's because of stigma/embarrassment); just temporize, show a lot of interest, and see if over time they will open up.

b. It's a matter of rapport—not realistic to expect to connect fully on day 1, but can help them understand you're trying to help, and you're not judgmental; look at their "specimen" and look at their skin.

c. Can give them a small treatment, like DuoDERM, etc., on first visit, and when they come back, reinforce they're doing well and are such a good patient; don't rush the topic of pharmacologic intervention.

d. Once there is rapport, shift away from etiology to treatment.

   i. *Can say something like,* "It's a mysterious syndrome. Nobody knows what it is, but most people who get it are [describe patient]. This is terrible. [Rehash all the ways it's been crippling their quality of life, not being able to help their family, fear of spreading to others, etc.]."

ii. "I want to know what is causing this as much as you do, but we will die of old age if we spend all our time trying to figure out what it is, and we just need to get you out of this ASAP."

iii. Remind them you're not an ID specialist, or parasitologist, but you know of some precious medications that seem to work but nobody knows how they work.

- *For example*: "If it works for you, I can't tell you why, but if you're willing to try it, then I'm happy to try it. If you still want to go for etiology, I've done all I could—feel free to go see a parasitologist, ID specialist, etc., and if they can't help, you're always welcome back here."

iv. They will probably ask if it's a psych med: "It's not. If any pharmacists tell you this is a psych medicine, they're wrong. All you have to do is look it up on the FDA website." (This only really works for pimozide, since it doesn't have FDA indications for psychiatric stuff.)

e. See them frequently (even if brief; don't make them feel like they can only get an appointment if they need something)—makes easier to build rapport.

i. When people are really depressed, it's easier for them to deny things; if they're severely depressed and don't even want to talk about it, may take multiple visits before they open up.

5. If they completely lack insight (delusions of parasitosis)—different ballgame; think about anti-psychotics. This will take proactive explaining.

a. Some basic questions and counseling before discussing pharmacotherapies:

i. "Do you feel like there's something in there that you need to get out?"

ii. "*Formication* is the fibromyalgia of the skin surface. Small nerve fibers sending signals to the brain. Need to break the cycle and prevent infection."

- Let them know there are two forms of formication—one is the psychiatric formication, where people think there are bugs in the skin and on the wall, and the other one is surface fibromyalgia (so tell them they have the latter—small nerve fibers in the skin [not the muscle/joints like regular fibromyalgia]).

b. "In dermatology, we steal meds from other fields to treat rashes. Doxepin 150 mg QD used for depression, we use 10 mg QD to block the histamine receptors in hives. MTX 20 pills per day used in the past for chemo, we use 10 pills per week and often even less than that to treat various rashes. And we use something called trifluoperazine (Stelazine), which at 40 mg QD is for insane people. We use 1/40th of the dose because it's amazing for skin fibromyalgia/formication—stops the tingling feeling—which no skin meds can really do. If you're willing to try Stelazine 1–2 mg QD, predict you will be 50–75% better in 1 month."

i. Stelazine much cheaper than pimozide, risperidone, olanzapine, thus doesn't need prior auth; explain very safe at doses we use (safety data is for psych doses).

ii. However, if they're completely against using Stelazine, can try pimozide, which is not FDA-approved for any psychotic indication—see more later.

c. Psychiatrists write the ethics articles about this, but they don't see these patients, so they don't appreciate the issues that dermatologists experience. The usual sense of ethics doesn't apply. The relevant ethical compass is what is best for the patient. In other words, you don't just tell them they are psychotic, there are no parasites, here's an anti-psychotic med—if you want to cover yourself and fail the patient, you can do this, but if you care about the patient, this is one instance where withholding the diagnosis is in the patient's best interest.

d. Never reinforce delusion (for example, don't give ivermectin, etc.).

e. Give them an out "small fiber neuropathy," get them confident in you, and then ask them to let you give the real medicine for 1 month and see if it works.

Most of DSM-5 doesn't apply. Many patients use anxiety/stress interchangeably; depression, psychosis, OCD are basically the breadth. If cosmetics, then personality disorder. If you can get through this psych ddx, you're in good shape.

2.1.10.2 Management

Non-pharmacologic:

- *Habit reversal/replacement therapy*: systematic way of addressing repetitive self-injurious behavior (some mental health specialists focus on this).

- *Cognitive behavioral therapy*: all of us have a certain pattern of aperture of thoughts. Accomplished people think positively; they work on mindset. Antecedence (something triggers their behavior), if trigger is negative thoughts, then more effective if CBT vs. purely behavioral therapy.

- *For people who pick habitually and unconsciously*: tell them to go buy a cheap digital watch, and set alarm Q 1 hour. If they find themselves picking or about to pick, tell them if they can wait 5 seconds, then they can pick (but if they can wait 5 seconds, then try to wait 8). If they can wait 20 seconds, the urge tends to go away, etc.—simple approach to behavioral extinction.

Pharmacologic:

More than half of psych meds prescribed are from non-psychiatrists (usually IM, PCPs, FM, peds), so don't feel weird about prescribing it.

1. Buspirone—anti-stress/anxiety med around since 1980s.

   a. *Pros*: minimal (if any) side effects, non-sedating, non-addictive.

   b. *Cons*: 1 month to see effect; not sexy because people want benzos (fast-acting); 5–10 mg BID to QID; if no response at 1 month, then uptitrate.

2. Alprazolam—old benzodiazepine.

   a. *Pros*: generic (cheap), quick-acting.

   b. *Cons*: possibly addictive, thus limit how much/how long you give (think like high-potency TCSs—not going to give a lifetime supply).

      i. Smallest dose 0.25 mg. If break in half, guarantee that nothing bad will happen, but also guarantee nothing good will happen. Can start here, then go up to 0.25 mg, then 0.5 mg, etc.; try to take off the stress without causing sedation.

    ii. Once controlled, don't keep on for longer than 2 months (usually, acute stress goes up and down). When you stop, taper down (don't stop abruptly).

3. Paroxetine (SSRI)—more relaxing, dosing is simple.

    a. Multiple FDA indications (not just depression); 10 mg (low dose) is good for anxiety, 20 mg is good for depression, and OCD might need 60–80 mg.

        i. If you have chronic psych patient, 20 mg might not be good enough, but many derm patients may not have had a psych med, so 20 mg is probably plenty.

        ii. Sexual dysfunction for men pretty rare; other nonspecific side effects; don't see weight gain as much in derm patients.

    b. SSRIs good if picking obsessively.

        i. If they say they tried to stop, usually they will either say they do it when they're bored or they say the more they try to stop, the more they feel restless/see things/have strong urge to pick—this is OCD picking; SSRIs beneficial.

        ii. *Cons*: benefits come 2 months later.

4. Doxepin—low dose has been head-to-head compared against diazepam (Valium).

    a. Most powerful anti-itch antihistamine (blocks 260× better than Benadryl, 62× better than hydroxyzine).

    b. But individual metabolism is hugely variable.

    c. If you're willing to titrate, then doxepin is just as good at controlling anxiety without being addictive; also helps with itching (even though there is no primary derm etiology, they scratch so much that the itch becomes real). Start 10 mg QHS, then adjust individually.

        i. Can get doxepin trough serum level (needs to be at least 12 hours after last dose); some people are ultra-metabolizers and might need up to 300 mg QD (as long as in therapeutic range, then you're fine).

5. N-acetylcysteine (NAC) (OTC)—sometimes causes GI upset, but generally well-tolerated.

    a. Dosing is on bottle; just start at the lowest dose and titrate up. Seems to be helpful for OCD type of picking.

    b. *Con*: supplement that patients have to get themselves; not covered by insurance.

6. Memantine (anti-dementia med)—if demented and chronically picking on skin, can try this; 10 mg QD for 2 weeks, then 20 mg QD for 6 weeks. Can reduce hair pulling, skin picking.

Psychotic patients (delusions of parasitosis) have crazy ideas why they pick their skin.

1. *Good news*: meds like pimozide, risperidone, work well.

2. *Bad news*: the problem isn't the med efficacy; it's connecting with these patients.

3. Both risperidone and pimozide come in 1 mg tablet; start with either 0.5 or 1 mg.

   a. Don't expect any benefit until getting to 3 mg (be patient; we go slowly). Increase half-tablet every 2–3 weeks until getting to 3 mg (patient will often say, "I think the bugs are dying, I don't feel it anymore," etc.). Keep going until symptoms are almost gone or are gone (clear or almost clear), then continue at that dose for 3–4 more months (if abruptly stopped or tapering too soon, it will recur and patient will get very discouraged).

      i. Most derm patients need 3 mg QD (+/–1 mg QD). Pimozide for Tourette's dosing often higher (around 10 mg QD).

   b. For tapers, lower by half a tablet every 2 months.

   c. Reason pimozide is great is that it has no anti-psychiatric indication (explicitly and proactively tell patients this); a lot of the other meds they will look up they will see are anti-psychotics for insane people (like Stelazine).

   d. Theoretically can get stiffness/restlessness (pseudoparkinsonism, akathisia), so have them carry OTC Benadryl 25 mg up to QID for stiffness/restlessness. But almost never happens, and if you stop the med, they will disappear anyway (but should still just use the Benadryl, though).

   e. Can also get cardiac side effects. (The cardiac complications occur in high doses in Europe for schizophrenics, not at derm doses; nonetheless, should probably get before and after EKG. If any abnormalities, ask PCP or cardiologist for their blessing to use it.)

   f. Tardive dyskinesia almost never happens and, when does, usually only if high dose for long time.

Other considerations and simple/topical options:

1. For formication on arms: can also wrap in Unna + say, "GOC are to heal open areas, but taking the Unna off will ruin everything. If you get a lesion, put a Band-Aid on it and come in."

2. Pramoxine is also good for neurogenic itch; can treat secondary lesions (prurigo nodules, LSC, etc.) with clobetasol.

3. Keep in mind, gabapentin, pregabalin, Stelazine—not great for fall risk.

4. If doing gabapentin, do very low dose if also on SSRI (can potentiate).

Most people who achieve remission never change their mind (they think the pimozide killed the bugs; only rarely do they say, "I know I don't have bugs").

2.1.11 Undifferentiated Pruritus

Chronic itch affects 40% of the world, increases with age (roughly 28% geriatric), and is also more common in Black skin.

1. Are there primary lesions? (Such as LP, AD, psoriasis, etc.)

2. If no primary lesions and just excoriations, for instance, start with very basic labs.

   a. CMP (looking for: LFTs, renal function, glucose).

b. CBC with diff (looking for hematologic dyscrasia and eosinophils [Th2 polarization or AD phenotype can have high eosinophils and high IgE]).

   i. If have Th2 polarization on labs (supportive but don't need them): dupilumab might work via downregulating IgE (Th2-modulating therapy).

   ii. Atopy is usually moderate eosinophilia.

   – If eosinophils are startlingly high, consider other things on NAACP ddx (neoplasia [CML, Hodgkin's], Addison's, connective tissue disorders/Churg–Strauss, parasite).

c. TSH.

d. Other things (depending on presentation).

   i. Can consider imaging for lymphoma (CT CAP, HIV—even treated HIV can have significant itch).

   ii. BNP (chronic itch biomarker—but hard to get approved indication).

3. Chronic itch.

a. IL31 = prototypical cytokine mediator of itch; also IL4, IL13, JAK–STAT pathway.

b. Th2 cytokines very important—can directly stimulate nerve fibers; others are less prominently involved, such as Th17 (psoriasis).

   i. Thus why new biologics resolve the itch first (before the inflammation).

   ii. Inflammation -> destroys DEJ -> less itch, but more pain (thus panniculitis usually not itchy, but painful; same with deep dermal infiltrates).

   iii. Scabies, bullous pemphigoid, others also associated with Th2 cytokines.

c. Need nerves; without nerves, you don't have itch (itch + pain can coexist; some PN patients have chronic burning pain too).

   i. Patients might say, "I put clothing on and felt more itch, change in temperature and felt more itch," due to neurosensitization.

   ii. Less nerves in epidermis in AD skin for some reason (counterintuitive)—possibly related to proteases that downregulate nerves (Wallerian degeneration) that cause neuropathy type of phenomenon.

MANAGEMENT

Most itch meds are off-label.

All itches have an immune side and neural side; on a spectrum.

No perfect drug that covers all itch, but management options vast now: dupilumab, nemolizumab, JAKi, IL17s, etc.

1. Upadacitinib and abrocitinib are most potent anti-itch, followed by dupilumab. Tralokinumab is least effective for itching; baricitinib also not very impressive.

2. Nemolizumab works rapidly; even one injection makes big difference. Many improve (itch, sleep disturbance, etc.) by 4 weeks.

   a. Has less robust effect on inflammation than IL4/13; thus, its potential in AD is less exciting (except for low inflammatory stuff like lichenification) but will be very strong against itch.

3. GABAergic drugs: good for neuropathic itch, CKD itch, idiopathic chronic itch, CTCL.

   a. Gabapentin (start low, especially in older patients, because can be sedated off other meds; can start 100 mg QHS, and can increase by 100 mg per day).

4. Beta-alanine (sports supplement) appears to work well for aquagenic pruritus.

There are also imbalances in μ- and κ-opioids in chronic itch (mu endogenous overexpression = more itch [just like opioids that work on mu agonist cause itch as side effect]; kappa downregulates mu).

1. Butorphanol (kappa opioid and mu antagonist) is an inhaler, good for intractable itch; doesn't cause addiction.

Miscellaneous itchy entities:

1. Notalgia paresthetica (unilateral scapular pruritus)—usually, notalgia is very focal and a specific spot (patients will say "Right there"); recommend keeping neck as straight as possible (might have pillow that is too hard or too soft). Yoga is good for necks. Can try Sarna Sensitive at night.

2. Pudendal dysesthesia: perineal itching in skinny elderly men with dry skin. When sitting, causes neuralgia (small impingements). Can try topicals, topical gabapentin 6–12% ointment, doxepin cream sometimes, or lidocaine (need to trust they will only put focally and won't put on large areas of body).

3. Scalp dysesthesia.

   a. Common after menopause; essentially, scalp nerve endings transmit itch signals.

   b. Itch is out of proportion to the inflammation, so hard to treat (anti-inflammatories not very effective; gabapentin rational but needs somewhat high doses, which can make older people sleepy).

   c. Stress, of course, makes it worse (just like stress makes blood pressure worse).

4. Itchy red scrotum.

   a. Red bag syndrome: caudal neuropathy nerves coming out of back (burning itchy is not a rash; it is a neuropathy, typically worse at night, an itch that rashes); treat with SSD QD, 0.025% TAC BID PRN when irritated, gabapentin 100 mg QD.

   b. For pruritus scroti 2/2 caudal radiculopathy: gabapentin 300 QHS; if no response in 4 weeks, then increase to BID. Second line is pregabalin, third is naloxone, fourth is TCAs, which are better for burning sensations.

5. Uremic pruritus (at least ~50% of ESRD patients)—*FYI*: Doesn't correlate with extent of uremia or Cr levels or duration on dialysis.

   a. Resistant to conventional anti-itch regimens (corticosteroids [both topical and systemic]/antihistamines).

   b. Phototherapy sometimes helpful but of course increases risk of skin cancer (consider if patient potential transplant candidate).

   c. Renal transplant most effective, but HD doesn't help.

   d. Generalized xerosis also very common (at least half-ESRD patients); more common in PD > HD, for some reason.

   i. Lipid-rich emollients, mild keratolytics (dissolves scales).

6. ESRD + lymphoma patients are always itchy, so they scratch deep -> damage follicles and collagen -> body tries to get rid of it -> perforating disease (such as Kyrle's disease, where body tries to transepidermally eliminate keratin).

7. Diabetes only causes localized pruritus (used to be thought to cause generalized).

2.2 GENERAL DERMATOLOGY—NEOPLASMS
2.2.1 Keratinocytic
2.2.1.1 Malignant

Skin cancers in setting of immunosuppression occur roughly 5–10 years after starting the immunosuppressive meds (so don't expect them to be growing NMSCs a month after their transplant, even though they will often be referred to you immediately after).

Transplant patients are at higher risk of SCC (65×), BCC (5×), and melanoma (3×), and they grow faster/more aggressively too. Not only because of poorer immune surveillance but also because of possible HPV co-infection.

FYI: This is relative to baseline risk (so a baby who had a heart transplant still shouldn't be sprouting NMSCs).

AZA + CsA are the worst; AZA metabolites incorporate into DNA and absorb UVB really well, which persists for 5 years even after cessation (keep in mind before prescribing). CsA causes more problems than tacrolimus because distributes into skin cells more extensively (hence why we don't really use Prograf for rashes [in addition to the need for monitoring, etc.]).

When immunosuppressed patients start developing skin cancers, they develop a lot and fast—very steep changes (so should almost think of their first skin cancer as a sentinel event in the sense it may be a foreshadowing of many more to come).

Heart and lung highest risk because rapidly fatal if rejected (so they immunosuppress them more).

Sirolimus and everolimus (mTor inhibitors) seem to be least problematic with skin cancers, so if patient having major issues with their skin, correspond with transplant to see about switching to these (or reducing doses).

Can also consider acitretin as NMSC prophylaxis in transplant patients (normalizes keratinocytes—particularly protective against SCCs; however, need high dose, which can be hard to tolerate [xerosis, etc.], and once you stop it, all the NMSCs that "were prevented" seem to build up and surface all at once). Niacinamide written about but doesn't seem super helpful.

2.2.1.1.1 Basal Cell Carcinoma (BCC)

Cancer is, of course, a scary word for patients. You can alleviate the disproportionate stress by telling them BCC is the most common cancer in humans, period (~20–30% of fair-skinned people get them), and doesn't tend to spread to liver/lungs or shorten life (only metastasizes 1/35k and usually only if they get huge and invade nerves/lymph nodes), but they will continue to grow (and thus can threaten cosmesis/function) so should be removed.

Often, patients will have scabs, from pets or something. If they have a reliable story, it's fine; if they're unsure, make sure you let them know NMSCs can look like scabs that never heal and often bleed for no reason (thus should RTC for biopsy if doesn't heal within a couple of months and/or grows).

Other clues:

- Feel the scabs; if they feel infiltrated, then more concerning for BCC.

- Sometimes itchy.

- Learn the dermoscopy features (look at pictures).

- Roughly doubles in size Q 6 months to 1 year on average (typically takes 10+ years unaddressed to metastasize).

Clinical and dermoscopic nuances typically correlate with histologic subtype.

- *Nodular* (most common) tends to have more arborizing vessels (often more pigmented in skin of color), rolled borders, smooth/shiny surface.

- *Superficial BCCs* (second most common) look more psoriasiform clinically, or like an SCCIS.

- *Infiltrative BCCs* (less common, more aggressive) tend to look ulcerated/ eroded/depressed, possibly with crust; usually not well-defined (can grow downward more than upward, so skin surface can sometimes be misleading as far as how big it actually is).

- There are, of course, several other subtypes you should know (albeit less common).

Ddx:

- *Spider angioma*: pulsates with glass slide, then disperses like a spider (BCCs don't do that).

- *Fibrous papules* can have telangiectasia but of course behave more innocently than BCC (don't really grow, don't bleed, etc.).

- *Trichoblastoma/trichoepithelioma*: less likely to be ulcerated than BCC, and more innocently behaved; also much rarer. Subtle dermoscopy differences. Realistically, probably best to biopsy if unsure.

- *Intradermal nevi*: usually more squishy than BCC but can have telangiectasias and look shiny sometimes. Can ask how long been there (if unchanged for many years, then probably OK, but sometimes BCCs can look a lot like benign nevi).

- *Has wobble sign* on dermoscopy (nevus can be moved side to side with the dermatoscope).

- *LPLK*: honestly sometimes hard to tell, and a few times biopsy of lesions that looked a lot like LPLKs turned out to be BCCs (albeit happened in patients who had track records of many BCCs—so should probably consider that).

Management options are broad and are generally dictated by histologic subtype, location (cosmesis or high-risk site), size, whether it's a recurrence, patient's immune status (in other words, if it's high or low risk—look up NCCN guidelines).

Would look up the Mohs Appropriate Use Criteria (there's a nice app, "Mohs AUC," that can calculate the score for you), and know the H, M, and L areas at least to start. Size cutoffs vary by location and histologic subtype.

Excision or EDC generally appropriate for low risk; LN2 and topicals (5-FU, imiquimod, etc.) also might be reasonable for some patients.

Mohs generally best for high risk.

For example, 5-FU wouldn't really be a great option for an infiltrative BCC (because tentacles go too deep), and EDC not great because tissue can be like a scar when gets deep (vs. the rotten apple stuff), so hard to tell when to stop curetting.

EDC less favorable for hair-bearing skin (tumor can track down follicular units). Also not great cosmetically (usually white circle scars, possibly hypertrophic scars).

LN2 not favorable for hair-bearing skin (alopecia) or legs (ulcers). Poor cosmetic outcome as well (scars are also usually white circles though don't tend to cause hypertrophic scars).

Imiquimod good for cosmetically sensitive areas—such as the genitals—or something like a confluent superficial BCC on dorsum of nose (wouldn't be desirable to do Mohs for a wide area and shallow tumor).

Intralesionals are also an option; intralesional 5-FU (have to numb before you inject) probably better because covers both BCCs/SCCs vs. intralesional MTX (doesn't really have as much evidence for BCCs).

Some patients may inquire about superficial radiation (they might fantasize about not getting scars, etc.). Advertised as something new but is an old technology. Would make sure rad-onc does it if patients are adamant. But plethora of options that are reliable/proven and would favor those. XRT also increases risk of future skin cancers, so don't do in young patients. Very expensive as well.

Procedures covered more extensively later; will cover med treatment options here.

All said, practically speaking, histologic subtype is important, but it's not everything. As long as you treat for an adequate duration with good instructions, you probably have an acceptable chance of clearing the cancer with topicals (particularly relevant for bad surgical candidates, older patients; in other words, wouldn't risk using topicals in a 50 year old on the face, for instance).

Topicals:

1. Good to outline the tumors (with desired margins) with a marker and take pics with the patient's phone so they know where to treat, because sometimes they can (understandably) lose sense of where the tumor is/was when it gets red/blotchy.

a. If doing imiquimod (usually Monday to Friday for 6 weeks), RTC at 8 weeks (2 weeks after finishing, so they have time to heal up/clear their reaction to the cream; otherwise, they will come in red/blotchy and you won't be able to appreciate their response [or lack thereof] as easily).

    i. Tell them to apply a thin layer with 15 mm margin Monday to Friday QD for 6 weeks after bathing.

    ii. Preface that imiquimod is pretty miserable; put gauze over it to avoid occluding itself.

    iii. If gets blistery, apply Vaseline.

        – *FYI*: Make sure they don't apply TCSs (want to encourage inflammation).

2. Combo treatment works well; some people do LN2, then wait for it to heal, but seems better to lightly LN2 (or CO_2 laser, etc.—same concept, basically poking holes in skin so creams penetrate better), then immediately do the creams.

a. Triple-therapy method works very well (for both BCC and SCC).

    i. LN2 lightly (only until it barely turns white, but get a margin too) at baseline and Q 2 weeks.

    ii. Combine tretinoin (highest %) imiquimod-5-FU on back of Telfa pad (don't need to mix it up; it'll spread out) and place overnight. Do Monday to Friday for 6 weeks (30 total applications).

When doing LN2 for cure, get the hard white all the way to the margin with LN2; thaw until white is gone, then do another two cycles. Usually, when you see recurrence, it happens on periphery of scar (suggesting the issue was a matter of width [vs. depth]). Remember to outline the lesion and the margin before spraying, because otherwise may lose track of the lesion.

Systemic options:

- Vismodegib—one cycle is 28 days of treatment; should assess at 1 month, see if they're responding, then decide if want to do another cycle. Not really used super frequently (but good for patients with innumerable BCCs, or BCC nevus syndrome). Not great for young patients.

    • Start 150 mg QD; see Q 1 month for first few months. Can take breaks, especially if having side effects (most commonly muscle spasms, dysgeusia)—if recovered from those side effects, can resume. Could pulse for a couple of months at a time then give a break (might help them avoid surgery if poor candidate).

    • Dysgeusia can be problematic, especially if they're frail/older at baseline (might lose weight from not eating) too, so follow frequently.

- Sonidegib 200 mg QD—can consider if can't tolerate vismodegib, though side effect profile somewhat similar.

- Cemiplimab (PD1 inhibitor)—can consider if failed the hedgehog inhibitors.

Using the systemics as neoadjuvant (shrink them before cutting them out) is a good tool for large tumors (theory is that tumors will shrink from the border [decreases size and depth, making it more primed for Mohs]), thus why you inject at the edges (edges are where the new vessels are formed, so likely where med is most distributed).

2.2.1.1.2 Squamous Cell Carcinoma (SCC)

Second most common skin cancer. Of course, can affect other organs, but focus here is on cutaneous SCC.

Risk factors: Radiation (total cumulative; usually XRs), HPV-related, chronically diseased/injured skin (radiation derm, ulcers, DLE, LSA, LP, blistering disorders, genoderms, etc.), immunosuppression (see earlier; 65× higher risk [relative to their baseline]).

Overall, ~10% of men and ~5% of women will get. Darker-skinned patients more often get in scars/non-healing ulcers. Roughly 4% metastasize.

Satellite mets are close to the primary tumor (within 2 cm).

In-transit mets are further away (>2 cm) from the primary tumor. Both essentially the same thing clinically (serious but haven't yet reached regional lymph nodes).

SCCs are categorized as low and high risk (with regard to metastasis and recurrence risk):

- *Low risk*, generally = small, well-defined, primary, on specific sites (such as neck/trunk/extremities). Low-risk SCCs generally have good cure rates, even with non-Mohs options (EDC, excision, LN2).

- *High-risk* tumors are essentially anything not low risk (large; quickly growing; a recurrence; immunosuppressed patient; arising within chronically damaged/diseased skin; on particular anatomic sites, such as ears, lips, scalp, forehead, temple, eyelids, nose, dorsal hands, genitals; etc.). Histologic features can also be high-risk (invasion to deep dermis [or below], poor differentiation, PNI, etc.).

Relative risks below are rough estimates (and subject to change, obviously), but just to give a general idea:

Bigger (>2 cm) SCCs recur (2×) and metastasize (3×) more often than smaller SCCs.

Rapidly growing SCCs and SCCs arising from chronically diseased/injured skin have ~3× risk of metastasis.

Deep dermis/subQ extension has higher recurrence (1.5×) and metastasis (5×) risk.

Immunosuppressed patients have ~2× higher metastasis risk than immunocompetent.

Recurrent tumors metastasize more often (~4–5×).

Poorly differentiated SCCs recur locally ~2×, metastasize ~3× more often than well-differentiated SCCs.

PNI (when the tumor hits a nerve fiber and then grows along it; if clinically apparent, then of course worse prognostically than if incidentally found on histology). Recurs and metastasizes ~5–6× more often than SCCs without PNI. Possible reason the rates are higher is that even if "margins are clear," don't know if there's noncontiguous tumor away from the surgical site.

For high-risk SCC, should do Mohs (or at least excision with appropriately wide margins). Can consider adjunctive medical treatment if very high risk.

Should know the BWH and AJCC staging systems. BWH basically stages the SCC based on the number of high-risk features (while also taking into account the presence of bone invasion). AJCC staging criteria is slightly more complicated but still considers essentially the same high-risk features. Usually best to actually consider both for all patients and take whichever gives them the higher risk.

Would also look up the NCCN guidelines (which are beyond just dermatology-specific [considered the gold standard across specialties, so nice to stay informed about updates which will better allow you to "speak the same language" when co-managing with other specialties]).

When looking at Mohs layers, SCCs tend to be less straightforward than BCCs (and sometimes you don't know they're high-risk until looking at the layers—particularly if the diagnostic biopsy was a small superficial portion of a larger and deeper lesion).

Should look for poor differentiation, whether invading subQ, PNI, intravascular invasion.

FYI: Regular excision layers are like a bread loaf (good chance that if it appears clear, you're just not seeing where the residual is). It's like having a moldy loaf of bread and only checking a few slices of the loaf.

Differentiating SCCs from AKs clinically can be difficult sometimes. *Some things to consider*:

- Ask if painful (painful is more concerning for SCC vs. AK).

- If noticeably more hyperkeratotic part of lesion in center, then more concerning for SCCIS vs. AK.

- If feels more infiltrated, then more concerning for SCC.

  - *FYI*: Cutaneous horns often have SCCIS underneath, especially if feel infiltrated (though cutaneous horn ddx also includes verruca, trichilemmoma, etc.).

FYI: If concerned for oral SCC, biopsy the red part, not the white part (red part is the cancer).

Work-up:

Many SCCs you see will involve the head/neck; may consider ordering imaging for high-risk tumors in these areas. Especially if large and fixed, may invade deep and need removed in OR.

- *CT with and without contrast*—lets you see bones + lymph nodes.

- *MRI with contrast*—lets you see PNI.

- *PET CT*—good for detecting hypermetabolic tumors (such as SCC). Can assess lymph nodes and distant organs but can't assess brain mets (so would need brain MRI for this). Usually used in context of post-op monitoring (scar tissue can make visualizing/assessing for recurrence on regular CT harder).

FYI: You get the imaging ~4 weeks after surgery, since the swelling, etc. make it hard to see tissue well.

Some use adjuvant radiation (optimally ~6 weeks after surgery) for high-risk tumors, especially with PNI, etc. Timing is crucial, so have to work closely with rad-onc.

Benefit of sentinel lymph node biopsy (SLNBx) controversial (usefulness has been called into question because even negative SLNBx patients have considerable chance of subsequent recurrence/metastasis, and patients who have positive SLNBx who undergo complete LN dissection still have higher rates of recurrence/mets). So basically, SLNBx may help elucidate prognosis, but management influenced by the info you get from it doesn't really change prognosis. And it's more invasive/uncomfortable for the patient than an excision.

Seems to have more of a role in mucous membrane areas (for instance, if have a mouth SCC and negative SLNBx, they usually don't get lymph node mets later).

MANAGEMENT

Not unreasonable to do topicals if have a very small and very thin SCCIS (but keep in the back of your mind that if the diagnostic biopsy was superficial/partial, then it may not be fully representative [and could actually be invasive]—particularly relevant to consider if on face or something).

Could do 5-FU QD for 6 weeks for SCCIS. Will reiterate that it is nice to outline the tumors (with desired margins) with a marker and take pics with the patient's phone so they know where to treat, because sometimes they can lose sense of where the tumor is/was when gets red/blotchy.

Obviously, excision/Mohs is often appropriate and commonly used options for SCCs.

SYSTEMIC TREATMENT

Can be used as neoadjuvant treatment before surgical resection (or adjuvant [post-op treatment]).

Newer drugs are immunotherapies (which empower the immune system to fight the tumor).

Idea: Cancer cells upregulate PD-L1 (ligand) to evade the immune system by binding to PD-1 (receptor) on T-cells.

These meds disrupt that interaction (and are also used for melanoma—see that section below in this chapter for a more in-depth explanation of the immune system and how these meds work).

- *Pembrolizumab* (binds to PD1 receptor on T-cell; AKA PD1 inhibitor).

  - FDA-approved for unresectable melanoma.

- *Cemiplimab* (another PD1 inhibitor): pretty fast-acting (response ~2 months) for both metastatic and locally advanced SCCs.

  - FDA-approved specifically for unresectable SCC.

- *Nivolumab* (another PD1 inhibitor).

- *Avelumab* (PDL1 inhibitor—still blocks the same interaction but instead binds onto a protein on the tumor cell).

An older drug is cetuximab (EGFR inhibitor)—sometimes works but can get acneiform rash. Not as good as the newer immunotherapies, but better than what was used before it (cisplatin, for example).

2.2.1.1.3 Keratoacanthoma (KA)

KAs and SCCs are often conflated, and arguable whether KAs exist as a separate entity, but they probably do.

Reasonable to separate because their behavior, management, and even histology are different (KAs do not have acantholysis; SCCs push their way into the dermis, while KAs pull their way into the dermis along elastic fibers; KAs have eosinophils rather than plasma cells).

95

KAs are capable of keratinizing themselves to death, but although KAs can spontaneously regress (exam answer), still better to excise (or at least EDC or inject chemo [such as 5-FU or MTX]). Reason is that they don't always go away on their own (some even say they commonly don't), and even if they do, it'll leave a scar. Also, a partial biopsy can't guarantee there isn't an underlying invasive SCC on the deep margin (which is obviously risky because fast growth of an SCC is a high-risk feature). In some ways, it might make sense to just excise or EDC or inject chemo without biopsying first (since they're so clinically distinctive and it would save the patient an extra office visit), but most surgeons will prefer biopsy confirmation first. *FYI*: KAs tend to explosively grow (sometimes within 1 week or so) after biopsy (vs. SCCs, which do not really react to biopsy), so if that happens, don't freak out (in other words, don't send them to head/neck surgery for extensive removal out of fear for a rapidly growing SCC).

Management can depend on context:

- If on an older guy's arm, can probably just cut it off.

- If big on a cosmetically sensitive area, can inject with 5-FU (50 mg/mL straight out of bottle—no dilution; hurts, so should probably numb with lidocaine first) or MTX (25 mg/mL straight out of bottle—no dilution; doesn't burn as much as 5-FU). Only time to dilute would be if the lesion is so huge that you need more volume.

  - Injecting KA is like a keloid; if you inject right into the middle of the keloidal collagen, don't really accomplish much (that's not where it's proliferating)—similarly, if you inject in middle of KA, you're just injecting into the keratin crater.

    – Want to blanch everything that is peripheral to the core (which helps you know you're injecting into the proliferative epithelium).

    – Also similar to keloids—should get softer after first injection, and you usually inject QW until clear.

- If too large to inject with 5-FU or MTX, can put on psoriasis doses of MTX (15 mg QW or something).

- Can also do 5-FU chemo wraps (slather with 5-FU, wrap in Unna boot, do QW until gone).

  - Chemo wraps work well after injecting in-office.

2.2.1.2 Benign
2.2.1.2.1 Seborrheic Keratosis (SK)

You already know them (thus good to practice dermoscopy on in the beginning).

From birthdays and genetics.

Of course, almost never actually the Leser–Trélat sign (though shouldn't completely forget about this and perhaps consider if covered in them and erupted all at once, with generalized pruritus and skin tags).

Can make patients feel good by saying there's 0% chance of them turning to skin cancer and thus no medical reason to remove them. Also can spontaneously fall off.

FYI: Patients may mention they put stickers on these lesions during mammograms (same with cherry angiomas).

MANAGEMENT

If highly bothersome either cosmetically or if irritated/inflamed/itchy, can remove; just make sure they know they may trade it for a white spot (from LN2) and also not 100% guarantee will work.

- Remember, LN2 not good for skin of color, so do electrodesiccation (then can scrape off with a curette).

- SKs take 2 weeks to fall off after LN2; scars if infected or picked at, so put hydrogen peroxide on cotton ball for first 1–2 days, pat dry, and put Vaseline on.

  - If on scalp, use Purell or something instead of hydrogen peroxide (will bleach hair).

- Topical options (none of which work super well):

  - *Diclofenac gel* (FDA-approved for AKs; don't really use much to be honest, not sure why it'd work).

  - *CeraVe SA*—might help decrust the crusty thick ones; no miracles.

    - Or T-Sal (salicylic acid) shampoo for scalp SKs, 2× weekly (regular shampoo all other times).

  - *AmLactin 12% lotion*—same as earlier (keratolytic).

You would think isotretinoin might work since it encourages epithelial turnover and SKs are epidermal growths, but they're probably just so continuous that it's not feasible to clear someone of SKs. Not sure if it's been investigated formally, though.

2.2.1.2.2 Actinic Keratosis (AK)

Pre-cancerous, although risk for transformation is relatively low. Have heard widely varying numbers (obviously hard to study), but reasonable estimate may be 1/1000 or so.

Feels gritty. Can look pigmented if solar lentigo and AK coexist.

If painful or feel infiltrated, then consider biopsy. Same if recur despite LN2 or if large.

If thin and diffuse, can do topical 5-FU BID for 10–14 days (or 5–7 days of BID 5-FU + calcipotriene). Need to achieve a red, irritated response (AKs will "light up" because 5-FU is specific for cells that are multiplying too fast, hence why it doesn't work for SKs). Always clarify with patients whether they achieved robust responses or not. *FYI*: You also don't want to biopsy questionable lesions when patients are still red from 5-FU (wait until 2 weeks or so post-5-FU; otherwise, interferess with the path read—will have atypia from the cytotoxic effects, in addition to the inflammation, so basically will look like an SCC).

If patient's entire skin has AKs, LN2 the thick ones and feel for deeper ones (consider biopsy vs. LN2 for those). Then can do field therapy (which also treats subclinical lesions, so more proactive than just LN2 at every visit). Remember to pick off the crusty part of the lesion before LN2 if you can (for better access to the problematic cells).

Peels Q 4 months. Work well for AKs.

2.2.1.2.3 Lichen Planus–Like Keratosis (LPLK)

- Essentially the immune system trying to get rid of AK, SK, or solar lentigo (usually, anyways).

- Thus can sometimes resemble a lot of those growths (NMSCs, iSKs, AKs).

- Arguably not even really pathological (evolutionarily advantageous).

- Typically take few months to go away (and if they don't, then consider biopsy).

2.2.1.2.4 Chondrodermatitis Nodularis Helicis

- Due to ischemia of ear cartilage from repeated trauma/pressure (ask if they sleep on their side or talk a lot with their phone on that ear).

- Usually middle-aged to older men with fair skin.

- Tender.

- Essentially a very small decubitus ulcer (and same line of thinking for management—offload pressure).

- **Management**: Sleep on other ear (or get donut pillow); can offer TCSs, LN2, or ILK if really painful.

- **FYI**: Nitroglycerin paste doesn't really work because won't get rid of the fibrin core (histologically is actually well-vascularized [granulation tissue], which is reactive to the ischemia).

2.2.2 Melanocytic

2.2.2.1 Melanoma

Most (70%) come from the sun (flat black dots on sun-damaged skin [background of solar lentigines], usually take 10–15 years to develop), while 30% come from pre-existing moles (usually junctional [flat] nevi, not compound/intradermal nevi [since mole cells are in the dermis for those vs. melanomas, which start in the epidermis; the raised moles have 0% chance of melanoma, although melanomas can, of course, be nodular, particularly if have progressed or if rapidly growing]).

Obviously good to avoid sunburn, but not necessarily enough. Genetics plays significant role. Not uncommon in younger patients (ages 20s–40s). If caught early, easily/consistently curable. If caught late, devastating. Thus, early detection is imperative.

Higher-risk patients include those with 50+ moles (also if 5+ atypical nevi), people with intermittent intense sunburns (more so than chronic low-grade sun exposure), fair freckly skin/red hair.

For people with 50+ moles (especially if also atypical), can be nearly impossible to know which ones to biopsy (and to some extent, it'll be tempting to want to biopsy all of them). However, shouldn't just biopsy all of them (you'll realize this once you see patients who have been through countless biopsies/excisions and have really disfiguring scars). For these patients, consider total-body photography (better monitoring and diagnosis). FYI: Insurance doesn't cover, and this is typically a couple hundred bucks [might have to repeat roughly every 10 years—or sooner if they experience major changes to their body, such as pregnancy]; patients will get a flash drive copy of the images if they transfer care [since the images won't be accessible by all their doctors]). Also good to ask about family history if they have 50+ dysplastic nevi (ask about pancreatic cancer, melanomas, etc.). Sometimes, genetic testing is appropriate (albeit rarely); if no genetic mutation, then may fall into the dysplastic nevus syndrome category. Make sure you also clarify/know where the previous biopsy sites are, as these can present as scar + pigment (if was compound nevus, etc.), which can both clinically and histologically resemble/mimic regressing melanocytic neoplasms (it basically tries to grow back through a scar). Thus, important to tell patients to remember where their biopsy sites are/were (previous moles can often be over-called as melanomas, especially in patients with histories of melanomas).

Patients might also question the dysplastic nevus concept, which is very nuanced, and even experienced pathologists may categorize dysplastic nevi differently. Moles can look "funny" or atypical clinically and histologically, but what ultimately matters is what it means biologically for the patient. Adding to the potential for "over-calling" things are special site nevi (moles with inherent site-specific atypical histologic features that can be confused for melanoma—such as acral sites, genitalia, ears, and several other body parts). But *FYI*: A lesion is either melanoma or not; some patients find it reassuring to learn there is no such thing as a pre-melanoma (in other words, can explain although pathology describes it as mild to moderate atypia, "mild to moderate" is still a normal mole).

A brief overview of the common subtypes:

- *Superficial spreading:*

  - Most common, ~70% of melanomas. Not classically photodistributed areas (rather tend to be areas that are burned from intermittent exposure, such as the back or lower legs).

- *Nodular:*

  - Second most common. Rapidly grow. Usually highly sun-exposed areas (trunk, head, neck). Most likely to ulcerate/bleed. Might be itchy/stingy.

- *Lentigo maligna:*

  - Usually sun-damaged areas (face). Takes long time to grow (grows outward before vertically); thus, patients may think it's a lesion that has "been there forever."

  - Tends to have subclinical extension (though not nearly to the extent of MACs or DFSPs), so regular excision with wide margins tends to have high recurrence rates. Can do slow Mohs (which is basically a staged excision with en face permanent sectioning—in other words, you're removing around the tumor, processing it like Mohs, but reading it under permanents), but this takes longer for the patient and has slightly higher failure rates than doing regular Mohs (with frozen sections that are read same day).

  - If covers a broad area, could potentially use imiquimod QD for 12 weeks, but caution, because will be amelanotic if it recurs (which is obviously terrifying, so not really treatment of choice).

- *Acral lentiginous:*

  - Not common (5–10% of melanomas), but disproportionately Blacks and Asians (and is actually the most common type of melanoma they get). Driven more by trauma to sites rather than sun.

Nail (subungual) melanoma:

- Rare; more common in Native Americans, Asians, Blacks than Whites. Rarely kids. Poor detection. Poor prognosis.

- Nail can be destroyed, may get ulceration.

- Hutchinson sign (pigment on skin surrounding nail) classically thought of as a hallmark sign but is common and can be in both benign and malignant lesions.

Ddx:

- Melanonychia—just means discoloration of nail; can be due to several entities which have subtle differences:

  - Melanocyte activation (not same thing as nevus, which is a benign hyperplasia): thin uniform gray lines.

  - Benign nevi—make parallel regularly spaced bands; basically a mole growing in the factory. Nail pulls it out, growing in a line (direction of growth lets you know if it is something to worry about); usually present for life.

  - The previous items are in contrast to melanoma (malignant hyperplasia), where the pigment characteristically extends to the cuticle/nail fold.

- If you see a dark line is moving with the nail and it's being eliminated, then probably due to trauma (dark blood stretching along the nail); no treatment needed (if a toenail, then buy half-size-larger [longer] shoes, or take out the regular insoles and replace with half-arch support insoles [helps keep the foot from sliding]). Let them know it will be a slow resolution; fingernails grow 1 mm per week, toenails 1 mm every other week. Can't just buy wider shoes, because it's not going to be wider where it needs to be (the toe box). *FYI*: They don't make arch supports for kids, so if it's a child, recommend they get the smallest women's half-foot Dr. Scholl's and cut it to size.

Amelanotic and hypomelanotic melanomas:

- Difficult to detect (in my opinion, at least); dermoscopy helps, just like the other melanomas. Some clues are the vessels (usually polymorphic).

Melanomas have similar concerning clinical features as NMSCs (sores that don't heal within a month or so, bleed for seemingly no reason, or "scars" that come out of "nowhere" and grow). Don't forget about hair (unexplainable repigmentation, for example).

When biopsying, obviously try to avoid partial biopsies (need to know Breslow for management/prognosis, so basically want the thickest and most abnormal part of lesion to be biopsied at the very least). Usually, shave is best (want to capture the peripheral margins). Hope to not see pigment underneath after you shave (if you do see pigment, then it's possible you may have transected it). It's obviously best if you avoid doing this, and can potentially avoid it if you shave a little, then look underneath, shave a little, look underneath, etc., so you can get it all in one intact piece. However, if you suspect it's a melanoma and you complete a shave and still see pigment underneath, you should repeat shave through the dermis until you no longer see pigment (won't really see it invade fat, anyway), because although it will mess up staging, you still need full histologic characterization (put the multiple specimens in the same bottle). It's also possible the pigment you're seeing is from melanophages (not nests).

As far as reading the biopsy report, some poor prognosis things:

- Thickness (Breslow, sometimes Clark level [issue with Clark's is people have different-sized skin, so a Clark 2 in one person might not be a Clark 2 in another person]).

- Mitoses per mm^2 (marker of activity).

- Perineural and lymphovascular invasion (self-explanatory).

- Ulcerated (can be a sign that it's proliferating very quickly and aggressively [so quickly that part of it runs out of blood supply and so aggressively that it destroys the epidermal tissue]).

- Tumor-infiltrating lymphocytes (if NOT there, then bad, because it means immune system basically not recognizing the melanoma as a problem).

- Regression (if immune system attacks and leaves stuff that looks like a scar).
  - Overall, actually bad prognostically (despite being indicative that immune system is recognizing it) because can mean the Breslow depth might be larger than what can be measured (since the assumption is that the regressed areas used to have melanoma).

- *Other things to consider*:
  - Patient's age, pagetoid spread (migration of melanocytes up in epidermis).

You should know the AJCC staging (AKA TNM staging).

If not in lymph nodes, then stage 1 or 2. If in lymph nodes, then at least stage 3, which is systemic and means you need to rule out stage 4 via imaging.

FYI: "N" in melanoma staging is not based on your clinical lymph node exam (which, of course, sometimes may not pick up on microscopic disease, for instance, that a nuclear scan would).

A slightly more detailed overview of staging:

- *Stage 0* = MIS (no risk for mets)

- *Stage 1* = early invasive; thin, low-risk recur
  - 1A = Breslow <1 mm
  - 1B = Breslow 1.1–2 mm without ulceration

- *Stage 2* = also invasive; higher risk for recurrence, but doesn't involve lymph nodes and doesn't qualify for adjuvant treatment (thus an important group, because they're sort of caught in the middle)
  - 2A = Breslow 1.1–2 mm with ulceration, or 2.1–4 mm without ulceration
  - 2B = Breslow 2.1–4 mm with ulceration, or >4 mm without ulceration
  - 2C = Breslow > 4 mm with ulceration

- *Stage 3* = most often means spread to lymph nodes (metastatic), but also includes satellite mets and in-transit mets (which both mean the melanoma has spread beyond the primary tumor but hasn't yet reached a lymph node; essentially the same thing but differ based on distance travelled)

- Satellite melanoma = spread <2 cm from primary tumor

- In-transit melanoma = spread >2 cm from primary tumor

- 3A = spread to 1–3 nearby lymph nodes

- 3B, 3C, 3D—somewhat detailed and nuanced (just look it up)

■ *Stage 4* = distant mets (liver, lungs, brain, bone, GI tract, etc.)

Of TNM staging, the biopsy only really tells you the thickness (nodes and mets, of course, require more extensive work-up). Obviously, thicker = higher risk for lymph node spread. If thick enough (>1 mm), NCCN recommends SLNBx (surg onc basically injects radioactive tracer near melanoma, which drains to the sentinel lymph node and highlights where the lymph node is, then it's excised in OR). Sentinel lymph nodes are the first ones the melanoma could travel to. (*FYI*: For a specific area of the body, the drainage occurs in the same sequence consistently—almost like a bus that drives the same route every day.) Different from lymph node dissection/lymphadenectomy (where they take out more, maybe like 10 or 15 [or even more]). But *FYI*: Can't do lymph node mapping/lymphadenectomy if already did WLE (because skin closest to the melanoma is gone, so skin lymphatics have been disrupted and flow to sentinel node may be altered).

Although SLNBx is best way to assess if node involved, utility somewhat controversial (elucidates prognosis/risk for distant spread [except for really young and really old patients] but doesn't impact survival).

Lymph nodes are probably a filter vs. a stopping place for melanoma (some cells probably catch through as they're disseminating systemically), at least for epithelioid superficial spreading melanoma. Spindled melanomas may be different. Desmoplastic melanomas definitely different (where plucking nodes might have a survival advantage). So just remember, there are nuances depending on the type.

In any case, SLNBx are very uncomfortable for patient.

If you're seeing a patient with a recent metastatic melanoma, remember to check their most recent scans. Usually, they'll do CTs ~Q 6 months for a couple of years after finishing immunotherapy.

MANAGEMENT

If they're early and shallow, can do excision or Mohs (never can do EDCs for melanomas).

If more extensive, then will likely warrant systemic treatment (which is usually a multi-specialty effort with onc, surg-onc, path).

■ *Neoadjuvant* = before surgery (beneficial because can see whether responsive or not for post-op treatment planning; also, if it makes the tumor shrink, can make for a less-morbid/extensive surgery).

■ *Adjuvant* = after surgery.

SYSTEMIC MED TREATMENT

This landscape is changing relatively rapidly, and we don't really use chemo much anymore. More often, use immunotherapies (such as PD-1/CTLA-4 inhibitors, etc.), which basically shut off parts of immune system to empower your body to fight the tumor. *FYI*: These work differently than other, somewhat-new melanoma therapies, like vemurafenib, trametinib, which decrease gene products (and are not immunotherapies).

- Basically, the cancer inhibits the T-cells from killing the cancer cells via immune checkpoints; the medicines (PD-1 inhibitors, CTLA-4 inhibitors, LAG-3 inhibitors, etc.) disinhibit the T-cells via inhibiting these checkpoints (thus creates inflammation intentionally—explains why they're associated with so many potential side effects, such as vitiligo, bullous pemphigoid, SJS).

  - Sometimes these side effects are profound and can be treatment-limiting; checkpoint inhibitors' adverse effects, of course, also extend beyond the skin (most commonly colitis, but also some that are hard to treat and not uncommonly fatal, like myocarditis). Familiarize yourself with these toxicities since will often see in patients on these treatments for other cancers as well.

  - Adverse events are graded 1–5 (which guides management based on severity of toxicity).

Remember that after a melanoma diagnosis, patients require more frequent FBSEs.

- *Stage 0*: Q 6 months for 1–2 years, then Q 1 year

- *Stage 1A–2A*: Q 6 months for 2–5 years, then Q 1 year

- *Stage 2B and higher*: Q 3–6 months for 2 years, then Q 6 months for 3–5 years, then Q 1 year after

2.2.2.2 Congenital Melanocytic Nevus

Should not change over time technically (but in practice, patients' caregivers will often mention the lesions are "changing," because the growth point is oftentimes below the surface, so it may seem to grow, get hairy, etc.).

Three sizes for birth moles (small and medium are essentially just cosmetic issues):

1. *Small*: 1/500k risk for melanoma—if want removed, usually better to wait until older so can do it under local (1/3,000 experience complications with sedation).

2. *Medium*: 1/200k risk for melanoma—same management consideration as with small.

3. *Large*: 2% risk for melanoma over lifetime (previously thought 7%); never grows out of the risk, and thus most people want to remove the lumpy spots.

   a. Main question is whether spinal cord lining has melanoma in it.

      i. Ask if patient has signs of abnormal development—such as trouble walking, etc.

      ii. Probably don't need MRI if baby is progressing well; just continue to follow until 3 years old, then refer to plastics.

      iii. Problem needs multiple rounds of sedation (which, when too young, risks learning disability and neurodevelopmental issues).

         – Better to wait to refer to surgery until actually ready, since if they see them, they will probably end up doing it.

- Ideal time for plastics to start removing is 3 years old (risks associated with sedation for a 2-year-old baby are same as adult's if you do one stage but needs to be 3 years old to have same risk as adult if doing 2+ stages).

- They usually can't feasibly remove the entirety of the large lesions, but they can remove the lumpy areas.

iv. In regular melanoma, start on surface (it's noticeable), but this is deeper, so impossible for families to monitor for/notice a melanoma, thus why we resect.

2.2.2.3 Epidermal Nevus

Sometimes only noticed later in life because might have just been below surface. Usually get darker and more warty over time.

- Two categories:

  - *Keratinocytic* (overgrowth only of components of epidermis—linear verrucous).

  - *Organoid nevi* (has components of entire skin); nevus sebaceus is a subtype, usually more orangish (browner in skin of color) and waxy, and hairless.

2.2.2.4 Acquired Nevus

- Most people are born with none (unless they are congenital nevi).

- People get new moles from 2 months to 75 years.

- Nevi are hamartomas.

- See Melanoma section.

2.2.2.5 Common Acquired Nevus

Dermal (raised), compound (raised), junctional (flat)—all benign.

Some teenagers will want benign moles removed for cosmetic reasons.

Should try to encourage long-term thinking and not do stuff that they'll likely regret later (especially teenagers who don't really understand long-term thinking yet).

Things you can say:

1. Their skin is amazing + healthy, and you don't wanna put a scar on it.

2. There's always a chance you don't get all the mole cells (especially for intradermal and compound nevi)

3. Don't want to do things that make them happy temporarily now and full of regret forever later.

Defining an atypical nevus is complex. Generally, people consider nevi with clinical atypia (asymmetric, irregular borders, color variation) to be atypical nevi. However, there is also the histologic diagnosis of dysplastic nevi. These don't always correlate. Best to explain lesions are either melanoma or they're not.

2.2.2.6 Spitz Nevus

- Can be pink/red, red-brown, or dark-brown (almost looks black).

- Usually children/young adults. If adults or has atypical features, should at least consider excision and closely follow up (higher risk for melanoma).

- *Ddx*: JXG, melanoma.

2.2.2.7 Nevus Spilus

- AKA speckled lentiginous nevus (has a lentiginous component and a nevus component).

- Some consider a congenital nevus subtype (localized defect in neural crest melanoblasts).

- Probably a blaschkoid segmental post-zygotic mutation that gives rise to the lentiginous area (coffee-colored), which is fertile ground for melanocytic lesions to arise (brown moles); sometimes can be bad soil (possible to get melanomas in them—albeit very rare).

2.2.2.8 Blue Nevus

- Dermal melanocytic tumor. Onset in childhood and middle age.

- Several subtypes.

- Ddx graphite tattoo (ask if got stabbed by pencil), venous lake, melanoma.

- Biopsy if rapidly grows or multinodular.

2.2.2.9 Halo Nevus

- Usually teenagers, but ages 10s–50s.

- Typically regresses but may take years.

- About 20% also have vitiligo.

- Often, patients will be concerned.

- If onsets at >40 years old (and/or if has personal or family history melanoma, etc.), have higher caution for coexistent melanoma (don't forget to look at mucous membranes and feet).

- If young, can probably reassure them it will eventually self-resolve (and explain the immune system basically saw a protein that it didn't recognize [not because there was something wrong with it] and lymphocytes went up and attacked to make white around the mole; the mole will lose its color and become just a bump after the process is done).

2.2.2.10 Combined Nevus

- Uncommon. Different from *compound nevus*.

- It has 2+ distinct nevi components in a single nevi (usually a compound + blue nevus).

2.2.3 Lentigines
2.2.3.1 Solar Lentigines

Onset ages 20s–30s. Persists for life (vs. freckles, which can fade).

You can actually reduce these with at-home products (basically DIY chemical peels):

- 2% salicylic acid QD or lactic acid

  - 6% (low concentration) lactic acid is more moisturizing (shouldn't sting).

  - 12% (high concentration) lactic acid is more of a keratolytic (might sting/burns).

This will encourage constant epidermal turnover (want because lentigines are epidermal growths) and make skin shiny, avoid dryness, and have less lentigines.

2.2.3.2 Lentigo Simplex

- Not related to sun exposure; present early, sometimes at birth (vs. solar lentigines).

- Doesn't evolve to melanoma.

2.2.3.3 Cafe au Lait Macule (CALM)

- Topicals don't work.

- Can use laser (outcome not always perfect—discoloration, scars, recurrence). Requires several treatments.

2.2.3.4 Freckles (Ephelides)

- Usually begin to appear within first 3 years of life. Fair-skinned patients.

- Only on skin and get darker with sun (marker of UV damage). Intense sun -> activates predetermined melanocytes.

- Ddx with lentigines (which can affect mucous membranes and stay same color).

- Can fade over time.

- **Management**: Photoprotection, tretinoin (not miraculous). Laser if really bothered. Hydroquinone too hard to make even.

2.2.3.5 Melanotic Macule

- Subset of lentigo simplex.

- Oral and genital.

- Usually onset in 20s–40s. Can grow over months to years.

- Can remove on lip without scar if doesn't involve vermillion border.

- Can remove without cosmetic fee because doing it to "rule out melanoma."

2.2.3.6 Linear and Whorled Nevoid Hypermelanosis

Explain this is from a small mosaic mutation in the gene that controls color that occurs when the body is a ball of cells. Not a mole; histologically look like CALMs (muddy feet).

FYI: Conditions that occur when the body is a ball of cells (which includes things like incontinentia pigmenti, for example) can have issues, such as seizures, cardiac defects, bony abnormalities.

So you should screen for these things (for instance, if the lesion affects the ears, ask if the patient has a hearing difference).

No effective topical treatment, can consider light LN2.

Can fade with age.

Hamartomas can have congenital tendency but not be fully evolved at birth (so don't be fooled if patients say "developing new lesions"—could also have a hypopigmented variant not noticed until in sun).

2.2.4 Adnexal Tumors and Glandular Disorders
2.2.4.1 Hyperhidrosis

Sweat more, and more often than normal.

1. Primary focal is most common.

   a. Axillae (often puberty) > palms/soles (often infants) > craniofacial (often middle-aged) > gluteal/inguinal.

   b. Needs 6 months total, with at least 2 of the following:

      i. Bilateral, mostly symmetric

      ii. Affects ADLs

      iii. 1+ episode weekly

      iv. Onset before age 25

      v. Most have family history

      vi. Improves while sleeping

2. Generalized, often secondary.

   a. Can be due to Frey syndrome, neuro trauma, meds/toxins, menopause, anxiety, hyperthyroidism, infections, neoplasms (lymphoma/leukemia, carcinoid, pheochromocytoma).

Intermittent, difficult to measure patient's sweat.
Can use the Hyperhidrosis Disease Severity Scale (very simple; scored 1–4).
Often, insurance will require secondary complications of their hyperhidrosis for treatment access.

■ For example, warts (2× more common in hyperhidrosis patients), pitted keratolysis (15×), tinea (10×), eczema (3×).

MANAGEMENT

■ *Topical antiperspirants* (go down to sweat ducts).

   • Drysol (patients don't tend to like, makes hydrochloric acid when they sweat, irritating), HydroSal (salicylic acid base; less irritating than Drysol), oxybutynin gel (prescription works but is hard to access [OTC Gelnique doesn't seem to work]).

      – Drysol = aluminum chloride (also used for hemostasis—precipitates salts to mechanically stop bleeding; so similarly for hyperhidrosis, plugs sweat ducts).

   • Can still use regular antiperspirant in am if they want scent.

■ *Miradry* (microwaves).

   • Permanent treatment; FDA-approved for axillae (not for palms).

   • Still will sweat (but essentially like a normal person); some say results not as good as Botox.

- Requires two treatments 3 months apart; some require a third treatment.
- $3k for two treatments total (but Botox is ~$1k per treatment if not covered).
- Trying to generate heat in the dermis, where the ducts/glands are.
- Risk brachial nerve injury in axilla.
- No compensatory sweating (which you get in endoscopic thoracic sympathectomy [ETS] surgery).
- Have to use local anesthetic (numb entire axillae).
  - Requires a lot; be careful about max lidocaine dosing (especially if they're small).
- Will get pain, considerable swelling, bruising (because using suction).
- Ask them to shave 3 days before (ideal to see some hairs), take ibuprofen before the procedure, then ice Q 1 hour after procedure.

■ *Iontophoresis* (usually for palms/soles).

- Time-intensive for patient: 15–40 minutes per treatment.
  - Start out more often, then titrate to QW once get benefit.
- Hurts if have breaks in skin (eczema, cuts, etc.)—apply Vaseline and treat eczema.
- Need ions in water to work, so if they have "soft" water, then add baking soda.
  - Can crush glycopyrrolate tablets (start with 2 mg, then add more) in the water.
- Devices last for decades, so an up-front cost for patient.

■ *Anticholinergics* (work on post-ganglionic muscarinic nerve receptors).

- Glycopyrrolate (cheap; works variably).
  - PO good if has palms/soles/axillae.
    - Can start low (1–2 mg QD), then uptitrate as needed; usually ~3 mg BID will be good enough.
    - Nice because doesn't cross blood–brain barrier (although oxybutynin does . . . unclear what long-term effects that has, but still something to consider).
    - Comes topically (Qbrexa wipes [multi-use, keep in ziplock bag so it retains moisture], or Secure wipes)—though still get some clinically relevant systemic absorption (just not as much as with PO, because no first-pass metabolism).
    - Also let them know, if they touch their face, they can get blurred vision/mydriasis, for instance (don't want them to think they had a stroke or something).
    - Can get via pharmacy.ca (Canadian pharmacy; comes in 1–4% glycopyrrolate—cheaper than Qbrexa).

■ *Botox*—approved for axillae.

• Works great.

• $$$ and will have to use a lot of units (50 per axilla, 100 per palm, 150 per sole).

  – Comes in 100- and 200-unit vials.

  – Neutralizing antibodies can form (albeit unusual), so probably shouldn't do both palms and soles same day (try to keep under 300 units total per session).

• ~50% insurances cover.

  – There is a patient assistance program, but only for axillae.

• Make sure you associate it with the correct ICD code (L74.510, which is for primary focal axillary)—in other words, don't use R61 (which is for generalized).

• Have patient shave 3 days before you inject, so you can see where the hairs are.

• Hurts but usually doesn't need anesthetics; can wrap ice in gauze and apply it to area before injecting (helps a lot, especially for palms).

• Inject aliquots in a grid—some people draw it out with marker (although it's a bit wasteful and messy, drawing out the grid may make it easier to calculate how much you'll need to dilute).

  – Aliquot volume depends on the dilution.

    – For palms, you might do 40–50 sites (20–25 sites per palm), so if you dilute a 200-unit vial with 4–5 cc total (for both palms), this would be roughly 0.1 cc per injection site.

    – For axillae, you might do 30–40 total sites (15–20 sites per axilla), so if you dilute a 100-unit vial with 3–4 cc total (for both axillae), this is again roughly 0.1 cc per injection site.

    – *FYI*: It can be challenging to inject small aliquot volumes (such as 0.05 cc) with 3 cc syringes, so if that's the dilution chosen, recommend using 1 cc syringes.

• Lasts longer than it does in muscles (try to get approved for Q 3–4 months, but some people only need Q 6 months); can get temporary muscle weakness in thenar eminence (1–2 weeks might have trouble pinching).

• Don't inject deep (not going into muscles)—try to stay dermal (should see a small bleb).

■ *Sympathectomy* (last resort, typically for palms; not as effective in axillae).

• Get horrible compensatory sweating.

■ *CNS meds.*

2.2.4.2 Sebaceous Hyperplasia

Can sometimes almost resemble BCCs/fibrous papules.
Usually have several lesions, though (be suspicious of other entities if solitary).

For removal with hyfrecation:

■ Needle special hyfrecator tip and comedone extractor.

■ Want low settings (1.2–1.4; make sure it's plugged into the low voltage [usually, it'll be plugged into high voltage]), which will do less epidermal damage and focus more where you want it (down in the sebaceous gland).

   • Same thing with DPNs and smaller SKs (pulse until it blanches gray, then wipe off with wet Q-tip [curette probably a bit aggressive]).

■ Can numb, but topical is probably most practical if they have a lot of them.

   • For example, BLT (bupivacaine, lidocaine, tetracaine), which has different % options.

   • Or EMLA 30 minutes before (supposed to be under occlusion, but not very realistic).

■ If just one lesion, can just have them ice it; won't hurt more than LN2.

■ For hyfrecating, bury the tip inside the central dell of the lesions (don't just set it on top).

   • Quick pulse it, stop when can see it bubble up, then press with comedone extractor and it'll all bubble out.

   • This way, don't have to curette, which gives them a lot of unnecessary downtime.

■ Can pulse low-dose isotretinoin on/off as needed—more for preventative/maintenance.

2.2.4.3 Nevus Sebaceus

■ Around 1/100 are appendage tumors, but generally no reason to remove for cancer prevention reasons.

■ Mole of oil glands, thus no surprise gets bigger with puberty.

■ However, must distinguish puberty growth (relatively uniform) vs. tumor growth (really odd disproportionate growth).

■ Would also defer removal until can make own decisions and also so they don't need conscious sedation (can just do under local).

2.2.4.4 Syringoma

■ Benign. Small papules, usually around eyes/on face. Can be elsewhere.

■ Removal is cosmetic. Can consider electrodesiccation, CO_2 laser, maybe LN2.

2.2.4.5 Microcystic Adnexal Carcinoma (MAC)

■ Rare. Roughly 1k per year.

■ High survival rates, but what you see clinically is not what you get histologically in terms of size (similar to DFSP). Thus, Mohs is the preferred management option, as it often necessitates deep and wide margins to clear the tumor.

■ One of the issues with this is that many MACs will only be diagnosed as a MAC while doing Mohs for a "BCC" (knowing the paisley tie ddx will help you understand why).

- This exemplifies why pre-procedure counseling is so important (making sure the patient is aware that even a small spot on the surface of the skin can sometimes require large defects for tumor clearance).

2.2.5 Vascular Tumors

2.2.5.1 Cherry Hemangioma

- Benign. More with age. Sometimes can be really dark brown to even black (almost resembling a nodular melanoma—biopsy if you're really not sure).

- Laser is the best treatment (see Section 6.2.3). Can do LN2 (not typically done/offered and because doesn't work as well as for stuff like SKs or AKs, though I've done LN2 once for them on a patient who specifically asked for it and it worked).

- *FYI*: Patients may mention stickers being put on these lesions during mammograms (same with SKs).

2.2.5.2 Infantile (Strawberry) Hemangioma

- Proliferation of blood vessel cells.

- Not present at birth; first couple months of life, rapid growth for 4–6 months, slow involution.

- Around 50% involute by 5 years, 90% by 9 years.

- Propranolol vs. topical timolol based on size of the lesion; best to shrink them as much as possible (because procedures to address poochy skin [plastics remove] and red dots [laser] are not covered by insurance).

- Ddx from capillary malformation (such as port-wine stain, nevus flammeus, etc.), which doesn't fade and is often present at birth; 0.1–2% of newborns.

2.2.5.3 Pyogenic Granuloma

- Rapidly grow. Benign. Possibly from infection, eczema, injury, hormones, or retinoids.

- Usually painless, but bleed easily.

- Recurrence is common (drug-induced more so than pregnancy-related). Shave off and desiccate the base.

- Recurrence less likely if excise with linear closure.

2.2.5.4 Venous Lake

- Basically looks like a bubble with purplish hue. Not always on lip; can be on face/ears, etc.

- Not a malformation, just weak collagen. Blanches (vs. melanocytic lesion). Benign.

- Make sure only on lip and doesn't extend to chin, for instance (which would be a malformation).

- Can laser (best) vs. LN2 vs. excision.

2.2.5.5 Glomus Tumor

- Rare, benign, painful.

- Usually on fingertips (highest density of glomus bodies) in women, 30s–50s.

111

- Look for red or bluish papule.
- Surgery curative—nail or hand surgeon.

2.2.5.6 Malformations

- May look like they're growing, but they're actually not growing; they're just filling.
- If vascular malformation is symptomatic, it's likely because of small blood clots forming and preventing smooth blood flow.

Three structural possibilities (relevant for management planning):

1. *Ectasia* (superficial dilation of vessels)

   a. Usually stays flat (such as port-wine stains, nevus simplex, etc.)

2. *Loopy in middle*

   a. If has flow on both ends, then can cut out the loopy part; start with ultrasound (75% are good) to characterize, MRI with flow if need definitive imaging if planning for procedural intervention.

3. *Arteriovenous malformation* (high flow)

   a. Tube area malformed and tube goes on—can do surgery to dam the flow.

2.2.5.6.1 Port-Wine Stain (Nevus Flammeus)

Birthmark, though might not be noticed first day of life.

Can explain they have a perfect baby with perfect blood vessels; the vessels are just a little pooched out, so looks darker, thicker, redder.

When on upper eyelid, can affect the eye.

Can be striking how thick they can get over time from chronic sludge (blood). So try to treat before it thickens; otherwise, will be much harder to laser (usually takes roughly three treatments when thin, at the very least two, because vessels are shaped like an hourglass).

- Plastics will need conscious sedation (like a colonoscopy), which can't do at all until baby turns 2 years old and can't do multiple times until baby is 3 years old, so explain that it's best to wait until baby turns 3 (since needs at least two treatments minimum).

2.2.5.6.2 Nevus Simplex

Ectasia, lighter than port-wine stain and supposedly self-resolves (though I often see them on older people, so may not be a guarantee).

2.2.5.7 Lymphangioma

Can be superficial or deep, so appearance is variable.

Can be gravity-dependent (water accumulates in tissues). Observing this is interesting and helpful. If on forehead or something, ask them to bend over and you'll see the lesion get bigger. Treatment is excision.

Lymphangioma circumscriptum (AKA microcystic lymphatic malformation) can be much bigger than you think based on what you see on the skin, so should feel obligated to get an idea of where it goes and its extent. Should do MRI with flow to find the pulsating cavernous cistern, which needs to be cut out by plastics; otherwise, will "keep coming back in different places" (so consider if someone has had LN2 + desiccation, etc., and lesions keep coming back or are "moving around" within a region). You may also be able to inject bleomycin to sclerose the problematic lymphatic area.

2.2.5.8 Cutis Marmorata Telangiectasia Congenita

Basically a malformation variant of livedo. Some people call it "physiologic livedo" but can be confusing to patients (because they'll look it up), so should probably avoid that term.

Looks like the mottled appearance normal babies get when they're cold (livedo), except it doesn't go away when they warm up (though still blanches).

Gets more dramatic-looking with temperature changes.

Typically only one extremity; usually always been there but sometimes not noticed until later.

Often persists until adulthood; can fade with time.

Usually harmless but sometimes has associated malformation of bone underneath—thus recommend XR (can ask PCP to order it).

No specific treatment (can't correct surgically).

Want soft tissue ultrasound to rule out other vascular malformations (it's not significantly distorted or high flow).

2.2.6 Spindle Cell Tumors

2.2.6.1 Dermatofibroma (DF)

- Firm, nodular. Characteristically dimple and have scar-like hypopigmentation in center on dermoscopy.

- Basically scar tissue; thought to be 2/2 previous trauma, such as a bug bite.

- Persist for life.

- Sometimes painful and patients want removed.

2.2.6.2 Dermatofibrosarcoma Protuberans (DFSP)

Most commonly on trunk and extremities in patients 20–40 years old but can, of course, be seen on other parts of the body in children and older patients, too.

Rare. Roughly 1200 cases per year in the USA. Incidence is stable (which is odd, as most other skin cancers [particularly the common ones] are rising in incidence) and is the only skin cancer in which Black patients have the highest incidence. Possible that it is not related to exogenous exposures (such as the sun, etc.), or maybe it's underdiagnosed.

High survival rates, but DFSP is notorious for its tendency to recur (likely because of subclinical extension [deep and wide] causing high frequency of positive margins on regular excisions). In other words, what you see clinically is *not* what you get (which is also characteristic of microcystic adnexal carcinomas). Further, the subclinical extension in DFSPs can be like tentacles; thus, margin assessments of regular excision specimens may be falsely negative (see Mohs section in Chapter 5 for explanation regarding tissue processing for Mohs vs. regular excisions).

This is particularly important and relevant to recognize if you think about surgical planning for DFSPs in kids. Obviously, it is not ideal to sedate a child, excise it, have positive margins, sedate and excise again, have positive margins, sedate and excise again, have negative margins (and it comes back anyway). Not only because of the repeated sedation and failure rate but also because of the tissue alterations and cosmetic outcome which obviously has significant implications on a child's development. Mohs in the OR is the most preferred treatment for DFSP.

Unclear whether imatinib could be used as neoadjuvant/adjuvant therapy to make for a less-involved surgery, because it is unknown whether these would shrink the tumor centripetally (turning a big sphere into a smaller sphere—what you want) or if these would turn it into multiple little puddles that are no longer connected (what you don't want—because essentially makes margin control meaningless).

2.2.6.3 Keloid

Commonly tender when ropy.

Also commonly itchy, usually the peripheral part; has increased Th2 cytokines, but also possibly periostin (from fibroblasts). Collagen so thick it damages the nerves, so probably that too.

Probably will be doing ILK, at least to start.

Need big enough needle (**FYI**: It hurts more) or won't get any ILK in there.

- A 25 G needle for body; 30 G probably too small.

- Inject into base (where it's growing, also easiest place to get the ILK in).

- Can do LN2 (freeze like a wart) before ILK 2–3x—the LN2 basically helps create more space (via edema) for the ILK, but higher risk of hypopigmentation.

- Can also pre-treat with clobetasol under occlusion if too firm to get ILK in the lesion or for chest keloids (very painful and hard to tolerate injections).

For ear keloids, if just one side, can shave, let heal (have them RTC 1 month), then do ILK.

- Could also do ILK same day but will, of course, heal slower.

- Dumbbell keloids that involve front and back of ear probably need excised.

After treatment, can have them wear pressure earrings at night when sleeping (probably not fashionable enough to wear during day).

- Can get them via Amazon (Delasco pressure earrings).

- Make sure not too tight (or can damage cartilage).

Some people also use imiquimod, but they may get the flu-like symptoms since they'd be applying on a wound (more absorption) (though could maybe try telling them to put on after they heal, but still needs prior auth, etc.).

If you cut them out, subcuticular suturing is probably best for patients with keloid tendency.

Don't cut out grapes; inject ILK (40 mg/mL) to turn them into raisins.

Excision without ILK ×3 rounds (2 weeks apart each) has 50% chance of recurrence; 15% chance if doing the ILK before (basically trying to suppress exaggerated wound healing to normal before cutting them out). Should inject ILK after too (some plastics people do post-excision ILK Q 1 month for 1 year).

If keloids don't respond to ILK, then can do W-plasty.

If thinking they need radiation (which probably has the best data but seems to scare patients), probably better to send to plastics, since they probably coordinate with the radiologists more often. Timing is important so needs good setup.

2.2.7 Fat Tumors
2.2.7.1 Lipoma

- Most common soft tissue tumor.

- Too much normal fat tissue in a normal location.

- Benign. Grow slowly to a stable size. Don't go away spontaneously.

- Can excise (see Section 5.4). If rapidly growing, perhaps better to excise when small.

- If has vascular component (angiolipoma), usually painful.

- Good to know painful ddx (BLEND AN EGG).

2.2.7.2 Nevus Lipomatous Superficialis

- Rare, benign. Essentially a herniated lipoma type of thing.

- Starts small, gets bigger with friction.

- Dermal deposition of mature fat tissue.

- Can shave vs. excise.

2.2.8 Cysts

- For most cysts, excision is curative (if not entirely removed, risks recurrence—see Section 5.4 on excisions).

- A lot of the nomenclature nuances are derived from histologic features.

2.2.8.1 Milia

Tiny epidermoid cysts (cells from top layer of skin break away like seed, grow into a ball, and sloughed skin gets trapped in dermis—so what they see is basically a hard ball of dead skin and oil trapped in epidermis).

Can get after cosmetic procedures (such as chemical peels, dermabrasion, laser, etc.) and trauma.

Patients may describe them as sweat blisters. Post-traumatic milia self-resolve.

Can also see after blistering disorders (EBA, PCT, BP, VZV, contact derm, bullous SLE, DH) after they heal.

Can occur in areas of TCS-induced atrophy.

Tretinoin (or even OTC adapalene) can minimize amount of milia that appear but doesn't help remove them; needs extracted (which becomes easier once on retinoid [the filling will come right out instead of having to dig for it]).

For extracting, incise (nick it really superficially) and express contents with comedone extractor.

FYI: Not same as miliaria (milia is the plural; milium is singular).

2.2.8.2 Epidermal Inclusion Cyst (EIC)

Very common. Essentially sacs with the outside part of the skin on the inside. Usually older patients (if pre-pubertal, then consider rare genoderms).

Due to trauma, eccrine duct or pilosebaceous unit occlusion, HPV infection, etc.

Sometimes can't really see the punctum (more on this in Section 5.4.1).

EICs are common on the scrotum and eventuate over many years into idiopathic scrotal calcinosis (basically start as EICs that calcify).

Benign, but because skin sheds, they tend to grow, and if ruptures, dead skin goes into live skin and gets inflamed and eventually infected, which is of course a bigger problem/annoyance for patients than having to get it cut out. But if it's small, not growing, and/or not bothersome, then don't really need to strongly recommend removal (especially if patient isn't willing to take it easy during the healing process—could get a fish mouth scar or something and end up disliking that more than they disliked the small cyst).

2.2.8.3 Pilar Cyst

Benign cysts from hair follicle.

Smooth, sometimes tender (suggestive of inflamed/infected).

Usually middle-aged women, on scalp.

Patients may fear it's a sign of something wrong.

Pretty much the only bad thing that can kind of look like these are a follicular lymphoma.

FYI: NOT the same as EICs (which are more superficial and more common) but clinically look similar, and management same (excision, though are more hardy than EICs and typically rupture less/blow up more with anesthesia than EICs). No punctum in pilar cysts (vs. EICs). More on this in the Chapter 5.

FYI: Not a sebaceous cyst (the only sebaceous cyst is a steatocystoma).

2.2.8.4 Pilonidal Cyst

Essentially from skin touching skin intergluteally (hair follicles on one side penetrate/clog pores on other side [and vice versa], which get occluded, then infected, then form balls of skin that continually get inflamed and grow downward [until get to anus, then circle around it], which ultimately results in them all becoming interconnected, which creates the sinus tracts/tunnels, etc.). Thus best to take out early if possible.

Tend to show up around puberty and start similar to HS but progress different. Often occurs in HS. May even look like intergluteal HS but won't respond to HS meds (so think about this in any HS patient).

Crease between butt cheeks is what the problem is. Only cure is to cut them out and make butt flatter. Hard because they can go deep and create tunnels. Usually need OR with plastics so can cut wide around and under to totally take them out. Usually, they will just take out skin the first time. If recurs (30% chance [yes, embarrassingly high]), can take back and go deeper (which you can also start with the first time but is, of course, more aggressive, more painful, more bleeding, etc.). Usually takes around 2–3 operations to be done with them.

Post-op is a drag; can't sit down for 2 weeks (have to either stand or lie down) because will pull on the closure. If they absolutely have to sit down for some reason (such as a truck driver, etc.), then they can leave the wound open and do wound care for several months instead (but that requires a lot of confidence in the patient to follow instructions consistently).

2.2.8.5 Pseudocyst

No epithelial lining.

2.2.8.5.1 Mucocele

- Usually lower mucosal lip or tongue.

- Salivary glands get blocked -> mucus accumulates, forms vesicle. Could be from trauma.

- Usually short-lived (resolves spontaneously) but often recurs. If doesn't resolve, may need excised (can refer to dentist).

2.2.8.5.2 Digital Mucous Cyst

- Usually dorsal distal fingers. Might see depression in nail plate distal to it.

- Unclear etiology.

- Can ILK or excise. Commonly recurs.

2.2.8.5.3 Ganglion Cyst

- Usually on wrist.

- Usually don't communicate with joint space.

- Can try few weeks of compression and/or aspirate + ILK.

- Can excise, but recurrences are common.

2.3 GENERAL DERMATOLOGY—MISCELLANEOUS COMPLAINTS AND CONDITIONS

This is a hodgepodge of topics patients ask about but don't really have a text-book diagnosis. Intermixed are some considerations for people with subpar skin quality.

- *Sensitive skin*: mild soaps/cleanser—such as Dove unscented, Cetaphil, Vanicream cleansing bar, etc.).

  • After showering, pat dry, put unscented moisturizer creams (Cetaphil, CeraVe, Vanicream; Aquaphor or Vaseline if super dry). Moisture everywhere, not just where rashy. Continue moisturizing even when not rashy—prevention is key.

- *Skin care*

  • Simple is key.

  • AM regimen: wash face with water, moisturize, then sunscreen.

    – Clinique high number face sunscreens good for females; face sun-screens aren't as sticky, so they wash off when put on body; body sunscreens are stickier (substantive), so people don't like putting it on their face.

    – If using spray sunscreen, needs to feel damp.

  • PM: wash face, apply a retinoid, then moisturize.

  • If using OTC toners, use in AM.

    – Clean up regimen if has rash! Tell them to stop all the garbage they're using, like shea butter ("skin diet").

- *Wrinkly skin*: AmLactin.

- *Aging skin*: tretinoin QHS as tolerated.

- *Solar purpura* (more from shearing between top and middle layers of skin, so not painful like bruises [because no hematoma causing mass effect])—takes several weeks to resolve; for the brownish-orangish discolorations, can try arnica gel (doesn't work miracles).

- *Thick, scaly skin*: glycolic acid.

- *Dry lips*: Aquaphor.

- *Stretch marks*: tretinoin helpful for striae if still purple (inflamed).

- *Large pores on face*: topical retinoids (takes 3–4 months) vs. chemical peels; can alternate tretinoin with hyaluronic acid.

- *Folding skin (from aging)*: alternate hyaluronic acid + glycolic acid.

- *Irritated skin where glasses rest on nose* (could be beginnings of acanthoma fissuratum if skin actually thickened or papular, etc.): recommend glasses with plastic nasal things (and/or wearing them as little as possible—to allow healing), and Protopic vs. dilute ILK to areas (for patients with inflammatory component). If no response, can treat as acne/rosacea.

- *Radiation fibrosis: vitamin E* (PO 100 mg TID) and pentoxifylline 400 mg TID (for 12 months starting 1–3 months after XRT); can also use pentoxifylline for radiation ulcers.

- *Getting more hairy* (for example, growing vellus hairs in beard distribution) after menopause.

  - Can explain hormone changes, estrogen protects against beard growth, so when they age, they start to get facial hair, etc.

- *Baggy eyes*: periorbital fat atrophy causes bags under eyes—caused by genetics + birthdays (can also be caused by latanoprost, or bimatoprost [Latisse]); can try filler to address volume loss (usually ~Q 6 months at most for under eyes). Lasers don't work great; if it's just fine lines/wrinkles, then lasers can help.

- *Darkness under eyes*: if due to visible vasculature, can try OTC Revision eye cream, which might be cooling/help shrink vessels; can also try Neostrata brightening eye cream.

- *Nail breakage* can be dryness and aging; recommend Elon nail moisturizer.

  - Can trial biotin 2–3 mg (usually comes in micrograms) for 3–4 months only; this is the only thing biotin is potentially good for.

  - Avoid nail polish/removal (desiccant—dries out nails).

  - Wear gloves when cleaning with chemicals, etc.

  - Being on HD can cause hair and nail changes; may improve on own.

- *"Nail fungus" without fungus.*

  - Traumatic nail dystrophy (onycholysis with traumatic hemorrhage): risk that gets wet under the nail with dead skin; can grow pseudomonas or fungus that sits in there like a yeast. Good to use Gold Listerine, put on Q-tip, put under nail (but don't aggressively cram because will further unzip the nail). Get half-size larger shoes, take out the inside soles, and replace with half-arch support insoles.

- *Hair breakage*: not many medical options; can occur after significant illness (ICU, major weight loss, etc.). Can try Nutrafol three pills daily. Avoid biotin supplements (don't work); stop coloring, henna, etc. (even if been doing for 30 years without issues, as this could actually be the problem—a chronic exposure). Rinses are most you can do but can be damaging as well (color basically pokes holes in hair shafts in order to get in; that is how it works). Stay away from semicolor, and avoid heat.

■ *Tanning bed addiction*: ask why they like it—is it the color or the feeling? Spray-on tans aren't the same but are obviously much safer. If they do it for self-care, it's safer to wear sunscreen and go to the beach if they like the warmth.

■ *Bumps on wrists*: piezogenic papules; when extend wrist, fat pops out between collagen (sometimes hurts). Comes/goes. Can't cut out.

■ *Irritated skin after shaving legs*: can recommend getting the Venus razors with the middle bar (that protects against the skin); for technique, the razor should keep contact with the skin while moving in up-and-down motion (not shaving in one direction, then lifting off the skin and putting it back on the skin before shaving in the same direction again).

2.3.1 Ingredient Labels for Cosmetic Products

You will inevitably experience patients bringing in their skin care products and asking for your opinion on a bag full of products. It can be intimidating, and some ingredients have more than one name (such as hyaluronic acid, which has multiple). While you might not necessarily need to be an expert on this subject, it's nice to at least have a general idea so you can answer basic questions from patients.

Products can claim a great deal (the rules are very loose). So don't pay attention to the claims or the product descriptions. The only truth is the ingredients (which you can find on the label on the product itself, the box, or if the product is in a tub, might have to peel a sticker back to find them).

As an aside, when a product is in a jar, it's best to recommend the ones that come with the pump (because if it's just an open jar, some ingredients [such as vitamin C] can get oxidized [won't work as well], and it's also less sanitary).

US law does require a few things for cosmetic products (which includes cleansers, lotions, lipsticks, fingernail polishes, makeup, hair color, deodorant, shampoo). They must do the following:

■ List all ingredients.

■ List the ingredients from highest % to lowest % (except the ingredients that make up <1% of the overall product, which can be listed in any order [within the <1% category]).

■ Must not have prohibited ingredients (such as formaldehyde).

• However, many products contain formaldehyde releasers.

There are many ingredient categories (absorbents, antioxidants, plant extracts, preservatives, scrub agents, silicones, slip agents, texture enhancers, thickeners, vitamins, cleansing agents, coloring agents, emollients, emulsifiers, exfoliants, film-forming and film-holding agents, fragrance [synthetic and plant extracts], humectants, moisturizers, minerals, skin conditioning agents, preservatives, keratolytics).

Moisturizers can be a humectant (attracts and holds water [hydrophilic], such as hyaluronic acid or glycerin) or an emollient (forms a protective layer over the skin [hydrophobic]—such as petrolatum). Glycerin is probably the most common humectant in decent products (also an emollient). Propylene glycol (gives things a slippery quality) is also a very common humectant (and emollient); it can be used as a preservative and is used frequently as an enhancer (such as in foods, in TCSs [because it improves penetration], etc.). You may encounter patients who are allergic to propylene glycol (for whom you may have to find propylene glycol–free TCSs).

Petrolatum is one of the most common emollients. Aquaphor is a mixture of emollients (petrolatum, glycerin, lanolin) and is essentially a fancy Vaseline. *FYI*: ~1% of people are allergic to lanolin (was the contact allergen of the year in 2023). It is commonly recommended to women who are breastfeeding (so think about a lanolin allergy if seeing a nipple dermatitis in a breastfeeding woman). *FYI*: The contact allergen of the year is not necessarily the most frequent contact allergen for that year; the American Contact Dermatitis Society basically chooses to recognize an allergen every year that they think warrants increased awareness.

Dyes are put in stuff to make things look good and smell good (includes tinted makeup). Neither of which our skin has a tendency to like. Dyes, of course, are used in foods/beverages, too, which are being banned in various places around the world.

Fragrances are appealing to consumers but irritating to skin. Products that state "no added fragrance" can be misleading because they can still contain stuff like limonene (which has a natural citrus smell). Camphor (in Vicks VapoRub, Carmex, etc.) is also not technically a fragrance but emits a fragrance. Other examples: eucalyptus oil, tea tree oil, peppermint, menthol—which patients have a tendency to emphasize are "all natural"; however, our skin doesn't like these things.

Preservatives can also be irritating. Formaldehyde (now banned) was the contact allergen of the year in 2015. Of course, appealing to manufacturers because cheap and gives products longer shelf life. Pathologists, of course, use it (formalin, AKA formaldehyde in water) to preserve our biopsy specimens. Paraben is another common preservative irritant. *FYI*: Vitamin E is an antioxidant, but when in tocopherol form, it's more of a preservative.

Surfactants are things like cleansers, bodywashes, detergents (things used to clean stuff). Many can be irritants, such as cocoamidyl-betaine. Shampoos that lather up (foaming action) tend to have sodium lauryl sulfate.

Terms that mean nothing (made-up terms that aren't regulated):

- "Hypoallergenic," "non-comedogenic," "unscented" (only means it doesn't have a smell but doesn't mean they didn't put masking fragrances in), "chemical-free" (doesn't make sense; everything in the products are chemicals), "paraben-free" (can be accurate but isn't regulated), "natural," "eco-friendly," etc.

Terms that are regulated by somebody (but not the FDA):

- "Organic" (ambiguous; what it means in the chemistry context [containing a carbon atom] is completely different than what it means in the food industry), "vegan," "cruelty-free," with the bunny rabbit symbol, means there was no animal testing of the product performed. But it doesn't mean that the individual ingredients are all free of animal testing.

Can see more details regarding what chemicals are safe vs. not safe on the EPA (government) website. Other websites to consider browsing include the FDA site and cosmetic info database.

If patients are looking for general recommendations, can just keep it simple and recommend safe, well-known options, such as CeraVe hydrating facial cleanser. Fine to use as hand soap, bodywash, for example (even though it's called a facial cleanser).

On a related note: eye creams, neck creams, and so on, are basically just marketing. Patients can use whatever moisturizer they normally use and apply it under the eyes. If they insist on needing an eye cream, then you can just recommend CeraVe eye cream or something that's well-known and easy to get (mass-produced, etc.). SkinCeuticals, EltaMD are also fine.

2.4 SUBSPECIALTY CLINICS

2.4.1 Complex Medical Dermatology and Connective Tissue Diseases

For patients with skin signs of internal issues, broadly speaking, there are a few possibilities:

1. Impression of rash unifies everything and solves what is going wrong on the inside (such as DM [why they're weak], sarcoid [why they can't breathe/see], CSVV, etc.)

2. Patient has a reactive dermatosis (associated with diseases associated with immune complexes [such as IBD, AICTDs, myelodysplastic disorders, etc.], infections, drugs [usually not; overstated], and 50% of time is idiopathic); vasculitis is a prototypical reactive dermatosis.

   a. Can't address unless working with a colleague to stabilize (if due to uncontrolled RA, need a more stable RA program; same with IBD, etc.)

3. They have something completely unrelated, but the steroid tapers for the internal stuff make the skin disease go on roller coaster along with the internal stuff and confuses providers (seb derm, rosacea, poikiloderma of Civatte, scabies, fibromyalgia, etc.)

If they present from outside with clinical-pathologic disconnect, would still try to get the outside biopsy (may be best chance for useful info since was most likely before on treatment) in case it just wasn't read correctly. Look at the words on it; the interpretation is sometimes wrong (not the pathologist's fault—pathologies can be similar, but the clinical subtleties are what make it—for instance, scalp with interface, LPP but the path read as DLE, or vice versa); so ask for your in-house pathologist to read the outside slide.

- Usually best to ask patient to bring the report with them, then the pathologists can request the outside slide with that; it's usually too much trouble to try to get in touch with the other doctors.

Will focus on the most common conditions you'll see/manage. Didn't include MCTD, which is very rare (and 20% of people with rheum disease have overlap; thus, most patients are overdiagnosed), but wanted to highlight here that distinguishing MCTD from other AICTDs matters for treatment because MCTD is very prednisone-responsive; if calling something MCTD, 100% needs U1RNP (50% of women over 50 have positive ANA).

2.4.1.1 Dermatomyositis (DM)

Basically an acquired autoimmune interferonopathy.

Orphan illness; one of few serious diseases without double-blind prospective placebo-controlled trials for treatment (except for IVIG, which is lifelong treatment and typically will not yield remission and probably won't even perfectly control it—albeit can save someone's life if not being adequately controlled on other treatments). More on management later.

Ddx:
Some patients may be referred for concern for SLE (poikiloderma sometimes misinterpreted as psoriasis), and people might be confused why LFTs elevated (when it's because of muscle enzymes in DM). DM is more purple, and lupus more red. Should also look at hands—DM lesions are over joints, lupus lesions between DIP/PIP. DM also confused for CTCL at times (which has the poikiloderma but won't have the photodistribution and nail fold changes that DM does).

Other characteristic features and considerations:
Mechanics' hands is essentially just eczema superimposed on poikiloderma.

The hand ulcerations (characteristic of MDA-5 but can also be seen in other variants when inadequately controlled) are an apoptotic reaction (not vasculitic, like you might predict); need to prevent infections of these.

If red rash and concern for AICTDs, look at cuticles—won't get those changes from AD.

Poikiloderma on scalp = pathognomonic for DM (and poikiloderma in general is a relatively important finding, as it can be seen in CTCL, lupus, radiation derm. Albeit there's also poikiloderma of Civatte, which is common and benign).

Three reasons DM skin can flare:

1. Muscle uncontrolled—can do MRI to rule out muscle inflammation.

2. Too much sun despite reasonable control.

3. Cancer.

Possible internal issues:
Dysphagia—patients with scary DM have cricopharyngeal dysfunction and can't initiate swallowing (it's not esophageal dysmotility). People with food catching have overlap with scleroderma.

About 10% of DM patients have a tendency to develop ILD, usually more of a low-grade subacute/chronic issue (very rarely rapidly progressive, even in MDA5 patients). Jo-1 predicts lung disease; many pulmonologists think MTX causes it (which it can, if given at chemo doses), but weekly MTX doesn't seem to actually cause interstitial fibrosis. The patients who get it have seropositive psoriatic arthritis (for example, RA in patient with psoriasis) or other AICTDs (thus not the drug but just a manifestation of diseases it's used to treat, such as DM, lupus, scleroderma, MCTD).

MALIGNANCY ASSOCIATION
There are case reports of children with cancer, but not above statistical norm (in other words, there is no association with neoplasia in children).

In adults:
Similar to BP, people thought DM was a cutaneous sign of malignancy, until they did age-matched controls (older people get BP/DM, older people get cancer). Probably overstated, because in referral setting, there's a lot of patients with cancer (so it's probably not even close to 15–20% that patients think).

Patients also think the "1/5 chance" of malignancy is lifelong—which isn't true; it's 2 years of risk (in other words, 2 years after the start of their skin disease, their malignancy risk returns to normal).

The most associated cancers are lung, ovary, breast, and stomach; the tumor association appears related to the skin (polymyositis don't have it, and amyopathic DM does).

Possible the overactive interferon response characteristic of DM is a good prognostic feature via increased anti-tumor immune response (somewhat similar to developing vitiligo on immune checkpoint therapy for melanoma) but not studied yet.

Juvenile DM:
Number 1 cause of death in kids is GI vasculitis. Look for that.

Before prednisone, 1/3 of kids died, 1/3 were crippled, 1/3 had delayed long-term illness that led to remission.

Calcinosis cutis is more common in kids, but if you control muscle disease aggressively, you will limit its formation. It looks like chalk coming out of skin (or big bricks if really uncontrolled). No viable medical treatment for calcinosis cutis because no blood supply there; have to get surgeon to cut out worst areas. An ounce of prevention worth a pound of cure; derm has special opportunity to suppress the disease early (skin precedes muscle). Need to obsess about disease control.

EVALUATION

When testing for proximal extensor weakness, neutralize the elbow (otherwise patient will push with deltoid—like squinting on eye exam when you need glasses).

FYI: If you ask a surgeon to biopsy a muscle, they might biopsy the deltoid (not what you want, because deltoid is the last muscle to go; biopsy should be of the triceps).

Hard to distinguish histologically from acute lupus (but is differentiable from SCLE and DLE lesions).

LABS/WORK-UP

Rheum tends to think ESR predicts prognosis, but probably not useful; reasonable to trend CK and aldolase (especially if symptomatic). The goal is to keep these enzymes WNL.

If you see DM late with CK 15k or something, you'll probably need to follow for 15 years.

If have DM for 8 years and develop rash when CK WNL, it means CK likely not reliable, or patient has cancer, or rash is from UV light.

Should consider antibody panel—especially the two that are strong for cancer (TIF1-y and NXP-2 [particularly useful for kids]). MDA5 also worthwhile to get because it's a very scary variant and presents a whole different management challenge (can infarct digits/skin lesions, ulcerative disease head to foot, severe lung/cardiac disease). Inverse Gottron papules, hyperkeratotic palmar papules, and lymphopenia are features consistent with MDA5 disease.

Around 10% of people with each AICTD have an overlap; if suspect has erosive joint disease (pain in am, takes 1 hour to warm up), get a CCP and RF (might have overlap with RA).

Should get DLCO; board answer is restrictive PFTs, but that's late-stage (first sign is gas exchange issues).

Can also consider high-resolution chest CT, particularly if complaining of shortness of breath. *FYI*: Different study from a regular chest CT, so make sure you order the correct study (otherwise, it won't tell you what you need). Should consider pelvic ultrasound in female patients.

MANAGEMENT

Derm has unique opportunity because we tend to see it first. Easier to treat if caught early.

Some providers tend to treat it like lupus, and although DM is also a serious multisystem disease, the prognosis and treatment are completely different from lupus. SLE is lifelong (goal for SLE management is to use the least amount of medicine for life while keeping major systems in check). DM patients have 85% chance of remission after two years of MTX or MMF (if control CK); 15% have for a lot longer (fail to clear, but typically don't need a lot of treatment and don't have complications like calcinosis cutis, etc.).

Although the MTX/MMF data comes from a study that's not controlled, it has longer follow-up than most studies (that are, like, 6 months' follow-up), and shows can get majority completely off treatment forever. Rituximab/IVIG can save someone's life but is usually lifelong (the studies are RCTs, so yes, it's evidence-based, but it's short-term evidence). DM needs longer-term studies, but the research that is done is the research that is paid for.

If failing MTX/prednisone (if can't get enzymes WNL with less than 40 mg prednisone QD) for hypomyopathic/myopathic disease, then can switch to MMF (would overlap the two for at least 3–4 weeks during the transition time MMF takes to kick in). If failing MMF/pred, can do IVIG vs. rituximab, or for MDA5, can consider pulsed cyclophosphamide (sometimes rheum drives the ship and derm's main job is to prevent infections of the ulcerations). Can use rituximab as rescue therapy if cannot get prednisone <40 mg QD. Rituximab also recommended specifically for MDA5 because rational to deplete their pools of pathogenic autoantibodies (like pemphigus).

Some AICTD patients may report stiffness while weaning their systemic meds and describe as weakness, but possible it's the chronic wear/tear arthritis they had before, which rebounds a little bit, so may need to explain MTX/prednisone is not the treatment for OA (don't want to hold up graduation from DM treatment because of noninflammatory arthritis).

Achy arthritis that gets worse throughout the day = wear/tear.

DM skin is hard to treat. Sometimes, when DM skin burns out, it scars the stretched-out vasculature (and just like rosacea, after you treat the inflammatory component, the redness stays). So can't just assume that any redness is active cutaneous DM.

There's a lot of inappropriate use of high-dose prednisone, IVIG/rituximab for amyopathic patients and should probably restrict prednisone to hypomyopathic or myopathic disease (probably not going to touch the rash and can rebound the muscle and skin disease if you taper too quickly).

Although poikiloderma commonly very itchy, some of the chronic late DM patients (ones off treatment or presented late and still on treatment for skin but muscles in remission) have some superimposed AD, so pruritus might go away with dupilumab (doesn't treat the DM rash of poikiloderma but may help the itchy, scaly stuff go away). Skin after 8 years of DM is thinner and more irritable (thus, be extra cautious with TCS atrophy).

Treatment ladder for skin: HCQ, then MTX, then MMF (will never get normal CK on just these things, thus won't prevent from picking up muscle disease when/if it comes up).

Topical tofacitinib might work for cutaneous DM but quite expensive; can offer if patients willing to pay out of pocket. Be mindful if history of cancer; another thing to consider is roflumilast (Zoryve), but hard to get.

Reportedly, 1/3 of patients with DM get morbilliform drug eruptions from HCQ, but we use HCQ quite a bit without issues.

Hydroxyurea can cause DM rash (one of the rare causes of drug-induced DM) but don't tend to get full-blown DM. Can cause ulcerations.

Statins are weird; can have a normal CK and not be able to stand up, a polymyositis-like illness, hypomyopathic, myopathic, or full-blown DM while on statins and thus should have all DM patients stop statins.

For pulm DM, usually eventually hand off management to pulm since MMF works well for ILD. Typically, a chronic low-grade issue if occurs in setting of DM (in other words, wouldn't use prednisone for it).

Be aware of immunostimulatory herbs and gummies which have gained popularity (and particularly forced into the Latino population). They flare DM (and thus probably actually do help people get over colds via interferon stimulation). Patients, of course, probably aren't aware of this and, in fact, sometimes may ask about ways they can stimulate their immune system (which is obviously opposite of what they should want to do). You can point out that if the "immune boosters" were framed as "pro-inflammatory" supplements, then they'd probably sell a lot less even though that's how they work.

FYI: Also never give imiquimod or similar to patients with DM (or lupus), because you'd basically be activating mechanisms in skin already aberrantly activated (also not great to use in patients with stuff like psoriasis).

2.4.1.2 Lupus

Obviously a very complex and poorly understood disease. Will focus on some things to think about regarding skin lupus here. Many clinical subtypes. The three main ones are based on morphology/distribution (acute, subacute, chronic [most often discoid]). Won't really cover the rarer chronic variants here (such as bullous, profundus, tumid, chilblain, etc.). There are also other rare skin stuff you may see, such as EM-like lesions in lupus (called Rowell syndrome—may see on consults). Bullous SLE and Rowell are different, because SLE has autoimmune destruction of BMZ and (+) DIF. Rowell has targetoid lesions, (–) DIF, and the bullous changes are secondary to intense inflammation rather than autoimmune destruction.

Following is an oversimplification, but to give you context of the main idea:

- *Acute*—classic transient butterfly rash on cheeks. If think has rosacea but unsure, then do ROS and check labs (for lymphopenia, etc.) with close follow-up; an acute lupus patient is bound to be sick.

- *Subacute*—photosensitive annular or papulosquamous lesions on sun-exposed skin. Can get dyspigmentation.

- *Chronic*—most commonly discoid (pinkish-red scaly plaques, sometimes atrophic, hyperpigmented borders; scar with pigmentary changes; commonly associated with scarring hair loss).

125

You should always ask yourself what the clinical-pathologic lesion you see is (vs. calling it an acute SLE rash, SCLE rash, DLE rash). Probably best to frame it as "subacute lesions with renal involvement," or something similar (rather than saying "has discoid lupus"). Exams tend to hone in on lupus band test/DIF results for lupus, but no one seems to really use it in practice (although could maybe help if trying to distinguish LPP vs. discoid lesion or something).

The rheum diagnostic criteria is what dictates the epidemiology and the numbers that come from it, such as risk of progression, and so on. Great contribution in terms of categorizing/organizing diseases, but the downfall is the overlap; if patient has a discoid lesion under their eye, that alone is three criteria—discoid lesion, malar rash, photosensitivity. So if they have that in addition to an elevated ANA (which 50% of women over age 50 have) or develop an aphthous ulcer or something, then they "meet criteria for SLE" (when they actually might just have chronic skin-limited CLE). You can see how this can muddy the waters with epidemiology, etc. If patient has an isolated discoid lesion, negative ANA, no arthralgias, normal WBC, normal platelets, normal UA, then they realistically probably have essentially 0% chance of progressing to systemic involvement (despite the exam answer: DLE having a 5–20% risk of progression to SLE). So it's obviously important to understand and be able to explain this when counseling patients.

For drug-induced SCLE, ask about Naproxen (very common cause, though not included in many sources; probably even more common than hydrochlorothiazide [the test answer]).

MANAGEMENT

HCQ a systemic mainstay. Can also use MTX or MMF (either as second-line or as adjunctive first-line).

Thalidomide, albeit reserved primarily for severe or recalcitrant cases, is miraculous for chronic CLE (works even when MMF + belimumab don't) but a pain to obtain (via REMS program, only dispenses 1 month at a time). However, they might not necessarily need year-round, and you can suggest storing it during the non-sun months to reduce number of visits since it's such a hassle to get.

There are newer systemics on the horizon, like anifrolumab, that will likely become more established and frequently used in the future.

If localized skin-limited chronic CLE, can consider TCSs or ILK (of course, be careful with overuse since already susceptible to atrophy/pigmentary issues; can use TCIs, but not as strong and less helpful for very scaly lesions).

Patients are different, and some flare in sun, others in winter. Regardless, they all need broad-spectrum physical mineral sunscreen. This context exemplifies the importance of understanding the differences between how mineral (physical blockers, deflects light) vs. chemical sunscreens work. Chemical sunscreens may make UV-sensitive conditions (such as lupus) worse because it doesn't block the UV light like mineral sunscreens (chemical sunscreens allow absorption of the photons into the skin, which probably isn't helpful).

You may be able to get lupus patients prescriptions for tinted windows.

Mindful also of UV exposures from fluorescent light bulbs.

Smoking flares lupus; take advantage of opportunity to counsel on smoking cessation.

2.4.1.3 Scleroderma

Idiopathic, high morbidity, variable mortality. Hard to treat.

Rare; annually, 2.7/100k, female > male, 30s–50s, increased prevalence/ severity in Blacks.

Interesting because has odd combination of immunologic aspects, vascular aspects, dermal sclerosis aspects, connections with other autoimmune diseases and connective tissue issues, etc.; so hard to target what the real problem is, and there's not really one therapy that actually works. So while waiting for effective treatments to come out, should focus on everything that is reversible (for example, put on anti-reflux regimen, something for Raynaud's, involve pulm if SOB).

Derm is at front line of recognizing/diagnosing.

- *Hallmark clinical features*: Raynaud's, nail fold capillaries changes (twisted tortuous, dilation, and dropout—can also see in DM but doesn't have as much of the ragged cuticle as seen in DM), sclerodactyly.

  - Later onset, asymmetric, and severe Raynaud's should make you think CTD (vs. primary Raynaud's [very common], which usually starts age 30 or younger and is just a vasoreactive phenomenon, not something that alone has consequences that compromise circulation).

    - Of the AICTDs, Raynaud's is often the worst in systemic sclerosis.

    - *FYI*: You can see nail fold capillary dilation + dropout from Raynaud's (so not pathognomonic), but be on lookout for tel-angiectasia/puffy fingers, etc. (puffy fingers may be the initial complaint).

- *Other common features of SSc*: skin not very mobile between DIP and PIP (fibrosis starts distally and progresses proximally); difficulty making fist, can't fully straighten fingers (prayer sign); matted telangiectasias often on hands, lips, face.

  - *Limited cutaneous*—stays distal to elbows, distal to knees; may get facial changes; increased rates of pulmonary HTN, primary biliary cirrhosis.

  - *Diffuse cutaneous*—extends proximally to elbows/knees; can involve trunk; increased rates of ILD, cardiac/renal involvement.

Differentiating limited vs. diffuse helps prognosticate, but not a definitive thing in predicting systemic involvement.

- Systemic sclerosis sine scleroderma: no fibrosis; won't see a lot of these patients but may come in with severe Raynaud's.

EVAL/WORK-UP

- SSc—skin exam + autoantibodies

  - First, determine disease phenotype.

  - Determine disease duration (first non-Raynaud's symptom).

  - Determine antibody status: ANA, anti-Scl70, anti-centromere, anti-RNA polymerase; sometimes you'll be surprised by which one is positive.

- Anti-polymerase III of diffuse cutaneous has increased risk for renal involvement, so get routine BUN, Cr, UA, self-monitor BP for first 3–5 years (crucial specifically for these).

- All SSc patients should get baseline high-resolution CT chest (*FYI*: Different study from a regular chest CT, so make sure you order the right one); all SSc patients are increased risk for ILD. Used to get PFTs + DLCO, but now understanding not seeing early changes with those tests. The PFTs can be used to track patients over time. Get imaging Q 6 months for first 3–5 years, then repeat if has additional symptoms.

  - Because of the interstitial fibrosis/change in pulm architecture, prefer MMF over MTX.

  - However, if you use MTX (which probably doesn't cause these issues at QW dosing), make sure you document if has any pulm changes before starting MTX; otherwise, will of course get blamed on MTX.

  - Same thing goes for DM, RA, lupus, MCTD, etc.—lung scarring is a big feature of AICTDs, many of which are treated with MTX.

  - More on management later.

- Echo + EKG Q 1 year for 3–5 years, then repeat as guided by symptoms.

  - Should probably also get EKGs in sarcoid and lupus.

- GI work-up guided by symptoms.

  - Esophageal dysmotility (basically patchy dead areas, dysphagia in middle of chest for both liquids and solids) -> need reflux regimen because LES becomes incompetent and gets the crow beak esophagus.

Management of rare diffuse scleroderma is much different than limited CREST-like stuff (which is way more common). Patients with limited sclero-derma (such as CREST) die *with* it, whereas patients with diffuse scleroderma usually die *from* it (typically from severe renal arterial disease). Early every-thing works; late nothing works (arteries become like stones, which is when they start losing digits). Thus, probably best to send diffuse SSc patients to a scleroderma center (most will still die but can at least live longer with good care).

- Should use more MMF than MTX in systemic disease.

- MMF non-inferior to cyclophosphamide for skin fibrosis and preventing lung remodeling in SSc (MMF less toxic too).

  - Normally, MMF takes ~3 months to take effect for most diseases but takes ~6 months for fibrosing conditions.

  - Start 500 mg BID, then 1,500 mg BID after 2 weeks if labs are fine (esca-late quickly because takes long time to kick in and fibrosis very hard to reverse).

- Rituximab may have benefit in terms of fibrosis overall, but more side effects than MMF, so would probably only use if don't respond to MMF; can consider IVIG as adjunct for refractory cases 2 g/kg per month, so usually 1 g/kg per day over 2 days per month, usually back-to-back or spaced out by 2 weeks. Might add on to MMF, for instance.

- Physical therapy—improve mobility, prevent contractures.

- Abatacept, toclizumab, nintedanib don't really work for the skin fibrosis (sometimes reached for in ILD).

- TNFs and thalidomide don't seem to work.

- Botox can help reduce early-onset ulcers.

- If really bad ulcers, can admit for IV vasodilators (prostaglandin analogues, etc.).

- Digital ulcers in CTD-associated Raynaud's are an emergency. Can progress extremely quickly because no reserves to open vessels up and improve blood flow to fingertips. Patients can get ulcerations -> gangrene -> autoamputation or surgical amputation.

- Botox much cheaper than IV vasodilators; need strong wording in documentation, such as "crucial for severity of disease," "risk of digital autoamputation," "risk of possible admission," etc.—maybe cite the PMIDs to help get covered.

  • Apply EMLA to interdigital web spaces.

  • Reconsitute 100 units of Botox with 2 mL normal saline (5 units per 0.1 cc).

  • Clean with chlorhexidine.

  • Inject 0.1 cc into each interdigital web space, almost like nerve block, at 45-degree angle until hit bone, pull back a smidge, inject 0.1 cc, and repeat for each web space. Skip thumbs unless they're bad (one of the side effects obviously is hand weakness). Other side effects: soreness, infection.

  • Takes 2 weeks for full efficacy (same as cosmetics). Will often take multiple attempts to get covered; probably will never get for Medicare patients.

- Raynaud's treatment ladder

  • Lifestyle modification.

  • Calcium channel blocker (nifedipine extended release 30 mg QHS—usually OK even with some patients with low BP).

    – FYI: Don't put topical nitroglycerin on hands. Was tested as agent for Raynaud's at such a big dose that people got rebound cardiac vasoconstriction, then introduced with a ruler to be put on chest for angina; so if choose to use, dose with ruler on chest so it's dosed properly. If don't know the dose, could get cardiac complications.

  • Phosphodiesterase inhibitor (tadalafil 20–40 mg QD, or sildenafil 20 mg up to TID).

  • Chemo-de-innervation: Botox.

  • Other adjunctive treatments.

  • Admit for IV vasodilators.

- Microstomia has profound quality-of-life impacts.

- If focal fibrosis in perioral area -> think local procedural interventions: CO_2 lasers, fat transfer, injectable fillers, IPL, and more recently, hyaluronidase (can all be combined with systemic therapy).

  - Hyaluronidase comes in 1.2 cc vial.

  - Dilute with 4.8 cc normal saline.

  - Sterilize perioral skin with EtOH or iodine.

  - Injections are painful, so may need infraorbital and mental nerve blocks to numb perioral skin; do extraorally, since decreased oral aperture.

- Go in at nasal ala and up to mid-pupillary line until hit bone. Try to reach for just below orbital rim and inject lidocaine + epinephrine there; count four teeth out from center for mental nerve (sometimes can feel the ridge), and inject lidocaine + epinephrine there.

  - Then inject hyaluronidase intradermally in two rows in a perioral distribution.

  - Side effects: nerve blocks numb for hours, bruising, soreness, anaphy-laxis with hyaluronidase.

  - Try for prior auth coverage; out-of-pocket cost is ~$93 per vial.

  - Injections are Q 1 month, until plateau; usually plateau at 4–6 months.

- Salt-and-pepper dyspigmentation (can be presenting feature) is hard to treat.

  - If no history of or past treatment for vitiligo, should think CTD on ddx; more common in severe disease and over trauma-prone sites. Increased frequency in skin of color.

  - Thought to be led by fibrosis around hair follicles themselves that leads to depigmentation (thus, topicals not going to do much; need to address the fibrosis with systemics).

  - MMF might work (anti-fibrosing dosing).

2.4.1.4 Morphea

Completely different from scleroderma, so don't call it localized scleroderma to patients (they will get confused). Emphasize that morphea doesn't progress to scleroderma and morphea generally has minimal risk for internal disease (risk depends on subtype, which guides work-up).

Biopsy/lab studies (antibodies) not needed to diagnose morphea.

Explain at the first visit that there are two parts to morphea: the inflammation (our job is to control this), and then the body has to remodel the inflammation (leather has to be chewed up over 3 years [will soften and become fine], and color needs to normalize). The disease is so deep if you look 3 months later, it looks the same (hard to assess treatment response), so what you should judge is whether there's redness, new lesions, or blips at border that're expanding. If body is finished with morphea, might be a little wrinkly but otherwise will have perfect skin.

Although for most people it goes away in 3 years with low-dose systemic, 10–15% recur within 5 years of stopping treatment and have to restart systemic treatment. Can taper MTX slowly at roughly 2-year mark if achieved sustained control of inflammation (meaning no erythema [went from red to brown], no blips coming out from patch, and no new areas of involvement). Want 2 years of stability before tapering (or higher-risk relapse).

MTX first-line in morphea (vs. SSc) because not worried about ILD. More data for MTX than MMF in morphea. Decreases flares, increases remission.

MMF second-line because more strongly immunosuppressive.

HCQ for mild disease.

Can consider JAKis, IVIG, infliximab, if highly refractory.

For burnt-out morphea, some people do fillers (but there is potential for reactivation of disease).

Variants, presentations, and considerations:

1. *Plaque*: <3 plaques, <3 cm.

   a. No work-up; probably don't need biopsy.

   b. Treatment: topical calcipotriene + TCIs (more favorable than TCSs, actually); if severe -> phototherapy (NBUVB), maybe MTX if bothered.

2. *Generalized*: >3 plaques, >3 cm, often 2+ body sites.

   a. No work-up; probably don't need biopsy.

   b. Treatment: phototherapy, MTX, then MMF.

3. *Linear*

   a. Craniofacial looks like en coup de sabre or happens temporally.

   b. *Extremity*: can cross joints, high risk for contractures; thus, get good range of motion by physical therapy or rheum to prevent progressive joint contractures.

   c. Treatment: if involving face or rapid or crossing joint, MTX + SCSs (to turn disease off quickly to prevent joint contractures, long-term cosmesis issues if face involved, etc.) + physical therapy; next line is MMF.

4. *Pansclerotic*—fibrosis extends from dermis to subQ and even fascia/muscle; circumferential around trunk or joint; more severe.

   a. Treatment similar to linear.

5. *Deep morphea*: may not get same epidermal color changes; may just be a step off deeper plaque.

6. *Keloidal*: early fibrosis.

7. *Bullous*: if pronounced early inflammation, can get blistering.

8. *En coupe de sabre*

   a. Clinical diagnosis: classically paramedian, can be temporal.

   b. Brain MRI (debatable).

      i. MRI brain would be to see if neuro involvement and need neuro referral (risk for neuro complications if can have foci of inflammation or neural morphea); however, have to be quite negligent for many years to get inflammation of bone/neural complications.

c. Ophtho—uveitis screening Q 1 year for 4 years.

d. Dental exam if extends down to involve dentition (can have dental anomalies).

e. No ANA needed.

9. *Morphea profunda*: may get additional imaging if concerned for involvement of deeper structures.

Management of mixed morphea: guided by most severe disease manifestation.

2.4.1.5 Eosinophilic Fasciitis (EF)

Usually symmetrical swollen legs (knees to ankles) > arms (but can have both) that feel like leather and are extremely tender to palpation (patient will essentially jump off the bed).

Inflammation is not in the epidermis, not in dermis, not in the subQ, but in the fascia. If have fascial edema on MRI and clinically it's not scleroderma/ morphea, then can say it's EF without biopsy. Biopsy of fascia can also be falsely positive in linear morphea or systemic scleroderma, so an MRI showing fascial inflammation is better, anyway.

Like an AICTD in the sense that can put patients into remission if keep their erythema perfect for 2 years. Thought to be on severe end of morphea spectrum.

Female > male in 60s, possible physical stress/trauma induces it.

1. *Hallmark features* (which help ddx from SSc [as they will often be referred for "scleroderma"]):

    a. Nice mobility of skin between DIP/PIP joints, with fibrosis elsewhere.

    b. Cobblestoning along thighs because fibrosis along the fascia.

    c. Puckering in of skin (groove sign) along the veins of forearms when raising hands above arms (because fibrosis sits along fascia, when raising hands above head, the veins drain blood back to the heart and get puckering).

    d. Absence of Raynaud's, nail fold changes, and microstomia also favor it not being SSc.

2. *Ddx* from scleroderma matters because of work-up, treatment, prognosis:

    a. No ILD, no pulmonary arterial hypertension; possible peripheral eosinophilia (not needed for diagnosis); hypergammaglobulinemia and monoclonal gammopathy can be seen.

    b. Think about joint contractures from fibrosis of fascia overlying joints.

3. *Work-up*:

    a. CBC with diff (eosinophilia), SPEP with immunofixation (monoclonal gammopathy), MRI of most active compartment (avoid deep wedge biopsy since fibrosed patients will struggle to heal); MRI can track progression/response to treatment.

4. *Management*:

    a. *Mainstays*: SCSs (probably start with pulses, then taper over 3 months), MTX (up to 25 mg QW), or MMF (1.5 mg BID) after 2 weeks of test dose; tell patients 6 months for response.

    i. For CTDs in adult patients: MTX 10 mg QW for 2 weeks, then 25 mg QW; MMF 500 BID for 2 weeks, then 1.5 mg BID; don't want patient to lose faith while slowly titrating up. For peds, it's weight-based dosing; get to goal weight–based dose quickly, too, though.

    ii. Doesn't respond to just MTX monotherapy; really needs prednisone to go into remission.

  b. *Poor outcomes*: delayed diagnosis, lack of systemic steroids.

2.4.1.6 Considerations in Skin of Color

1. If very dark skin, harder to see violaceous erythema, often gray or brown (such as the heliotrope rash in DM; Gottron's papules and V-sign/shawl sign usually look hyperpigmented or poikilodermatous).

2. Higher predisposition for dyspigmentation; catch early, so don't get.

3. Wear broad-spectrum tinted mineral sunscreens with iron oxide.

4. Vitamin D supplementation (Black patients at higher risk for deficiency at baseline, but also likely avoiding sun because of their AICTDs, so important to be extra-cognizant).

5. DLE very common; frequently causes dyspigmentation + scarring alopecia.

6. DLE lesions can resemble vitiligo (erythema can be clue it's not vitiligo [unless it's inflammatory vitiligo]).

7. Rare comedonal variant of DLE often misdiagnosed as acne.

2.4.2 Hair

Set expectations. Stability is, in some ways, a response for the non-self-limited/chronic conditions (in other words, we're better at salvaging/preserving hair than turning back the hands of time).

As always, counsel on treatment response timeline; regardless of med they use, will take ~9 months to see a noticeable impact (thus, RTC ~Q 9 months [for non-inflammatory hair loss] is generally reasonable). Take pics (at same angle, if possible) at every visit or it will be hard for them to know/appreciate their progress.

2.4.2.1 Evaluation
2.4.2.1.1 Clinical

- Distribution/shape of hair loss.

- HPT (hair pull test): need to pull harder than you think; if it's (+), specify where (vertex, temporal, parietal, etc.).

  • >4 hairs of 40 pulled is (+)—helpful for determining whether certain conditions (such as TE/AA/etc.) are active.

2.4.2.1.2 Trichoscopy

Be comprehensive, but also make sure you're intentional with where on scalp you're looking. For example, if they're wearing box braids, look at the base, where the hair likely has the most pull, etc.

Want to assess the following:

- *Hair shaft thickness*

  • For example, AGA has miniaturization, which can also be in some inflammatory disorders.

    – Miniaturized hairs = previously large terminal hairs which shrank over time to become size of vellus hairs (vs. true vellus hairs, which have always been small).

- *Follicular openings*

  • Examples of findings:

    – Decreased openings (follicular dropout) in scarring alopecias (openings are replaced by scar tissue)

    – Hyperkeratosis (scaliness)

    – Erythema (darker in skin of color)

    – Fusion (multiple hairs emerging from one hole—feature of inflammation)

    – Pigment incontinence

- *Follicular epidermis*

  • Examples of findings:

    – Scaling/hyperkeratosis

    – Erythema

    – Disrupted pigmentary network

- *Vessels*

  • For example, lupus, DM have increased thickness and number of vessels.

There is overlap in some of the findings, so you really have to appreciate the subtleties and correlate clinically (for example, the lymphocytic scarring alopecias [CCSA, LPP, DLE] all have perifollicular hyperkeratosis, erythema). So if looking for specific stuff, search for red dots and interfollicular keratotic plaques in DLE, follicular fusion in LPP, peripilar gray-white halos in CCSA, etc.

Neutrophilic alopecias are a lot more inflammatory—a lot more compounded hairs (look like "doll hairs").

Tufted hairs = 6+ hair shafts from same opening—specific for FD. Severe inflammation at infundibulum and isthmus. Aggressive, widespread, need to be precise and prompt with treatment. Some people group folliculitis decalvans with acne keloidalis nuchae and call it tufted folliculitis.

Dissecting cellulitis—starts deep; can see non-scarring findings (black dots, broken hairs, slower-growing hairs, etc.) on scalp in beginning (almost like AA or trichotillomania, etc.) because not destroying hair follicle but is interfering with its growth (so get broken/slower-growing hairs). Make sure you include this info in the path order.

When progresses can see more aggressive inflammatory findings (3D yellow dots, hyperkeratosis that looks greasy).

Ddx from folliculitis decalvans—doesn't have the tufted hairs.
Acne keloidalis nuchae, similar histology to folliculitis decalvans (thus why some people think they're on a spectrum and group them together)—a lot of inflammation and hair destruction.

- *Frontal scalp*: FFA, traction, scarring alopecia in an FPHL distribution.

- *Traction (chronic)*: decreased terminal hairs and increased vellus hairs + follicular dropout + perifollicular erythema + sometimes perifollicular hyperkeratosis; also, sometimes in beginning, see miniaturization, and people think it's AGA.

Chronic traction = fringe sign vs. FFA (decreased vellus hairs in beginning; mostly just have terminal hairs—get lonely hair sign [lonely terminal hair on frontal line]).

Trichoscopy very helpful also for picking biopsy site. For instance, if trying to rule out LPP, want to assess an area with loss of follicular openings, follicular fusions, with erythema, and/or with white structures.

Can guess the histologic correlation; perifollicular hyperkeratosis (white scale around hair follicle) corresponds with infundibular inflammation around hair follicle.

Use lidocaine-epinephrine, then wait 10–15 minutes ideally before punching (want the vasoconstriction—less bleeding). Try to locate the bulb and cut at least 1 cm below that.

Want two 4 mm punch specimens (one for horizontal, one for vertical).

Horizontal cuts give you better view of the follicles—can see how they're structured, their size, count the vellus and terminal hairs (so basically more info).

Vertical cuts (only see maybe ~5 hair follicles at most) are useful if thinking seb derm or psoriasis or DLE and want to see basement membrane zone.

Black scalp patients:
Erythema harder to appreciate (compared to redness on white scalp). So if erythema is visible in skin of color, then should think anti-inflammatory treatments.

DLE—diffuse disrupted pigmentary network in perifollicular and interfollicular epidermis, dilated vessels, hyperkeratosis (in all lymphocytic cicatricial alopecias), interfollicular scale.

LPP has less interfollicular inflammation (is mostly targeted to the hair follicle), so pigmentary network should be mostly normal (except around hair follicle, if at all—usually look like targetoid blue-gray dots).

Red dots = inflamed and dilated vessels type of hair follicles; specific for DLE, so biopsy those lesions.

Vessels are also very thick in DLE, and thinner in LPP (if don't see much of this stuff [if you don't have a strong concept of what is thick/thin], then compare it to hair shaft).

Persistence of pink/white dots; should be regularly distributed (good example is in AA, but in CCSA has irregularly distributed pinpoint white dots that are different sizes).

Inflammatory happenings are in the non-renewable parts of the follicle (the isthmus, infundibulum); isthmus has the stem cells, so if gets persistent inflammatory destruction, there will have a scarring alopecia.

Peripilar gray-white halos are most specific for CCSA (94% of patients with these have CCSA). So take biopsy from those sites.

2.4.2.2 Hair Medications

1. *Topical minoxidil*

   a. Apply QD; don't need if already on PO minoxidil.

   b. Promotes growth phase, helps increase hair diameter, thus improves density.

   c. Foam (less liquidy/less EtOH) vs. solution (less crunchy after dries).

   d. Tell them to get the men's (5%) version (cheapest at Costco or Amazon— Kirkland brand).

   e. Can get in the way of styling hair.

   f. Can cause discoloration (graying, other color changes).

   g. Warn about possible shedding (starts 3–4 weeks into treatment; may last for 2–4 weeks while the hair growth synchronizes). Doesn't happen in everybody, but should be aware so they treat through it (instead of stopping it due to thinking it made their hair loss worse).

      i. Make sure they rub it into their scalp and don't wash it out after application.

   h. Have to stay on treatment indefinitely (because results are not sustained upon discontinuation [hair will revert back to where it would be if never treated]).

2. *PO minoxidil*

   a. Same mechanism as topical, obviously; slightly better (more effective, less messy) than topical (and patients adhere to pills better than topicals). Probably best hair loss med we have.

   b. Technically a BP med but shouldn't impact their BP at doses we use (we start at 1.25 mg QD for hair loss vs. BP control might be like ~20 mg QD).

   c. Possible side effects: lightheadedness, fatigue, maybe ~30% getting hair regrowth in less-desired areas (usually vellus [peach fuzz] hairs—better to frame as "won't grow a beard or anything," but good to consider when thinking about increasing dose, especially if has more facial hair than wanted already at baseline [which some women get after menopause]).

      i. Some can get LE edema + sometimes facial edema (occurs even with low dose, but both are temporary).

   d. Same warning about shedding and lack of sustained results if discontinued as topical minoxidil.

3. *PO finasteride*

   a. Reduces DHT in scalp (DHT damages hair follicles); usually start 2.5 mg QD (1.25 mg QD not enough to do much).

   b. Improves regrowth, but not as much as minoxidil; would think of it more as stopping/slowing progression.

   c. Don't use if has history of breast cancer (especially if within past ~5 years or so); benign breast cysts (common) are fine.

   d. Must avoid if pregnant (abnormal male genitalia/hypospadias).

   e. Warn about libido, possible gynecomastia (both resolve upon discontinuation), not really associated with depression, like bicalutamide.

   f. Topical finasteride may be minimally helpful if patients refuse PO, but not very preferable.

4. *PO bicalutamide*

   a. Been around for a of couple years; blocks male hormone receptors.

   b. Cousin of flutamide (which only was used when desperately needed because of its association with liver toxicity; thus, manufacturer went out of business, and it was used for men with prostate hyperplasia, but derm adopted it for FPHL).

   c. Warn about possible decreased libido, depression (because testosterone works in this way).

   d. Need baseline LFTs + 6 months later (don't need for finasteride).

5. *Spironolactone*

   a. Probably the least-effective of the FPHL treatment options, but can be a good adjunct.

   b. Would think of it as similar to finasteride in the sense that it primarily hinders progression.

   c. Rational if have coexistent acne/PCOS type of stuff.

   d. Avoid if history of breast cancer (especially if recent).

   e. May make periods more irregular.

6. *ILK*

   a. Nice if actively inflamed, which can be subtle clinically; if having symptoms of inflammation (itchiness, burning, pain), then would offer.

   b. Be mindful of concentration, as always; can generally do 5–7.5 mg/mL for frontotemporal scalp, 7.5–10 mg/mL for vertex, etc.

7. *TCSs*

   a. Instructions say to wash out Derma-Smoothe oil every morning after application, but skin-of-color patients don't need to (and shouldn't) do that.

8. *Ketoconazole*

   a. "When get into shower, rinse hair, apply ketoconazole to entire scalp [not the hair—it's a lousy "shampoo"], let sit for 5–10 minutes [do rest of shower], then rinse thoroughly."

   b. See considerations in the Skin-of-Color section.

9. *Non-pharmacologic options*

   a. Nutrafol (can do 2–3 pills QD instead of the 4 pills recommended to save $$).

b. Pumpkin seed oil for TE.

c. Good shampoos: Head & Shoulders, KeraCare Dry & Itchy (basically Head & Shoulders for skin of color), Royal Oils (good for skin of color), John Fritos for Frizzy Hair.

d. Use a lot of conditioner to prevent shaft damage.

e. Revian cap ~$945 after discount.

f. HairMax laser comb—maybe ~$300.

   i. Consider stability a response with these; for instance, if same as a year ago with low-level laser therapy (LLLT), that's a good thing.

g. Also, remind to augment overall health (diet, vegetables, organic foods, increased protein; supplements aren't absorbed same way as actual diet).

10. *Miscellaneous things*

   a. Avoid rosemary and lemongrass oil "treatments," etc.—aren't effective and can dilute medication absorption (oils can be OK as long as not placed on scalp—oils should be applied to hair, medications to scalp).

   b. Overuse of chemical relaxers, permanent waves, hair dyes, or bleaching can result in significant hair shaft damage (so always ask, especially at new patient visits).

2.4.2.3 Procedural Options

1. *Hair transplant*: impossible to give specific success rate; even with non-scarring alopecias, there isn't 100% salvage of grafts.

   a. If patients ask, probably ~75–80%, ~60% for scarring (which is pretty good).

      i. The percentages are in context of continuing treatment after.

   b. Need enough space on scalp to put hair transplant, so if have pretty good hair (but not satisfied), then can consider platelet-rich plasma (PRP).

2. *PRP*: concept is regenerative medicine; can be injected intradermally.

   a. Maybe 60% effective for hair (at best).

   b. Issue is variability, not only in how it's spun, but also with how platelets are taken out, the patient's baseline health status (can be on steroidals, can be sick).

   c. Exosomes are an emerging new thing which might offer more consistency.

      i. Concept is capturing microvesicles (normally facilitate communications between cells; contain similar growth factors as platelets) and applying topically (not really injected, yet, at least).

        – Can apply right after resurfacing (for wound healing), burn care, hair restoration, etc.

      ii. Can retrieve exosomes from adipocytes or plants.

3. *Micropigmentation* (basically pigment placed in dermis on scalp in small dots to help camouflage areas with follicular dropout).

2.4.2.4 Scarring Alopecias

Generally early in disease = signs/symptoms of active inflammation (erythema, scale, itchiness, burning sensation, tenderness, active hair loss, etc.).

Late = scarred follicles (can be hypo- or depigmented).
Thus, important to arrest inflammation before damage already done.
Not uncommon for them to have coexistent non-scarring conditions, so address the inflammatory stuff and promote growth of whatever is still there.

FYI: Hair histology not as well-defined as skin histology, so oftentimes patients are sent in wrong direction. Beneficial to consider taking a step back from any previous histology reports or diagnoses by other providers and trusting your clinical impression (sometimes patients with dreadlocks look like CCSA, and their biopsy will show CCSA, but they actually have traction); can start with treatment for non-scarring processes to elucidate what is left over after scarring.

Biopsy if concern for lupus; if can't tell has LPP vs. CCSA, can also consider biopsy, because matters if want to try MMF. Though the majority you should feel comfortable with clinically diagnosing.

2.4.2.4.1 Lichen Planopilaris (LPP)

T-cells target antigens in follicles (bulge) -> kills stem cells.

Whites > Blacks; usually ages 40s–60s, with ~50% having coexistent LP elsewhere.

Characteristically very itchy. Burning/tenderness common too. Increased hair shedding (positive hair pull test).

Perifollicular erythema and scale (usually at periphery of alopecia patch) = active (thus, think ILK/anti-inflammatory).

Can see interfollicular erythema as well (may be confluent—same with scale).

Sometimes, seb derm can even resemble LPP if severe; seb derm tends to affect frontal scalp.

MANAGEMENT

1. *Local treatment*

   a. TCS solution QD for flares, then 3–4× weekly (clobetasol or Lidex or betamethasone dipropionate).

   b. Offer ILK at visit if actively flaring/symptomatic. Inject superficially. Warn about hypopigmentation. Hurts.

2. *Systemics*

   a. Anti-inflammatory

      i. HCQ 200 mg BID

      ii. Doxycycline 100 mg BID

      iii. MTX ~10 mg QW

      iv. MMF ~1 g BID

v. Would only do prednisone or CsA if highly aggressive/progressive and, of course, only temporarily

vi. Maybe pioglitazone (PPAR-y agonist [PPAR-y anti-inflammatory, so when lose expression -> get inflammation -> destruction of sebocyte and stem cells with scarring])

– Haven't seen a ton of patients on this.

b. Augment hair growth for existing follicles.

i. Minoxidil

ii. Finasteride

Pseudopelade of Brocq:

■ Basically end-stage presentation of a scarring alopecia (classically LPP).

■ "Pelade" = AA (so basically it looks like AA but is scarred [doesn't have active inflammatory findings and usually asymptomatic]).

■ "Footprints in the snow" pattern (can see in LPP, other scarring alopecias, etc.).

■ Typically women, 30s–50s; either insidious (slowly progressive) or waxes/wanes.

■ *FYI*: Term doesn't apply if definitive diagnosis of another scarring alopecia established.

2.4.2.4.2 *Frontal Fibrosing Alopecia (FFA)*

LPP variant. Classically White patients, but can also happen in skin of color (who tend to have more itching and facial hyperpigmentation). Usually 50s–60s.

Unclear whether sunscreen actually can cause FFA (and why), but people who tend to apply a bunch of facial products seem to get more issues such as FFA.

The sunscreen belief is because in the 1990s (when it was first starting to be put in makeup, moisturizer, etc.), someone lost their hair and when they stopped the sunscreen the hair came back. But the case report looks more like ILK-induced atrophy (which can make you lose hair), so might be due to that. Seemingly more associated with chemical (> mineral) sunscreens.

Noninflammatory facial papules, eyelash loss, body hair loss = possibly severe course.

Eyebrow loss—possibly milder course (more common); usually don't really get erythema (if have broad scarred pink areas, then try to entertain DLE on ddx, which tends to leave a lot of dyspigmentation and surface changes).

Lonely hair sign (isolated, uninvolved hairs on frontal hairline). Perifollicular erythema/scale = active.

MANAGEMENT

Very similar to LPP (HCQ 200 mg BID, particularly for pre-menopausal women; can use finasteride/dutasteride in post-menopausal women).

Hard to treat; the end point is essentially stabilization (which is a win). TCIs can be good for eyebrows (not strong enough for CCSA/traction). Can also do ILK/TCSs.

2.4.2.4.3 Central Centrifugal Scarring (Cicatricial) Alopecia (CCSA)
Usually early middle-aged (late 30s, early 40s) Black women. Quite common 3–6%.
Incompletely characterized pathogenesis. Genetics (PADI3); studies have actually found no association with relaxers/hot combs/braids/weaves/etc. (in other words, hair care practice modification is not a sufficient management strategy, and CCSA is not something that patients bring onto themselves).
Usually starts at vertex, expands centrifugally; but can also involve other areas of scalp and take on other patterns (albeit less commonly).
Some patients may seek eval after noticing "hair breakage."
Look for peripilar gray-white halos (fibrosis) and black dots (broken hairs), though may not see peripilar gray-white halos in CCSA if burnt out, and sometimes inflammatory features can be subtle (especially early on, since normal hair will be intermixed).
Can be clinically diagnosed, but if opt to biopsy, use dermoscopy to guide where to take specimen from (don't biopsy the scarred area).
Sometimes hard to tell if active based on exam. Ask about symptoms. Typically tender, burns, itches when active (ddx from FPHL).

MANAGEMENT
Keep in mind there is probably always some undercover inflammation and most all patients should get a maintenance anti-inflammatory.
Also make sure to assess for coexistent hair conditions (FPHL, seb derm, etc.) and treat what you can; for example, seb derm probably makes CCSA worse (usually, seb derm has hair loss on frontal hairline).

If early and active:

1. ILK Q 8 weeks for 6–8× (7.5 mg/mL for vertex, 5 mg/mL for frontal hairline) to areas of hair loss and surrounding areas (where scalp looks seemingly uninvolved); injections should be 0.5–1 cm apart.

   a. Some also do Q 4–12 weeks for 6–9 months or longer.

2. TCSs (start off with Lidex or clobetasol ointment QD for 2–3 weeks [if symptomatic], then Derma-Smoothe or similar 3–4× weekly for maintenance [start with this if not symptomatic]).

   a. If first visit, can do clobetasol QD for 12 weeks, then BIW to TIW for maintenance.

3. Doxycycline 100 mg QD or BID for 6 months.

   a. Some do 100 mg QD–BID for 3 months, then 40 mg QD for 3+ months.

4. Possibly +/– seb derm treatment and AGA treatment (minoxidil can, of course, optimize whatever salvageable hair remains, so is almost always a good option if can tolerate).

5. Can also consider LLLT (such as Revian Red Cap 10 minutes QD [typically used for AGA]).

If late, consider suggesting hair transplant or wig. Maybe PRP.
Even though not associated with hair practices, still good to encourage gentle hair practices (for example, discontinue hot combs, relaxers, excessive heat). This will help avoid additional issues and help with overall hair health.

If unwilling to stop relaxers, tell them no more than Q 10 weeks and to avoid the scalp and avoid applying with other agents.

2.4.2.4.4 Traction (Late = Scarring)

From prolonged and repetitive tension from hair practices such as wigs, weaves, tight braids, cornrows, tight dreadlocks, tight rollers/elastic bands, tight ponytails, using hair buns or wearing turbans, hijabs, excessive brushing, extensions, etc. Especially if chemically relaxing hair too, though someone with natural hair (who doesn't know how to style hair) might be more likely to wear extensions over entire course of the year (bad) because takes them more time than someone with relaxed hair. So although relaxed hair technically at higher risk for traction, they might be less likely to be doing other things that add to the risk.

Also consider length of braids/cornrows/locks—longer = heavier -> more damage potentially.

Will see in kids (possibly from their parents styling their hair).

Usually bitemporal (fringe sign helps ddx from FFA) but can be anywhere (involved areas can resemble other conditions, such as the back of scalp looking like ophiasis AA).

Look also for broken hairs at different stages. Scale (AKA casts, hyperkeratosis [stuff that coats the hair follicles coming out, indicative of damage]) + erythema possible (helps ddx from AGA). Sometimes have pustules perifollicularly early on. Can also have tenting (scalp literally being lifted up).

Whether early (non-scarring) or late (scarring), management similar (better hairstyling practices + anti-inflammatories). These recommendations could apply to optimization of hair care in general. Full recovery possible if caught early.

You can think of management of traction like pre-diabetes (cheeseburger OK) vs. diabetes controlled with metformin (watch what you eat) vs. diabetes with insulin (point of no return—do you want to wear wigs?).

- For example, for someone without or with mild traction alopecia, tell them OK to get box braids; make sure braids themselves are thick, and take them out after 4 weeks. Don't have to avoid everything, but they need specific instructions.

Clarify current hair practices:

1. If they don't know the type of conditioner, tell them to avoid anything that makes hair dry/crunchy, stiff, straight, or hard—because it changes the physical properties of the hair that makes it more likely to come out.

2. Emphasize traction areas are fragile while recovering, so be extra careful to avoid high-tension practices.

   a. Don't twist locks close to scalp; tell them to tell their locktician (if they have one) to leave at least 0.25–0.5 in from root of hair (in other words, there should be zero pulling on hair, even if it doesn't hurt [some patients will say it doesn't hurt but will have perifollicular erythema and can see their root sheath being pulled out, so not a reliable judge]).

      i. Be cognizant that it will cost the patient more to do this (because have to get them re-done more frequently)—nice to acknowledge that you're aware of that.

      ii. For locks/braids/weaves/cornrows, try to have shorter than shoulder-length.

b. Take breaks from potential tension hairstyles, like braids, extensions, and definitely sewn-in weaves.

   i. An example of an OK hairstyle are crochets (not much tension).

c. Patients who wear hijabs often wear undercaps (to hold hair in) and wear hair in tight ponytails—so loosen ponytails and avoid undercaps, as well as volumizers (such as scrunchies/clips).

d. Patients who wear turbans often wear ponytails and twist/tightly knot their hair (including beard).

   i. Keep in mind they sometimes wear their turban 24 hours a day, and the material can be very stiff.

   ii. So recommend softer, non-starched turbans, avoiding wearing it when possible (such as when sleeping) and, when wearing it, to wrap it as loosely as possible at the base (and of course, tie hair loosely under the turban).

e. Must avoid gels, sprays, intense brushing/combing; haircuts are fine.

f. Also avoid glue-in stuff (see later sections on skin of color and hairstyling practices).

3. Slap cap at night (many will say they wear bonnets).

4. Silk satin pillowcases.

PHARMACOTHERAPIES

1. ILK ~Q 2 months ×3 rounds if inflamed.

2. May need to continue fluocinolone oil indefinitely 3–4× weekly to prevent recurrence in traction (similar to psoriasis, may have active inflammation but be asymptomatic).

3. Can consider doxycycline if has papules/pustules.

4. Topical minoxidil to traction areas (PO minoxidil fine too)—will help bolster strength of hairs as they come in.

2.4.2.4.5 Dissecting Cellulitis

Part of follicular occlusion tetrad (with HS, acne conglobata, pilonidal cysts).

Follicles occlude, rupture; keratin promotes inflammation with secondary staph infection -> dramatic neutrophilic inflammatory response to staph antigens.

Typically Black men, 20s–40s. Prominent boggy nodules; pus might come out if push on it. Pretty distinct appearance. Painful, but less tender than you'd think by looking at it.

Chronic. Waxes/wanes. Late stage = fibrosis, sinus tracts, hypertrophic scars with alopecia.

MANAGEMENT

1. Doxycycline 100 mg BID.

2. If can't tolerate, can consider TMP-SMX double-strength BID.

3. Dapsone rational given neutrophilic, but pretty weak in comparison to the problem, so probably not good as stand-alone therapy.

2.4.2.4.6 Folliculitis Decalvans

Suppurative folliculitis possibly an immune response to staph.

Perifollicular erythematous pustules and papules; if chronic, scarred alopecia plaques. Painful.

Any time after puberty (usually middle-aged). Earlier onset associated with severe course.

Usually has tufted hairs (6+ hairs coming out of single follicle).

MANAGEMENT

1. Topical anti-staph antibiotics: Clindamycin 1% lotion, for instance.

2. TCIs.

3. ILK 5–10 mg/mL Q 3 months if actively inflamed.

4. PO doxycycline 100 mg QD to BID if actively inflamed.

5. Can also consider isotretinoin (0.5 mg/kg QD for 6 months), dapsone (100 mg QD for 6 months, then 25 mg QD).

2.4.2.4.7 Acne Keloidalis Nuchae

Misnomer; not true acne, not really a keloid. Similar pathophysiology as pseudofolliculitis barbae (ingrown hairs). Some people just get bumps; others get progressive alopecia (in whom their pathophysiology overlaps with folliculitis decalvans, and they get crops of pustules and crusts).

Usually affects young Black men's occipital scalp. Some mention they think it's from getting hair shaved or from wearing helmets.

Painful. Commonly itchy and bleed.

May see tufted hairs. Don't see ingrown hairs.

MANAGEMENT

1. Avoid picking, wearing tight collars.

   a. Some people say shaving makes worse, but the actual problem might be how often they shave and their shaving technique.

      i. Shaving somewhat frequently is preferable (3× weekly or more) because it may prevent hair from growing long enough to cause irritation.

      ii. If they shave in the shower, they should do it first (the warmth and steam from the shower will swell the skin, so the shave won't be as close and the hairs can dig back in and cause irritation).

      iii. Patients should pre-treat before shaving with a gentle cleanser like Gillette or Aveeno.

      iv. Can recommend Gillette Labs razors. The Art of Shaving products are also nice

2. Clindamycin 1% lotion BID seems to work better than TCSs (but can do both).

3. If no pus, then ILK Q 4 weeks (especially if mild to moderate).

a. Give doxycycline 200 mg for 2 weeks, then 100 mg QD to sterilize before ILK.

   i. If really inflamed and thick, can do doxy 100 mg BID for 2 months and ILK 20 mg/mL.

   ii. The first ILK may soften it up and reduce itchiness/irritation, but probably takes about three treatments before starting to see flattening (make sure to mention the hair may not grow in those areas, but the goal is to at least not have to do with the bumpiness [and can still get growth around the areas, so will be easier to cover up if the plaques aren't sticking out]).

b. After ILK, can consider 50 mg QD maintenance + possibly clindamycin.

2.4.2.5 Non-Scarring Alopecias

Follicular ostia intact. Thus, of course, more reversible than scarring alopecias.

2.4.2.5.1 Telogen Effluvium (TE)

Prototype diffuse non-scarring. Typically asymptomatic. Usually just scalp.

Hair essentially gets lazy (something going on that makes body realize it has other things to take care of besides make hair).

Happens 3 months after a stressful event (examples follow) since each telogen cycle is ~3 months; TE lasts 6–12 months. Thus, best to say TE in setting of something in particular (such as an underlying condition, health event, etc.).

- *Review past medical and past surgical history.* Endocrine disorders, autoimmune diseases, high fever, illnesses/infections, surgeries under general anesthesia, pregnancy, fad/crash dieting, sudden weight loss (and bulimia/anorexia).

- *Common drug-induced offenders*: psych drugs, anticoagulants, beta-blockers, antibiotics, interruption of long-term estrogen-containing OCPs.

Always get TE after hair transplant.

If no clear trigger, ask about thyroid issues. Consider possible low iron, zinc, vitamin D, nutritional hypoproteinemia.

Hair pull positive if active.

MANAGEMENT

Reassure hair will come back with time.

Warn may happen again if get sick, have surgery, etc. (in other words, could be related to weight loss first time, then next time can be related to stopping tamoxifen, next time could be due to hospitalization, etc.).

If related to diet, consider dietician referral.

If has deficiency, start supplements.

Although biotin is in hair shaft to make it not split, supplements don't work.

1. If super distressed, can recommend minoxidil (though may get more shedding 3–4 weeks in).

2. If TE is active, can recommend Nutrafol (no miracles; can do 2–3 pills per day instead of the 4 recommended [given the $$$]).

3. If really against pharmacotherapy and still adamant to try something, can recommend pumpkin seed oil (some people say it works; perhaps they just naturally recover, but if it reduces stress, then a placebo is effective in some ways).

2.4.2.5.2 Alopecia Areata (AA)

Autoimmune, genetic predisposition to lose immune privilege to hair follicle -> IFN-y goes crazy, pulls in WBCs, starts cataclysmic reaction around hair follicles.

WBCs stay in the hair follicle (they just become inactive via treatment—thus easy to understand why AA recurs upon treatment discontinuation).

Usually 1–2 patches on scalp. But check body, eyebrows, eyelashes.

Eyebrow AA more common in thyroid disease (usually lateral brows).

Nail pitting = active. Positive hair pull test from patch periphery = active.

Exclamation point hairs (thinner closer to scalp) means their hair is being attacked.

Chronic, unpredictable course. Duration/extent variable. Recurrence is common.

Ophiasis pattern more recalcitrant.

Ask about symptoms of thyroid issues; look for vitiligo.

Might have family history of vitiligo, pernicious anemia, Hashimoto's thyroiditis, T1DM, etc.

Good to document SALT score (0 = no loss; 100 = complete loss).

AA score also good for approvals (categorizes as mild/moderate/severe, but more all-encompassing than just SALT score—because it allows you to use things that can move them up a severity category via consideration of additional factors (eyebrow/eyelash involvement, quality of life impairment, significant worsening, inadequate responses to other treatment, etc.).

MANAGEMENT

If localized, not bothersome, and recovering, perhaps can consider no treatment.

If localized and bothersome, can do ILK Q 6–8 weeks (7.5–10 to scalp, 5–7.5 if near frontal hairline) and clobetasol BID weekdays to edges (not center); stop when the AA patch is gone.

Make sure for AA eyebrows: inject ILK in straight line so doesn't grow back weird.

For extensive (totalis or universalis), probably systemics. Can use MTX. PO JAKis probably give the best results (baricitinib; could also use ritlecitinib [especially for peds], tofacitinib, or PO ruxolitinib), but usually responses aren't sustained when discontinuing the JAKi. May also flare if transition from JAKi to another JAKi. So from a cost/sustainability/long-term side effects standpoint, MTX is probably more favorable.

Make sure you keep them on the med long enough; sometimes it takes a while to see response (should keep on for at least 9 months to 1 year).

If been stable (at 20 or less SALT) for a while, then can trial dosage tapers.

Can always use adjunctive minoxidil to promote growth.

Topical JAKis don't seem to work well (despite reports of them working for eyebrows, eyelashes).

2.4.2.5.3 Androgenetic Alopecia (AGA)

Can happen any time after puberty. Birthdays and genetics. More common in men. Chronic, worsens with age. Women are protected by estrogen until ~50.

FPHL sometimes can be bitemporal (if strikingly MPHL in female, try to rule out virilizing tumor).

If also has hirsutism, irregular menses (hyperandrogens), try to rule out PCOS (and late-onset congenital adrenal hyperplasia).

Anisotrichosis (miniaturization—terminal hairs look thinner, then eventually become vellus [peach fuzz] hairs).

FYI: Sometimes TE episodes can unmask AGA (make it more noticeable). Otherwise, hair shedding usually isn't super prominent (hair pull might be positive in actively shedding areas, though).

MANAGEMENT

Need to stay on treatment indefinitely (until a cure or better medicine comes out) because is chronic problem.

Need 6–12 months of true adherence to determine whether working or not. If discontinued, will revert back to state where it was without treatment.

1. Topical minoxidil (get the men's version, 5%—same molecule, just stronger than women's 2.5%)—warn about possible initial shedding ~3 weeks in.

2. PO minoxidil is probably best hair growth drug (PO slightly better than topical; if doing PO, then don't really need to also do topical)—warn about initial shedding ~3 weeks in.

3. PO finasteride (make sure no history of breast cancer, etc.).

4. PO spironolactone (make sure no history of breast cancer, etc.).

5. Consider Nutrafol (2–3 pills QD) if has fine hairs.

6. Low-level laser light devices (such as Revian red cap 10 minutes QD, or HairMax comb, etc.)

7. PRP maybe.

8. Remember sunscreen, especially for men with bald scalp.

9. If not looking to spend money or do prescriptions, can change where their part is to make it not the midline and use a shampoo that makes the hair fluffier.

2.4.2.6 Hair Shaft Disorders

Don't forget about hair shaft disorders, which, of course, cannot be diagnosed via scalp biopsy. Should do a hair mount (can use oil on the slide; some people just tape the hair to the slide).

Acquired trichorrhexis nodosa: recurrent breakage of shafts (not a predominantly scalp disease) from poor hairstyling habits. Often occipital scalp.

- *Common culprits* (anything that weakens hair): chemical relaxers, thermo hair coloring.

  - Some patients stop taking care of their hair after receiving certain diagnoses (such as CCSA—especially if coming from other providers whose biopsies showed CCSA [which, remember, CCSA histologically only shows pauci-inflammatory scarring, so easy for pathologist to call it that if they think that's what the clinician wanted]).

  - Retention hyperkeratosis = sign of not washing hair.

- *Telltale signs of hair breakage*: looks dull in light, dyed tips.

- *Management: start on healthy hair path*: see hair care in skin of color.

- Use chelating shampoo *if have calcium deposition from no-lye relaxer* (they contain acids that chelate the mineral ions to wash it away).

Hair care for swimmers (all skin types):
Water rushes into hair and can burst it from the inside out (similar risk as with frequent washing).

So if swimming and rinsing hair every day, ask them to bring conditioner to the pool to apply after rinsing (in other words, OK to rinse hair, but just don't let it dry by air). This is analogous to swimmers with eczema—letting skin air-dry is bad (evaporates into air and takes moisture with it) vs. applying Vaseline right after getting out of water (good—because basically pushing moisture into the cuticle).

2.4.2.7 Considerations in Skin of Color

Oftentimes, patients will say it runs in the family, but poor understanding of hair care practices runs in families too (thus, quality counseling/education can be a life-changing paradigm). Example of good regimen: wash own hair ~QW (many never wash), leave-in conditioner, protein treatments, regular trims. See more in Hairstyling Practices section.

- Ketoconazole shampoo is best treatment for seb derm, but limited use in patients with long curly hair (very drying). Black men can use it; patients with straight hair can use it. If they color their hair, then regardless of race, better to avoid ketoconazole shampoo, because of stripping of weak hairs.

  - Should generally also avoid salicylic acid, coal tar shampoo in curly hair—meant to strip as much sebum as possible (curly hair is sebum-poor state).

    - Instead, can recommend OTC zinc-pyrithione shampoos that are made for skin of color (such as KeraCare Dry & Itchy, Head & Shoulders Royal Oils anti-dandruff shampoo, Pantene Gold shampoo + conditioner, Design Essentials Almond + Avocado, or Pantene Gold Intense Oil Moisturizer—albeit they are less effective than ketoconazole), ciclopirox (less drying than ketoconazole shampoo).

    - Still should apply to scalp.

    - Great for patients with seb derm that isn't hugely bothersome.

    - Aim for 1–2× monthly as realistic goal (can do less often if hair gets crunchy).

  - Can still make ketoconazole shampoo work in skin-of-color females, but may need to avoid certain hairstyles, such as braids, to be able to wash frequently enough (minimum QoW to be effective; QW is pretty good).

    - *FYI*: Braids are OK for washing; main thing is washing the scalp (so let them know the whole thing doesn't need to be wet). *FYI*: Apple cider vinegar doesn't count as washing.

- Any shampoo (ketoconazole, ciclopirox, an OTC, etc.) is just a wash on/off product; patients will also need a leave-in medication (such as Derma-Smoothe).

  - Package will tell patients to wash Derma-Smoothe out—warn skin-of-color patients about that, and tell them to ignore it. Should leave it in overnight and make one of the nights of application the day before washing.

- Minoxidil foam builds up too much if only washing QW or QoW; instead, use solution. If treating frontal scalp, then apply solution, then oil after (solution evaporates, but drying, so moisturize after using it).

  - Can compound it in an oil or ointment to circumvent these issues.

- Ask about vehicle preference (as for everyone); usually, Black patients like ointments more (solution better for straight hair).

  - Foam is lighter than ointment, but more watery, thus can mess up hair; betamethasone lotion also watery.

- For night: Grace Eleyae satin slap cap at night is better than wrapping in scarf and/or polyester bonnets; doesn't need to be at same time as silk pillow.

- Satin hair clips and satin-covered sponge rollers.

- Avoid derma rollers (can damage hair follicles and not a pleasant experience).

2.4.2.7.1 Hairstyling Practices in Skin of Color

Some basic science for background:

- Shiny/soft—characteristics of cuticle.

- Strength—characteristic of cortex (has disulfide bonds and weak hydrogen bonds).

  - If want to change appearance of hair (color), have to break disulfide bonds.

  - If want curly hair and have straight hair, have to break disulfide bonds.

- Sebum coats hair shaft, protects hair, is potent attractor of dirt (thus, straight hair gets greasy fast and feels like needs washed more often); curly hair takes long time to attract dirt, thus only have to wash Q 1 week.

  - *FYI*: Sebum in Whites and Blacks is the same, but the ability to coat the hair shaft is different.

- Physical properties of hair differ between races.

  - Tightly curly (African American) hair: sebum has difficult time traveling down hair -> more susceptible to damage and harder to grow longer.

    - Routine grooming of curly hair is dangerous.

    - Thus, many avoid daily grooming (by braiding hair, relaxing/straightening hair [takes less grooming to achieve longer lengths], etc.).

- Patients will often call tight braids a "protective hairstyle" because they were taught these things (protecting from regular grooming), not realizing that tight braids can cause traction.

- Taking care of curly hair is very time-intensive; the best way is to wear hair the way it is.

Relaxers (work via alkaline ingredients that break the disulfide bonds)

■ Important to use lye relaxer (contains NaOH).

• Supposed to be used by professional stylists only.

• Higher risk of ICD, but less risk of calcium deposits over time (non-lye relaxers work via chemical reactions that deposit calcium on scalp [which will break hair—can fall out in clumps]).

• Can tell patients to get boxes that say mild (lower concentrations) or texturizers (same as relaxer, but lower concentration [hair won't get as straight but will maintain hair integrity better because breaking less bonds]).

• Many non–skin-of-color women use chemical relaxers too.

Coloring

■ Alkaline agent (NH3) restructures the position of hair (for 15 minutes), then an acidic agent (hydrogen peroxide) brings pH back to 7 and kills the melanocytes, then color gets laid on.

Weaves

■ *Pros*: can get full appearance (increased density, length); can wear 2–3 months at a time.

■ *Cons*: common cause of traction alopecia; can't wash scalp while weave is in (except for the fusion), and thus, they wash hair Q 3 months, which is setup for scalp inflammation.

Weaves can be installed many ways

■ Hair braided down into cornrows, then portion of weave sewed to a track, and a needle used to connect the two.

■ Net installation (hair is cornrowed, but weave not directly on braid; it is sewed onto spaces between braids)—good because less tension on hairline; good if have traction and trying to limit tension.

■ Fusion technique (more common in non-Blacks, expensive; instead of linear track, take pieces of hair and glue to patient's hair, reapplied Q 2–3 months)—most damaging form of weave; hard because can't take it out at home and have to go back to stylist (who will tell them it is safe and won't lose hair, because they have financial motivations).

If feel strongly about a certain hairstyle, suggest wearing wig (which are really good nowadays) and taking it off at night to apply the meds.

■ Lace-front wigs: have lace covering that makes it look like wig growing from scalp.

■ Younger women sometimes glue to their scalp, however, because they just want to get up and go in the morning.

• Some get ACD.

• Some look like end-stage FFA (like immediately after) because so traumatic when removed, and accelerates formation of traction; before with braids took 10 years to develop end-stage traction, now patients can get in 1 year if they're gluing hair to scalp.

• Important to not use adhesive if wearing a wig, so ask them how they keep it in place, not leading questions like "Do you use glue?"

• Wigs are good for end-stage disease or those who have spent most of life doing camouflage techniques (braids, weaves, etc.) and need to get off those because have traction alopecia; wigs can be used temporarily to transition while treating.

Straightening

■ Thermal straightening (flat iron, blow-dryer, hot comb)—high heat can break disulfide bonds.

• *Cons*: it's repetitive -> cumulative damage; over time, much more damaging than relaxer.

– If patient wants to go straight for the long term, then better to use relaxer than to flatten hair repetitively.

■ Keratin treatments—another option to make curly hair straight.

• Contain mixture that, when applied to hair, cross links with keratin in hair and forms a bond, which is held in place when activated by heat. Hair remains straight for several weeks; however, mixture contains formaldehyde, which, when heated, releases formaldehyde gas (known carcinogen).

• In April 2024, the FDA banned formaldehyde/formalin/methylene glycol (which turns into formaldehyde when mixed with water) in products.

• If people have slightly wavy (not truly curly) hair and want to go straight, can use ingredients ammonium diglycolate, glycolic acid, glutaraldehyde, which are true formaldehyde-free temporary straightening ingredients (though don't straighten hair as well as formaldehyde).

Sister locks

■ Popular style.

■ People like because when you lock hair, you never have telogen hair; instead of hair shedding, it gets locked into your hair (trapped in hair shaft), so women can achieve longer lengths. If can only achieve long lengths of relaxed hair, people feel this is natural, plus requires minimal styling effort.

■ But sister locks cause rapid end-stage traction alopecia (not the usual along the frontal hairline—which is the classic presentation, because we have fewer follicles there and that is where they braid).

- Patients with dreadlocks, we used to think were CCSA best responders, but the reason they had traction; dreadlocks cause traction that looks like CCSA. If patient able to decrease how often refreshes locks (to Q 8 weeks) and apply topical minoxidil, can improve (doesn't need ILK).

- So in short, sister locks can cause traction alopecia that involves entire frontal hairline and central scalp; better prognosis than CCSA, but have to cut their locks. Regular dreadlocks cause less damage because parts are larger than sister locks with smaller parts (same concept as braids).

2.4.3 Hidradenitis Suppurativa (HS)

Female > male, Blacks disproportionately, but largest population impacted are Whites. Fairly common (6% of population). Usually post-puberty for adolescents.

Essentially, apocrine glands get plugged up (like a dam that collects green stuff like algae, leaves, etc.), which makes a nice home for staph germs to grow, so have to keep skin surface clean; otherwise, get buildup of stuff and get boils. Can get HS wherever skin touches skin.

Pathogenesis somewhat reminiscent of cutaneous Crohn's and often over-laps (can be quite difficult to differentiate them, and if you biopsied a fistula from a Crohn's patient and biopsied a fistula from an HS patient, they'd look the same).

From a high level, HS has a medical arm and a surgical arm. Medicine is to control flares and stop progression (spreading/growing). Surgical management is to remove the diseased tissue (scar tissue and sinus tracts) that have already formed (insurance almost always covers). Cutting out the tissue is relatively easy for surgeons (especially if small and focal [spread-out and deep ones are harder to remove]), but getting it to heal well afterward is the challenge (because HS is so inflammatory, which makes the body not want to heal; thus, need inflammation to be at rock bottom before surgery to avoid flaring nearby HS [achieve quiescence with meds]). Ideal if patients lose weight before surgery (decreases distance between blood vessels and the skin, so the skin gets more blood and heals better [basically like a rubber band—when you stretch it, it gets thinner—and when vessels are smaller, they don't let as much blood through and the skin gets starved of nutrition]). The extra/redundant skin from the weight loss also makes it easier to reconstruct/close them up after surgery (basically like an arm lift, where the part they cut out is the HS skin). So surgeons often have a weight or BMI threshold (usually minimum BMI 37) that they require before operating (the more weight loss, the better, obviously—and if patients are on a roll with weight loss, they will likely let them continue the momentum and then do the surgery when their weight plateaus). Of course, smoking hampers healing, and thus, most surgeons will make them commit to stop smoking before operating too (good to let patients know about these expectations before referring them for plastics eval). Also, be cognizant that HS often hurts so bad that exercising is very difficult; further complicating things, they need to be eating enough meals to be adequately nourished to heal properly (so can't just lose weight from eating less, which you should advise against patients doing, anyway). May take some coordination with PCP to get them on weight loss meds like Ozempic, Wegovy, etc. Bariatric surgery is also an option if meds don't work (though, of course, has its own package of implications/qualifications).

Follicular subtype is more superficial and usually heals better than nodular subtype (but downside is, they spread wider). Longstanding nodular lesions can be wide, though, too (and characteristically are deep).

■ If drains pus out of multiple places -> think PO doxycycline, etc.

■ If chronically backed up -> think opening procedurally.

■ If recently opened up procedurally, keep areas sterile (Theraworx Protect).

More details in what follows.

2.4.3.1 Evaluation

1. Have you had outbreak of boils in the past 6 months? Where and how many?

2. Activity: drainage, number of sinus tracts, new nodules, pain.

   a. *Questions you can ask to see how they're doing*: Peak pain in a week? In a month? Daily pain? What is the drainage like? How often do you have to change clothes (daily, weekly, monthly)? Then PGA. Because disfigured skin, can't use clearance as an end point.

3. Hurley 1: nodules.

4. Hurley 2: discrete sinus tunnels—have to palpate them to find them.

5. Hurley 3: no normal skin between sinus tunnels.

6. Patients will often ask about pathophysiology: complicated, but at least five areas (microbacteria attracts neutrophils, genetics, immune factors [response to biologics, SCSs, mediators of immune cell function], mechanical stress [tight clothes], lifestyle factors [2/3 of patients have high BMI, risk of metabolic disorders like DM, HLD]; if to address those, HS improves to an extent).

   a. So basically not precise enough to have definitive management algorithms. Similar presentations but triggers are multifactorial; thus, treatment should be individualized. Different stages have different chemokines.

7. Check the skin for psoriasis (gives you more treatment options). Ask about low-back pain (spondyloarthropathy); if they GI discomfort/bloody diarrhea, work them up for IBD (other specialties), and look for metabolic syndromes (check A1c, encourage PCP and nutritionist).

2.4.3.2 Approach

1. If treated early, can usually prevent progression, but some rapidly progress.

2. Stabilize with medical treatment.

3. Once stabilized, then sinus tunnels can be source of activity, so want to eliminate those surgically.

2.4.3.3 Management

1. Hard to characterize outcomes; thus, data hard to interpret.

2. Goal is to reduce number of nodules (stabilize, prevent progression) with medical treatment, reduce number of sinus tunnels (more remittive) with surgical treatment.

3. Cosentyx (IL17) approved for HS but honestly might have been better if they went for IL23 approval first since treats Crohn's, etc. IL17s could potentially be problematic if they have coexistent IBD, which many do, because IL17s won't treat their bowels.

   a. A reasonable way to approach this is to screen. Ask: What joints? Is it axial vs. peripheral arthritis? Do they have canker sores? Do they get neutrophilic dermatoses? If yes to any of those, then would probably be more careful with the 17s. Same approach with psoriasis.

4. Hair removal at beginning can be helpful in preventing progression; might not be able to do the whole series (insurance cares more about short-term profits than long-term prevention) but get maybe four treatments covered (out of 8–10).

5. Smoking cessation is good but doesn't always improve HS.

6. GLP-1 agonists/bariatric surgeries may help but may also have severe flares with the redundant skin after significant weight reduction.

2.4.3.3.1 Medications

1. Mild to moderate HS.

   a. Topical clindamycin solution QD to affected areas.

   b. BPO wash 2.5–10% wash, Hibiclens.

      i. BPO may be preferred because keratolytic, but Hibiclens is anti-microbial (BPO isn't); try to get 5 minutes of contact time with whatever wash they use. Some people use product called Cln.

   c. Bleach bathes QW, mupirocin for nares to eliminate staph carriage.

   d. Levicyn gel (basically a dilute bleach—hypochlorous acid).

   e. PO doxycycline 100 mg BID for first 2 weeks, then QD—generally do up to 3 months (goal is to have a few weeks with no new lesions).

      i. If doesn't work, then rifampin 300 mg TID + clindamycin 300 mg TID (RTC Q 3 months) or triple therapy (clindamycin, rifampin, and metronidazole or quinolone).

         – With rifampin, be careful with OCP decreased efficacy (because they may be doing more intimate things once they improve); check LFTs monthly.

      ii. If too young for doxycycline, can also do TMP SMX.

   f. PO dapsone—especially if coexistent PG.

   g. ILK to active areas/migratory papules (10 mg/mL if initial lesions, or if severe nodules that are indurated, consider TAC 40 mg/mL).

      i. If abscess that doesn't connect with skin, put small volume of ILK 40 mg/mL to diffuse into it.

      ii. If it's a draining sinus tract or interconnecting draining sinus tract, do higher volume of lower concentration (basically to flush out the sinus tracts), and put on antibiotics.

iii. Topical resorcinol (15% compounded into cream) BID PRN for active lesions is a good rescue.

iv. If recurring same area, can punch deroof and curettage down to viable tissue.

- Same concept as wound debridement (turn static non-healing granulation tissue [red stuff] to an active healing wound). Need to curette away all the anaerobes, inflammation, granulation tissue, all the gunk, etc., to create an active wound that will heal.

- Can take a small curette; use it as a probe, push it through to see where the sinus tracts interconnect, then cut across the top of the probe to open it up, then curette everything out, then can heal by secondary intention or another closure, if appropriate.

For antibiotics, plan for 3–12 months for maintenance; for flares, use Augmentin in addition to baseline antibiotics.

2. Severe HS (or if see any tunnel formation, want to stop at all costs).

a. Adalimumab 40 mg QW (rarely clear with it, though can dose escalate—30–40% chance will improve with this, but consider infliximab 10 mg/kg Q 4 weeks if no response to high-dose adalimumab).

i. More succeed with infliximab, but higher rate of allergic reactions (urticaria, even airway issues).

b. Secukinumab Q 2 weeks vs. Q 4 weeks not much different unless on PO antibiotics before (presumably recalcitrant disease).

c. Usually takes 6 months for response; if switch too early, may miss late bloomers.

d. Can also consider finasteride 1–10 mg QD.

e. Prednisone 20 mg QD for 1 week is good for flares.

f. Also, some evidence for IL1 inhibitors.

3. If presents as part of follicular occlusion tetrad (HS/acne conglobata/dissecting cellulitis/pilonidal cysts), management:

a. TMP-SMX for 1 month, bleach baths, Hibiclens, mupirocin to nose, Theraworx Protect, Listerine for mouth (AKA anti-staph program), then isotretinoin for 16 weeks for acne conglobata/pilonidal cysts (because stratified squamous epithelium) or adalimumab (Humira) for HS.

i. Be careful of pilonidal cysts—have tendency to go deep (thus usually don't remove in office). If they recur once, then it's probably quite deep; if recur twice, then likely need OR because likely goes to bone and need to move muscles to cut out the cyst. Pilonidal cysts typically originate higher up and tend to move down and make tunnels; feel for induration until can feel wall of cyst to determine how big.

4. *Pain management (get ahead of it)*: topical lidocaine, NSAIDs/acetaminophen (1–2 tablets 325–650 mg Tylenol, 200–400 mg ibuprofen, combine); if severe, consider gabapentin, duloxetine, venlafaxine, tramadol, or refer to pain clinic.

2.4.3.3.2 Procedures

1. Don't do when actively flaring (control with meds first); do surgery to reduce flares and make biologic work better.

2. If lesions are inflamed + large, more prone to adverse events, so pre-treat with ILK and RTC 10 days for procedure; roughly 33% recur after deroofing (though some people say much more; I've heard all the way up to basically guaranteed recurrence), up to 68% after excision.

   a. Deroofing—need a 10 or 15 blade. Probes are great if you have them. Hydrodissect, then see if any areas extrude out. Wear goggles and gown (might be messy). OK to do in smokers. Maximize protein intake.

   b. CO_2 laser

      i. Ultrasound to find sinus tunnels, the hypoechoic areas (darker), if pulsates on Doppler, then vessel. Trying to go to dermal–subQ junction; use in continuous mode. Basically ablating down to subQ (ablate through dermis, because that's where most of the sinus tunnels come back). After that, probe with probe to make sure got it all out. This costs $1800 vs. a biologic that's $32k (and is not a $25k OR procedure); probably not good in smokers (long wound healing process).

   c. Excisions

3. Laser hair reduction—consider for early-stage disease (basically want to destroy their hair follicles and sebaceous glands before they become problematic). May need Q 1 year.

   a. Protect eyes. Do cold compresses before laser. Helpful to have air-cooling device, but if you don't have that, then contact cooling is fine (helps with pain).

   b. Want to vaporize hairs and double pulse nodules (two quick pulses at the same time). Good for nodular stage 1. Settings: usually 10 mm spot size, 20–30 ms pulse duration (20 for lighter skin, 30 for darker skin), 30–60 mJ/cm² (don't need to have dark skin for Nd:Yag).

4. If have painful ulcerations, consider biopsy. Make sure not an SCC.

2.4.4 Vulvar and Male Genital Derm

Obviously err on side of being overly sensitive about their privacy (even if some patients say they don't care, should always offer gown, step out of room when they change, pull the curtain, never seem rushed, give explicit fore-warnings about what you're doing and why, wear gloves, etc.—all very intuitive but worth re-emphasizing).

If teenager, can say something like part of growing up is assuming responsibility for their own health, and ask if the patient would like to practice answering questions on their own without their parent in the room (instead of just asking if they're OK with their parent being in the room, which can be awkward).

Probably should offer exam of genital area to all patients—though definitely should be particularly cautious with HIV+ patients and immunosuppressed (much higher risk of HPV-related SCC, and SCCs in general).

Get specific symptoms (itch, pain, dyspareunia).

Ask about prescriptions (obviously), but also non-prescription stuff, since many will likely have tried treating themselves before seeking eval (and probably have been increasingly using these things as the rash worsened—unknowingly potentially propagating the rash further).

Some examples: OTC analgesics, anti-itch stuff—important because some contain benzocaine, which is a common contact allergen. Soaps, baby wipes (have methylisothiazolinone), cleansing agents/douching products also commonly used. Ask about other exposures, menstrual pads.

Inflammatory rashes are probably most common (of course, includes psoriasis, LSC—see those sections). Will be using TCSs a lot—helps to show them exactly where to apply them (and where not to apply them—for example, don't want to apply to outer surface of labia majora, unless have LSC or psoriasis or something). Also demonstrate how much—for example, half a pea-sized amount for LSA, since the ointment spreads so much. In genitals, TCS overuse typically manifests mostly as striae (not so much tearing/purpura/telangiectasia); mucosal surfaces tend to handle well (still need to be careful), but be very careful about the hair-bearing skin, even the thighs.

FYI: Penile skin is different than vulvar skin (vulva has more mucosal surface)—thus, TCS practices are different (penile skin less tolerant of potent TCSs).

Labia majora are analogous to *scrotum*; *labia minora* are analogous to *urethra* in male (in terms of what you'll see as far as conditions).

Will also see secondary candidiasis. If severe and resistant, think about diabetes. Can also consider HIV (but obviously less common).

Don't forget about malignancies.

2.4.4.1 Lichen Planus

About 50% of women with OLP have genital LP. Usually features vaginal discharge, pain, burning, itching.

Sometimes, erosive (most common form) vulvar LP can look pretty similar to early LSA (might question if you think you're not seeing a lot of classic white changes). However, erosive LP usually painful > itchy (tends to be well-demarcated red eroded patches). Also look in mouth.

Non-dermatologists might say patient with oral and genital lesions has LSA, but LSA doesn't go in mouth (and would be bizarre to have OLP and genital LSA, so if this happens, should question the diagnosis).

Similar to OLP—need to avoid erosions (associated with vulvar cancer risk).

- *Treatment*: TCSs (clobetasol) if localized; systemics (MTX vs. MMF) if generalized or local refractory.

2.4.4.2 Lichen Sclerosus (LSA)

Pre-pubertal girls and middle-aged women.

Usually very itchy (rarely asymptomatic). Painful intercourse.

Typically a clinical diagnosis (biopsy often has too many secondary changes), but should consider biopsy if patient mentions pain and has an indurated/ulcerated lesion (could be an SCC). If has a thickened area resistant to treatment, or if red-appearing, then can also consider biopsy (could be pre-cancer vulvar intraepithelial neoplasia [VIN]).

Sometimes have to look hard to see the porcelain white stuff if early—look everywhere, but especially around the clitoris, in the crease between labia majora/minora, and the perineum (where it's most commonly found).

Shouldn't affect the inside of vagina. If it does, it's associated with an increased risk of vulvar cancer—so routinely follow.

Important to treat early to avoid permanent scarring and anatomic distortion (clitorial and labial fusion).

Ddx from LSC: LSC usually asymmetric and on hair-bearing surface of labia majora (vs. mucosal surface). Also, LSC won't have architectural changes. Can use medium-strength TCSs for 1–2 months for LSC (until not itchy and the hypertrophic skin has nearly normalized).

PsO also itchy—can use low- and medium-potency TCSs, or vitamin D derivatives. Check for inverse psoriasis if there is genital involvement (in addition to classic locations).

TREATMENT

Typically, genital area (male and female) should use ointments.

Goals of management: control symptoms, preserve anatomy, prevent progression to SCC (thus, can't just stop treatment once symptoms are gone—important to explicitly explain to patients).

- TCSs (clobetasol), including in kids—can start BID (depending on how bad it is) for 1–2 months, then taper to QD for 1–2 months, then consider a maintenance (perhaps betamethasone) and re-eval in a few months, and keep tapering to lowest potency that controls their disease (can also decrease the frequency).

- TCIs are fine for maintenance but might not be effective enough and can cause irritation.

  • Also consider the black box warning of TCIs being "associated with SCC" (which it doesn't [and would actually decrease risk of SCC, since you'd be treating/avoiding chronic inflammation, which—if unaddressed—would risk SCC]).

- If controlled and mild, can probably hand off management to PCP if they're willing.

- If severe, should probably follow.

2.4.4.3 Atrophic Vulvovaginitis

Not uncommon in peri- or post-menopausal women not on hormone replacement therapy. Basically low estrogen.

Can be itchy or painful.

Can be a secondary condition along with LP, psoriasis, LSC, etc. So think about if only partially respond to anti-inflammatory treatment.

Topical estrogen improves integrity of tissue, thus will probably make the anti-inflammatory stuff work better (same as moisturizing in an atopic). Would still start TCSs first, though (if, for instance, doing clobetasol BID for LSA), then when wean to QD, can add the topical estrogen.

Can use intravaginal estrogen if complaining of vaginal dryness, or creams for the actual mucosal surface of vulva. Localized, so no systemic side effects (as long as used appropriately—same concept as TCSs and systemic side effects). Should still be mindful of post-menopausal bleeding, history of breast cancer, etc.

2.4.4.4 Various Benign Vulvar Dermatoses

■ *Fordyce spots*:

- Sebaceous glands visible, small yellow papules.

- Can be mistaken for milia or warts.

■ *Angiokeratomas*:

- Benign vascular growths.

- Small red/purple papules.

- Some patients may be concerned are skin cancers; sometimes can look like melanocytic lesions—look with dermoscopy.

■ *Bartholin's gland cyst*:

- From blocked Bartholin's gland.

- Can form abscess if secondarily infected.

2.4.4.5 Malignancies to Consider

SCC and pre-SCC will probably be the most common. May have pruritus, pain with intercourse, or burning. But many are asymptomatic.

Don't forget about melanoma (ddx from labial melanosis), EMPD (which can resemble LSC, typically on labia majora), and other adenocarcinomas (anatomic location of lesion [periurethral, four and eight o' clock of vestibule, etc., comment which structures are normal] is key).

The VIN terminology can be confusing but important to distinguish.

There's HPV-associated VIN (which can be either LSIL or HSIL) and non-HPV-associated VIN (includes differentiated VIN and others).

HPV-associated (most common, more often benign):

■ LSIL (low-grade squamous intraepithelial lesion) includes stuff previously referred to as condyloma acuminatum and usual type VIN 1.

■ HSIL (high-grade squamous intraepithelial lesion) includes stuff previously referred to as Bowen's disease, Bowenoid papulosis, erythroplasia of Queyrat, SCCIS, and usual type VIN 2–3.

■ Can use imiquimod (though maybe not in immunocompromised patients).

Don't confuse "usual type" VIN (associated with HPV) with "differentiated type" VIN (not associated with HPV [is a p53 issue]). Differentiated VIN (dVIN) is 2/2 chronic inflammation (such as in LSA).

■ Although dVIN is much less common than HSIL, it's harder to diagnose histologically (and actually has histologic overlap with HSIL), clinically more aggressive (more rapidly progresses to SCC compared to HSIL), and more likely to recur.

- Thus, important to emphasize to LSA patients to RTC urgently if developed pain.

  – Can refer to gyn onc (especially if unsure if invasive and thinking WLE involving clitoris or urethra).

2.4.4.6 Considerations for Male Genital Dermatoses

Most common inflammatory things: psoriasis (1/3 of psoriasis patients have genital involvement), contact derm, lichen planus, lichen sclerosus. Can also see zoon's balanitis.

Warts, tinea, herpes probably the most common infectious stuff you'll see.

Much of management is similar to female genital dermatoses. Careful with potent TCSs (probably only use high potency for lichen sclerosus, and only for 1 month max—don't give refills). Low- to medium-potency TCS or TCI for long term.

If uncircumcised, ask them to retract their foreskin (could have an underlying SCC, but skin can look normal without you asking them to do that).

Penile LSA similar to vulvar LSA—can have scarring and fusion (foreskin to glans), anatomic (frenular) damage, etc., which can occur before seeing the large white plaques. Ddx from zoon's balanitis, which doesn't have the scarring features.

Circumcision an option for LSA of foreskin.

■ *For biopsy:*

• Doesn't take much anesthetic at all (maybe 0.1 cc).

• If do punch, do very shallow (not even close to the entire punch). Use absorbable sutures (less uncomfortable than non-absorbable).

• Can also do snip biopsy instead of shave (basically pull up skin and snip with scissors).

• If have luxury of choice for biopsy location, choose inside of foreskin (not glans, which will scar more). Avoid biopsy around frenulum (risk fistula that is hard to repair)—work with urology.

Don't forget about herpes if has an erosion/ulceration (may not have the typical vesicles). Can generally stick to scraping scaly stuff to see if tinea and swabbing erosive/ulcerative stuff to see if virus.

Genital warts hard to treat. LN2 + imiquimod probably give best results. For LN2, be careful about hypopigmentation. Give explicit end points for imiquimod (want a little red, sore, irritated skin, but if too much, then take a few days off). Cover scrotum in gauze or Vaseline or something so the imiquimod doesn't get on there.

For intraurethral warts (in meatus or fungating out of it), take a tube of xylocaine jelly (which comes with an installation cone for urethroscopy that fits the thread of a 5-FU tube which they squeeze until the urethra is full [they will know when it's full], try to leave in for 1 hour or so, then void and make sure none drips on the scrotum [can produce a dramatic dermatitis and erode the scrotal skin—warn them about this]). Repeat daily until start to get sore/eroded/uncomfortable. If really sore or hurts to urinate, then can use the xylocaine jelly without the 5-FU. When they appear clear, then do urethroscopy (don't do early; otherwise, will seed the virus deeper and deeper into the urethra), and make sure they look at the bladder, too, for papillomas.

FYI: Condoms are protective against warts, but only the area it covers, and HPV so common, so of course can still get them.

Lesion features to potentially worry about (re: malignancy or pre-malignancy risk): single, fixed lesions, with palpable infiltration, may be persistently eroded or fissured (for instance, one area that is always cracking, bleeding).

Bowen's disease of the penis (from high-risk HPV types): need to treat patient but also partner (cervical pap, anal pap); examine vulva and perianal region for erythematous and pigmented lesions.

Can use imiquimod or 5-FU (works well if uncircumcised because contains the 5-FU; the issue with 5-FU [more so than imiquimod] is the dermatitis that can erode scrotal skin, as alluded to earlier).

■ *Common benign things*:

- Pearly papules (AKA angiofibromas—which are more monomorphic, symmetric, typically on corona—vs. warts). Female corollary of pearly papules are vulvar vestibular papules (which are also often mistaken for warts). Can remove with LN2 or CO_2 laser.

- Angiokeratomas (can be on both scrotal and vulva; benign capillary ectasia; can remove with cautery, LN2, or vascular laser).

- Idiopathic scrotal calcinosis (calcified cysts). Best way to remove is excision.

2.4.5 Cutaneous T-Cell Lymphoma (CTCL)

Often more eczematous > papulosquamous—tend to be diagnosed with eczema for ~6 years before being diagnosed with CTCL.

Primary cutaneous (originates in skin; what we'll typically see) much different than systemic lymphoma, with secondary skin involvement.

Should try to have a sense of indolent ones vs. scary ones.

MF is most common subtype of CTCL and, although it's classified as indolent, can really run the gamut; many patients can have aggressive MF (although board answer is that it's indolent).

CD30+ lymphomas tend to be indolent and treatment-responsive, reminiscent of PLEVA clinically.

Sezary is probably the most common aggressive CTCL you'll likely see; you may see some other rare ones like gamma delta lymphoma, which is invariably fatal. Other lymphomas with cytotoxic features (necrotic eschars) have a bad prognosis (will die of sepsis because can't survive the tissue breakdown—can basically look like SJS patients within a few months).

The most common cutaneous B-cell lymphomas you'll probably see are primary cutaneous marginal zone or follicular center lymphomas (both pretty indolent; usually can make one spot go away, then another pops up, but doesn't kill people).

For new patient, visits with biopsy-proven MF or concern for MF.

1. *Do full skin exam.*

   a. Need to look at groin + buttocks + underarms; often involves these areas (non-sun-exposed areas). But some still get lesions on head/neck (sometimes even the only place or the most severe place).

   b. Folliculotropism (fine milial-like/pebbly textural change) = marker of follicular involvement/more aggressive disease; can look like acne/rosacea if on face.

   c. Tumoral MF can often present as an ulcer; can look like PG or vascular ulcer.

d. A lot of immune dysregulation/shifts in MF skin, get a lot of staph secondary infections, get bacteremic very easily; can use bleach baths and PO antibiotics if needed.

e. Erythrodermic patients can develop diffuse furunculosis.

2. *Do good lymph node exam.* Lymphadenopathy doesn't necessarily mean involvement—could be reactive—but if they do have lymphadenopathy, that might get them an excisional lymph node biopsy (preferred over fine needle aspiration) to appreciate the architecture (see if preserved) and immunohistochemistry (see if dermatopathic or if involves lymph node or not).

a. If LAD, a PET CT is probably best thing to get. (See if lymph nodes are hypermetabolic or not; usually relatively low [only light up a little bit] if dermatopathic [standardized uptake value, SUV, is usually <3]. If true, lymphoma involving lymph nodes SUV usually like 4–7 [higher metabolic uptake of glucose].)

b. Usually onc orders the PET CT; PET CT better than plain CT and will probably end up needing the PET anyway (so better to avoid radiation ×2 and just wait).

c. Radiologists usually hedge ("with clinical correlation could be a marker for lymphoma," etc.), unless the SUV is super high ("very concerning for malignant process"). Usually, if <3, onc is "meh"; if diffuse, small enlargement 2–2.5 that's usually dermatopathic LAD. So usually don't do excisional biopsy; just treat and repeat the PET CT later. If you PET CT every erythrodermic patient, they will almost always have hypermetabolic nodes, regardless of erythroderma etiology. If you have 1–2 nodes, then it's more concerning, and obviously if they're more highly metabolic and/or one huge lymph node.

3. *Basic labs.*

a. LDH (poor man's marker of cancer burden; onc likes it, so good if co-managing with them [patients with severe or widespread disease tend to have high LDHs vs. lower disease-burden patients typically having LDH WNL]).

b. TSH, free thyroxine, lipid profile (if think bexarotene possible, need to monitor while on and have baseline labs).

c. Flow cytometry (screens for peripheral involvement and gives a Sezary cell count).

   i. Dogma is that if limited skin involvement, no reason to get flow on the blood (in other words, people believe patients should be erythrodermic if they have Sezary, but this is not always true; patients can have 10% patch and have Sezary >1000).

   ii. If 10% BSA of patch, probably reasonable to check flow (but don't check everyone, because it's not an inexpensive test).

   iii. If high Sezary count, life expectancy is in danger; send to onc—they'll start them on hard-hitter chemo.

   iv. The silver lining (of potentially overdoing work-ups) is that these patients are the best ones to transplant if you can get their Sezary count down while they still have limited skin disease (they don't have the skin breakdown/infection risk of someone who's erythrodermic or has diffuse tumoral disease [which, in the context of the level of immunosuppression you have to do to transplant somebody, is of course highly risky]). So best to transplant quickly—gives them the highest chance of survival long term because they're in the best health state they'll be in.

    v. *FYI*: All of us have Sezary cells (normal range <270); sometimes patients have MF with Sezary count around 500 (which doesn't meet criteria for Sezary [>1000]), so it's hard to know if transforming into Sezary or if they just have increase in Sezary cells because they have a lymphoma. If anything abnormal, probably good to refer to onc.

       – Gray zone Sezary counts—possible patient is an outlier vs. related to cell turnover/degree of inflammation vs. they are evolving to Sezary; thus, these are patients you follow closely with low threshold to recheck. Usually, they monitor disease activity with Sezary counts via flow, anyway.

    vi. *FYI*: The CD4:CD8 ratios are just eyeballed by pathologists (the stained slides), not formally counted (albeit they are good at estimating).

    vii. If you have a strong mixture of B-cells and a lot of T-cells, argues against CTCL; start thinking of pseudolymphoma, reactive lymphoid hyperplasia, and so on.

       – Histology for pseudolymphoma usually unhelpful; will say something like "favor benign infiltrate, follow for lymphoma," even though it's benign reactive lesion and can do ILK; similar thing if doing a lymph node biopsy in AD patient—will say "dermatopathic LAD, follow for lymphoma." Generally, the cells in the blood will be in the skin biopsy too.

d. Biopsy: do broad-scoop shave (not a punch) because need a lot of epidermis to diagnose MF.

    i. Can do T-cell receptor (TCR) gene rearrangements studies in addition to IHC to look for clonality.

       – TCR gene rearrangement—tells you if clonal population or not (vs. peripheral flow telling you what clonal population looks like).

          – *FYI*: It's not black/white (can get clonality in reactive conditions, such as chronic inflammatory disorders; can also have MF and have polyclonality).

          – Clonality can be requested by clinical team or path team; usually, clinical teams don't request clonality, because if you get a good shave and get IHC, that's usually enough, but if path team is on fence, then sometimes they add TCR gene rearrangement studies to look for clonality. If path comes back as sponge derm but you're highly clinically concern for CTCL, can ask them to go back and do clonality studies.

- IHC—looking at markers on cells to see whether normal or not; usually check like 5–6 of these. As one develops CTCL, often lose normal markers (such as CD5/CD7 in MF); CD30 not in present in normal T-cells but can have gain of expression—important for treatment options.

- Epidermotropism = how much the cancer cells stick to epidermis; somewhat oddly, boards questions emphasize that plaque stage has most epidermotropism (even though patch is least likely to spread to lymph nodes, etc.).

Non-Hodgkin's (T-cell and B-cell) lymphomas are service-connected malignancies at VA (Vietnam, Agent Orange) (but *FYI*: MF and CTCL as diagnosis codes are not).

Usually, PET CT is covered if they have a diagnosis of lymphoma; but if they're in gray zone and they have LAD, will be hard to get PET CT covered by insurance. Same with meds (if clinically looks like MF and not responding to PO agents and want interferon or gemcitabine, hard to get approval for those drugs without a path diagnosis of lymphoma).

MANAGEMENT

Stem cell transplant (SCT) only way to potentially cure MF, though have high incidence of relapse after SCT; management usually focused on symptom control and preventing progression (keep localized, flat, not itchy). Sometimes patients are really itchy, even after cancer improves.

Topicals (patch/plaque):

TCSs, topical bexarotene (very expensive, $30k monthly) or PO bexarotene, phototherapy, local radiation to hot spots on skin, imiquimod, topical mechlorethamine (very expensive, $2–3k monthly). If very widespread (diffuse patch/plaque), can do both phototherapy and low-dose MTX in beginning to sort of boost things for a few months, and if that gets things quiet, can try to peel them off one (whichever one they like less). *FYI*: Phototherapy only makes them slightly more tan (not insanely darker, which some patients may worry about).

PO options (tumor stage):

MTX, pralatrexate, interferon (Pegasys is weekly subQ injection of interferon alpha), total electron beam therapy (rad onc), extracorporeal photopheresis (especially if some degree of blood involvement; also used post-transplant as a GVHD treatment modality), vorinostat, pembrolizumab (usually onc manages), brentuximab, mogamulizumab (especially for advanced stages), gemcitabine (soft chemo; good if they can't tolerate more traditional chemo); can do combos, but not much data on adjunctive phototherapy—be careful combining UVB/PUVA with bigger-gun chemos. Unclear whether light therapy on newer systemics is safe (like mogamulizumab, for instance).

Historically, CTCL patients would get decent doses of radiation, but now standard of care much lower (sometimes 6 gray, in comparison to breast cancer, which is 60 gray)—great because can do it more than once. One of the best parts is, can radiate acral skin, can't do it over and over again, but if they have refractory acral skin involvement (fissuring, pain, can't walk well, or use hands), which is common, can do low-dose radiation and it melts it away; sometimes people will do same to face/scalp.

For phototherapy, consensus is to use NBUVB in people who have higher risk for skin cancer (narrow band, by definition, is supposed to be the rays that don't cause skin cancer to the same degree as UVB in general). PUVA for less risk of skin cancer or more aggressive CTCL.

For PUVA, can soak in bath of psoralen, apply topically, or take PO (most common is orally). Take 1–2 hours before UVA exposure. Biggest side effect is nausea. Weight-based dosing. Can do PUVA 2–3x weekly; most just do QW.

Excimer laser (handheld UVB) and PDT have also been reported.

For CBCLs, excision not really preferred because they'll just keep getting them (so would basically just be a Band-Aid); probably better to do IL rituximab—relatively noninvasive, melts away, no scar.

CAR-T is the hot new thing. Everyone wants to try it for everything (like immunotherapy), but issue is, you're modifying the cells to recognize abnormal markers, so if you have abnormal T-cells, hard to use CAR-T for a T-cell process. But they're looking at CAR-T for CD30 lymphoproliferative disorders because they have a distinct enough IHC profile/genotype that may be successful for that; immunotherapies haven't shown success yet for CTCL.

Late-stage CTCL—no great options.

2.4.6 Pediatric Dermatology

Most peds-specific content for boards is knowing genoderms (not covered in this book).

Focus here is mostly on miscellaneous practical tips (many conditions you'll see in kids are covered in other sections, so this is pretty brief).

1. LN2 vs. cantharidin. Usually LN2 only if 12+ years old; consider trying cantharidin on just one lesion first (causes scars, so wouldn't go too crazy with it, especially the first time).

2. If need to biopsy, mostly read the room/patient's maturity, but some things to consider:

    a. Make sure the parents know it's not just a skin "scraping" and that you'll be creating a wound with a blade that will leave a scar.

    b. Can do with patient sitting in parent's lap (if they're really young). Try to pick a lesion out of sight (not only for cosmesis, but also so they can't see the needle [though obviously should still verbalize to them what you're doing and when]).

    c. Can have nurses set up tray outside room (and bring it in the room still covered with a chuck or something).

    d. Can communicate with patient's caregiver via writing (saying need a biopsy) to get them to sign consent form.

    e. Can apply EMLA for 30 minutes under occlusion before, but sometimes better to just get it over with.

3. Ointments and creams more favorable than oils for kids (which are messy and can cause acne-like rash); also usually easier for them to apply in AM.

4. Discussing removal of benign lesions: no medical reason to remove, so better to wait until kid is old enough to make own decisions; plus, if old enough to make own decisions, can likely be removed with local.

5. If procedure requires one round of conscious sedation, needs to be 2 years old to have same risk of adult undergoing conscious sedation; if multiple stages, then needs to be 3 years old for it to be just as safe as it would be for an adult from anesthesia standpoint (risk related to learning disabilities, etc.).

6. Be mindful of giving sedating meds (such as hydroxyzine [Atarax])—don't want them to be sleepy during school and have it affect their academic/intellectual development.

7. If a kid comes in with parvovirus (slapped cheeks), having them stay home is not enough, because there are likely still several carriers (who don't yet have the rash) who can give it to people at risk of complications (such as pregnant women and people who have shorter-than-normal RBC lifespans [risk for aplastic RBC crisis, which can be fatal to a fetus, dangerous to sickle cell or someone with chronic hemolytic anemia, etc., because they count on their RBC production to support their hematocrit]). *FYI*: Every child who gets parvovirus has their bone marrow shut down production for ~1 month (which is fine if they're normal and have an RBC lifespan of 120 days).

   a. You should protect HIPAA by calling the principal, saying you have a student (no name) who has fifth disease, and that you understand the teacher is pregnant so she needs to see OB-GYN, get her parvovirus titers drawn, and because other kids might be shedding in the classroom and she's at risk for miscarriage, she needs to be out of the classroom until the titer comes back.

   b. Remember, adults get arthritis, purpuric gloves and socks, and miscarriages if pregnant.

8. Give kids enough meds if they split time between households (may not need to ask specifically if the parents are divorced, but can ask if the kids routinely spend time elsewhere or something, like a day care, etc.).

3 Inpatient (Calls/Consults)

3.1 GENERAL PRINCIPLES

■ Usually, the topicals they're using are at bedside—look at what they're using. Sometimes it'll be a tube of 1% hydrocortisone for something like erythrodermic psoriasis! It's the nurse's responsibility because it's a medication, so make sure they're applying it.

■ If cancer patient, know the type of cancer they have. Are they on chemo? What stage (induction, consolidation, salvage)? What agents? What antimicrobials? Common cause of drug rashes; see when they were started. Febrile? Neutropenic? Low platelets? What lines? History of skin disease?

■ For patients with complicated immune statuses (such as cancer patients, chemo patients, etc.), realize we are trained to recognize conditions as they occur in normal immune systems (so when patient's immune system is not normal, there can be a lot of clinical variability, and our recognition skills are less reliable/trustworthy, so very low threshold to biopsy anything).

• Also keep in mind they often also have other issues, so be explicit about risks/benefits discussion (low platelets, bleeding, neutropenia, infection risk).

– Also prepare yourself for these issues; if they have 3 platelets, make sure you have Drysol and pressure dressing materials in the bag.

■ Look at IV sites, port sites—highest-risk places for infection in cancer patients.

■ Should pretty much always look in the mouth for all inpatient evals.

■ If solitary lesion, do one punch and bisect with a razor (like the stuff you use for shave biopsy) to send one for H&E and one for tissue culture.

• For tissue culture, like doing a regular punch, but **FYI**: Don't put them in regular H&E containers; you should get a container without liquid (for instance, a urine collection cup), place a thin layer of gauze inside, squirt sterile saline and/or lidocaine on the gauze so that it's damp, and then put the tissue culture sample in that.

• Issue is, yield for tissue culture is low (uncommon for them to speciate and are slow to result), so helpful to get periodic acid–Schiff (PAS) on H&E.

■ Any vesicles, do a Tzanck; herpes good to have on essentially any ddx for inpatients. Mucosal lesions are common in immunosuppressed patients, who can also get chronic ulcerative herpes (thread-like pearly border, scalloped at edge).

■ Probably better to avoid doing outpatient stuff (like biopsying non-urgent skin cancers, removing cysts, etc.) when patients are admitted (liability if can't get hold of them after discharge; sometimes patients will disappear, so just get them in as close outpatient follow-up).

■ If the primary reason for admission is a derm issue, then of course follow more closely/assume more responsibility for discharge planning.

- Rush biopsy usually available next business day—let primary team know; problem is, if overnight or weekend, then there likely isn't a histotechnician on-site to stain the tissue (can usually get them if an emergency but probably have to pay them overtime and also need pathologist to come in and read it—so probably only do if it's weird-looking SJS or if patient is super sick [not just a regular drug reaction, etc.]).

- Make sure bag is actually stocked with everything you need (and more) before leaving the room. The most commonly used things are usually in there, but other things to think about: consent forms, sterile saline, lidocaine, Drysol, pressure dressing materials.

3.2 DIFFERENTIAL DIAGNOSIS BASED ON "CALL"
3.2.1 "Concern for SJS"
3.2.1.1 Stevens–Johnson Syndrome (SJS)/Toxic Epidermal Necrolysis (TEN)

1. *Figuring out if they have it.*

   a. Need drug culprit (primary teams sometimes don't even have this!).

      i. Ask about OTCs, NSAIDs, etc.

      ii. HIV has 1000× risk.

   b. Usually if with flu-like prodrome, almost always have mucosal involvement.

   c. Rash **starts as painful skin** due to keratinocyte death (if itchy, likely not SJS), few targetoid lesions, mucositis, conjunctival erythema.

      i. If caught this early and treated, can avoid even denuding.

   d. Blisters on macules are characteristic (blisters usually by day 3); worse days are 3–6.

      i. Classically **face, chest, back, shoulders** look terrible; hands/feet look fine—may have scattered lesions but usually don't coalesce.

      ii. Legs are oftentimes spared (except plantar skin).

      iii. Pretty dusky; sometimes can look targetoid.

   e. Usually **turns corner by day 7 of rash**; can sometimes even be re-epithelized in 2 weeks or less (can be a few days if you catch it extremely early).

   f. If involves mouth, may involve throat (pharynx)—clues: gagging, spitting up vs. actual swallowing.

   g. Nikolsky—basically telling how necrotic the skin is; if lightly rubs skin and it basically falls off, then (+).

      i. The ED/primary teams seem to love to mention this but is perhaps more useful for dictating management rather than diagnosing (letting you know if they're actively sloughing/necrosing or not).

   h. Need to biopsy; should get a DIF, too, to rule out LABD.

2. *Management recs.*

   a. Overall impression.

      i. If SJS/TEN been at OSH for too long and not having blistering anymore, sometimes right call is to do nothing (even though it's hard to do for transfers).

      ii. If not actively inflamed and skin doesn't hurt anymore, trunk likely already done, so don't need to unwrap if they're in burn unit dressings; just look at arms/legs, which usually aren't wrapped. If getting new targetoid lesions on arms/legs, could treat; if not, then just supportive care (keep clean, make sure not to aspirate, etc.).

   b. Role of immunosuppressives.

      i. **Benefit** of immunosuppressive management **depends on stage of disease**—usually better if early in disease (**if still rashy, then probably good to give**, but if they've been sitting around at OSH for a week and present 95% sloughed, then risks/benefits of immunosuppression likely not favorable; just wrap them and let them marinate in non-stick dressings, prevent infection).

         – Main players:

            – Etanercept 50 mg subQ 2–3 days apart, sometimes third dose (especially in EM major). Safe, works well, but hard to access.

               – Need within first 48 hours of symptom onset (so probably only if your hospital has on inpatient formulary/easy access).

            – If can't do etanercept, can try CsA 5 mg/kg for 4–6 days, no taper (works well, affordable, but more toxic—not great if has HTN/kidney issues or if concerned for infection).

            – IV steroids (pulse high dose 250 or 500 mg or even 1 g).

               – For rescue therapy: IV methylprednisolone 1 g over 30–60 minutes (~1,300 pred) for 1–5 days (can be tough to tolerate for patients).

            – IVIG—not good as monotherapy.

               – Usually 2–4 g/kg/day for 3–4 days.

               – Risk vascular sludging, pulmonary embolism, etc.

            – Expediting re-epithelialization is key because won't get superinfections or need pain meds -> aspirate -> PNA; so the morbidity is primarily from these things.

      ii. **If past the blistering phase, then basically manage as a burn patient.** Derm management matters most in early phases because therapy limits the blisters that form.

      iii. If post-erythema desquamating, then Fas-Fas-L not even happening; so more drugs is probably not better. When in burn phase, don't let scar.

3. *Role of antibiotic prophylaxis.*

   a. Prophylactic antibiotics are controversial and individual; usually, they spike a fever (systemic response, not usually local; usually bacteremia).

   b. If they present early and get appropriate management, usually won't give prophylactic antibiotics.

   c. If they come transferred and already on vanc/Zosyn, can consider continuing if very high BSA.

   d. If lower BSA, then don't have to give prophylaxis.

4. *Other considerations/involving other teams.*

   a. Important to document BSA, look at all mucosal sites.

   b. Most widely used criteria: SCORTEN—seems to overestimate mortality if at a facility with inpatient dermatology. Age also not considered, and older patients tend to do worse.

   c. Mouth mucosa takes long time to heal from SJS—like, 2–3 weeks; might not respond to CsA in first few days.

   d. Many times will need Dobhoff tube because they struggle to eat.

   e. Will see a lot of oral candidiasis -> probably PO fluconazole, nystatin swish/spit, and magic mouthwash usually not enough.

   f. Ophtho and urology involvement (only if they have symptoms); if female, then gyn instead of urology (many times will need foley, so probably better for uro/gyn to do it).

   g. Keep room warm.

   h. Immunotherapy-induced SJS/TEN behaves different. Sometimes heal faster; sometimes inflammation is turned off and doesn't respond to anything. Unclear what to do with these; often not impressive morbilliform for multiple weeks (and this is an exception—typically, morbilliform rashes don't turn to SJS). Blistering can go on and on. Onc literature states steroids are the choice, but really unclear what to do.

3.2.1.2 *Erythema Multiforme (EM) Major*

1. *Figure out if they have it.*

   a. Associated with infections (HSV, mycoplasma) >> drugs (vs. SJS).

   b. EM major **much more prolonged than SJS** and still worsening by day 7 (blisters usually by day 7–8); whole process 10–14 days.

      i. Hands/feet more involved; trunk not as confluent as in SJS.

   c. Juicy lesions that are **itchy before painful.**

      i. Usually, **juicy papules with blisters on top = EM** (vs. **flat macular erythema with dark purpuric areas = SJS**).

         – Papular not because of blisters; the actual rash is papular (run hands over it).

– EM blisters don't coalesce as much, but mucositis can be bad and take long to heal; can have a lot of rash with less blistering (but blistering may get worse than in SJS).

d. If you can feel the rim = a lot of inflammation (thus, EM and NOT SJS because no inflammation in SJS—it's just full thickness necrosis).

e. *FYI*: Sometimes outside facilities may say "biopsy-proven SJS."

f. **Hands/feet/face look bad**, but **trunk** doesn't **look that bad** (might have some stuff going on, but not as confluent).

g. The **mucositis is indistinguishable, might even be worse in EM** and take longer to heal.

2. *Work-up/management recs.*

a. Etanercept—psoriasis dose—sometimes ×3 doses (48–72 hours apart); sometimes steroids.

b. Respiratory virus panel, HSV, swab HSV, maybe mycoplasma; ask about vaccines.

c. See Chapter 2 if recurrent EM and not due to HSV and can't find trigger despite thorough ROS; sometimes put on low-dose MTX/MMF or intermittent prednisone/CsA PRN for flares. May be some virus that can't be tested for or something.

3.2.1.3 RIME (Reactive Infectious Mucocutaneous Eruption)

1. Tends to affect young patients; can almost look like SJS, but only mucous membranes (limited skin involvement, if any).

a. Vesicles/bullae and erosions/ulcers commonly.

b. Classically lips, sometimes buccal mucosa and oropharynx.

c. Can have similar symptoms; if involves mouth, may involve throat (pharynx)—clues: gagging, spitting up vs. actual swallowing.

2. Usually mycoplasma, but can be due to reaction to other viruses (FluB, parainfluenza 2, rhinovirus, enterovirus, adenovirus, chlamydia pneumoniae, COVID), and some we can't test for (and that if others caught that virus, they wouldn't have the same response).

a. Prodrome (~1 week prior): cough, fever, malaise.

3. Don't usually biopsy; histology hard to distinguish RIME vs. EM vs. SJS/TEN, anyway (but can get a DIF if think might be vesiculobullous).

4. Generally good prognosis (3% mortality, mostly if significant respiratory complications).

5. Steroids benefit is debatable; probably more helpful if instituted early on.

a. Can do prednisone (or prednisone equivalent) 1 mg/kg per day, for 3–5 days (mainly to arrest process, so don't really need to taper).

   i. Can add CsA (3–5 mg/kg QD split into BID dosing) if having an inadequate response to steroid monotherapy.

b. Mucositis mouthwash if mouth pain.

c. If have wounds, dressings (wrap Xeroform in SSD cream, change BID); ensure enough protein (maybe protein boost supplements).

3.2.1.4 Generalized Bullous Fixed Drug Eruption

1. Might be the best SJS/TEN mimicker (in fact, the original describer of SJS/TEN accidentally included a couple of cases of generalized FDE in their original report).

2. Still sick; LOS and mortality rates only slightly less than SJS/TEN.

3. Large **dusky** lesions with generalized bullae + erosions **separated by large areas of normal** skin.

   a. Very **short timeline** after drug **exposure**—rash onset can be minutes to 1–3 days ([vs. **SJS 1–3 weeks** for most part]).

   b. Because resident memory T-cells in skin, activated by drug (different pathogenesis from SJS/TEN).

4. **Tend to not have fevers; mucosal involvement less common and, when occurs, is usually not extensive.**

5. SJS/TEN more central; **FDE more in flank/folds.**

6. Rash + blistering **onsets fast, heals slow** (maybe because denudes so much or because TNFs don't work as well as they do in SJS/TEN).

7. For some reason, super rare in kids (whereas EM quite common in kids).

   a. Might not necessarily need to be given the drug before, but possible need multiple hits (from other drugs/viruses, etc.) that prime one to generalized bullous FDE.

3.2.1.5 LABD (Linear IgA Bullous Dermatosis)

1. Bad annular rash with blistering (central clearing with edematous ring), no mucositis, vs. SJS, which has central purpura (annular and targetoid are not same).

   a. Bad annular rash: ddx AGEP that hasn't formed pustules yet, Rowell syndrome (EM major in setting of CTD), bad SCLE that hasn't gotten scaly yet, and LABD.

2. Long lead-up: ~9 days of rash before start to blister.

3. Could be a two-hit thing: get a virus, then get an antibiotics; or start a drug, then get a vaccine; etc.

   a. Could get rash first at site of vaccine.

   b. Less mucosal involvement in drug-induced cases.

4. Probably biggest takeaway: can mimic SJS; thus, **always get DIF when biopsying for SJS.**

3.2.2 "Concern for DRESS"

3.2.2.1 Drug Reaction with Eosinophilia and Systemic Symptoms (DRESS)/Drug-Induced Hypersensitivity Syndrome (DIHS)

1. *Figuring out if they have it.*

    a. Conventionally 2–6 weeks after exposure, but timing is variable; can be several months or even years.

       i. Can be after dose escalation (not necessarily new drug).

       ii. Common med culprits: same as SJS, anti-epileptic drugs, antibiotics, allopurinol.

       iii. Sometimes triggered by viral infection.

    b. No hallmark cutaneous eruption, but classic things: diffuse lymphadenopathy (usually head/neck), swelling of face + helices of ears, CBC issues (high or low; obviously don't need peripheral eosinophilia [classic example of why it's confusing to have pathologic terms in the clinical designation]), almost invariably fever, usually some sort of organ involvement (kidney/liver/aseptic meningitis/ARDS-type picture).

    c. LFTs most common lab abnormality; fulminant liver failure leading cause of death.

    d. Facial edema poor prognostic factor.

    e. RegiSCAR criteria (don't biopsy; not helpful [at best 0 points]).

2. *Management recs.*

    a. Get primary team to trend CBCs with diff, LFTs (by default, check Q 1 week, but get them to get with diff and CMP QD).

    b. Can check viral serologies: HHV6, CMV, EBV.

       i. May impact management if cause was viral vs. a med (that might want/need to be continued).

    c. Need thyroid function tests at follow-up to assess for hypothyroidism (risk long-term thyroid dysfunction).

    d. Patients may also mention their skin is more sensitive/easily irritated/flushes randomly after recovering—probably because the dramatic inflammation damages blood vessels and they become more easily dilated.

    e. IV steroids.

       i. Oftentimes, need second agent in addition to steroids (IVIG or CsA or rituximab or MMF); usually need longer taper sometimes over several months (because higher risk of reactivation) vs. SJS, where they usually only need a few days.

3.2.2.2 Exanthematous Drug Reaction

1. Similar to viral exanthem but has more of a tendency to be itchy; maculo-papular erythema.

2. Usually dermal-based lesions (can range from areas that look like morbil-liform erythemas to urticarial lesions, to lesions that are evolving toward urticarial lesions).

3. Usually 1–2 weeks after exposure (sooner if re-exposure).

4. DRESS can also start as mild macular erythema; thus, ask to trend CMP, CBC with diff every few days.

5. Usually, AGEP also starts as macular erythema or looks like morbilliform drug, so must RECHECK on them to see if develop pustules.

6. Sites of pressure are accentuated in exanthematous reactions (don't be fooled by duskiness/purpura).

7. TAC BID PRN, can do wet wraps, antihistamines, +/– systemic steroids if not fevering from illness.

8. If patients are bedbound for chronic issues, chucks at hospital can be occlu-sive, so also consider heat/sweat rash (miliaria), if only on back.

   a. *For miliaria*:

      i. SSD (risk for infection).

      ii. Calamine lotion can be drying, FYI.

      iii. Mild TCSs are fine if itchy.

      iv. Usually resolves in couple of days.

3.2.2.3 General Checklist for Drug Reactions

1. Timeline.

2. Culprit?

   a. Allopurinol, TMP-SMX, carbamazepine, phenytoin, phenobarbitals, aminopenicillins, cephalosporins, quinolones, vancomycin, abacavir.

   b. Don't forget OTCs (NSAIDs, etc.).

   c. Ask about herbal medications and complementary alternative treatments.

   d. Consider inpatient exposures (contrast dye, dialysates, etc.).

3. Previous med allergies?

4. Recent URI symptoms?

5. Asian (Chinese, Thai)?

6. Derm history? History of lupus/autoimmune conditions?

7. Past medical history? History of cancers?

8. Family history?

9. Mucosal (eyes, mouth, genitals)?

10. Fever?

11. Diarrhea, nausea, vomiting?

If truly a SCAR, management:

1. Stop culprit med; calculate SCORTEN (SJS) or RegiSCAR (DRESS).

2. May need ICU/burn unit (vitals Q 4 hours for first 2–3 days). Keep room hot; contact isolation.

3. IVF (NS) in view of increased TEWL.

4. Decolonize nares; oral + genital mucosa TID with mupirocin.

5. Make sure no yeast in mouth—can inhibit healing.

6. SSD to all eroded skin (can wrap Xeroform gauze in SSD and place on patient rather than rubbing SSD on skin, which will hurt), or burn shirts/rubber burn sheets if in burn unit.

7. Aquaphor or similar healing ointment for lips/nares, etc.

8. Consult ophtho + urology (if symptomatic, need foley, etc.).

9. Consider liquid/pureed diet to mitigate esophageal trauma (especially if gagging/spitting more than swallowing, etc., suggesting esophageal involvement).

10. Nutritional replacement key; needs protein to re-epithelialize (can recommend BOOST protein shakes).

11. Consider stool softener to mitigate anal mucosal trauma.

12. Depending on stage of process, systemic immunosuppressives may be rational (if still in inflammatory phase).

    a. TNFs ×1 dose if can get within 1–2 days of rash onset.

    b. Consider IVIG if early in process, but $$$$; doesn't help if past the blistering phase.

    c. CsA 5 mg/kg in BID dosing, if still worsening after systemic steroids and need additional affordable/accessible fast-acting agent (check BP and Cr; can't do if HTN or if kidney issues).

    d. Likely will only use CsA to arrest process, for ~5 days, so probably don't need to monitor Mg (though, of course, needs if on chronically), and probably doesn't need a taper.

13. Obviously, pain control, nutrition, non-stick dressings, IVF.

FYI: Most drug eruptions are not violaceous and usually are itchy.

3.2.3 "Concern for Bullous Pemphigoid"
3.2.3.1 Bullous Pemphigoid

1. Urticarial base, tense blisters, usually generalized.

2. Almost invariably itchy.

3. Sometimes recent vaccine (or other immune stimulation).

4. Immunotherapy-induced BP more unpredictable.

5. See BP Chapter 2.

3.2.3.2 Edema Bullae

1. Basically acute on chronic edema; sterile blisters.

2. Tense bullae, no urticarial base, surrounded by edema.

3. Consider patient population (CHF, hypoalbuminemia, cirrhosis, DVT, on calcium channel blockers, or other water-retaining meds).

4. Management: address underlying etiology (diuresis perhaps), compression; can drain the blisters for comfort (take a syringe and suck out the fluid/ push the fluid out of the hole made with the syringe onto a gauze pad or something, then leave the blister roof).

5. Will get worse with systemic steroids (more fluid).

3.2.3.3 Coma Bullae

1. From pressure/friction/local hypoxia (lesions are at site of pressure).

2. History? Did they have loss of consciousness? Neuro disease? Prolonged immobilization? (Don't have to be comatose to get them—people also call them neurogenic blisters).

3. Management: Mepilex AG or Xeroform (change daily) or SSD QD, posture changes.

4. Spontaneously resolves in 1–2 weeks.

3.2.3.4 Friction Blisters

1. From repetitive rubbing (such as walking long distances or something).

2. Management: Mepilex AG or Xeroform (change daily) or SSD QD, posture changes.

3.2.3.5 Post-Burn/Graft Blisters

1. Tense, only involve injured skin.

2. Delayed; develop weeks to months after injury (second-degree burns, STSG donor sites, etc.).

3. Management essentially the same as earlier; dressings +/− drain sterilely.

3.2.3.6 IV Infiltration vs. Extravasation

1. Basically when the IV med leaks into tissue outside vein.

2. If ever suspect this, should always clarify what was going through IV.

   a. Infiltration = non-irritating (such as LR, etc.).

      i. Management similar edema bullae; dressings, compression +/− drain sterilely.

b. Extravasation = irritating (such as Levophed, etc.).

   i. Obviously, discontinue the infusion, aspirate any remaining fluid in catheter, irrigate with saline, and elevate the area. Some report that phentolamine injections into the area may help (basically opposes vasopressor action via vasodilation); also reports of subQ terbutaline and nitroglycerin ointment (covering entire affected area).

3.2.3.7 LABD

1. Recent vancomycin?

2. Usually otherwise well-appearing.

3. See LABD in "Concern for SJS" Section 3.2.1 (also LABD in Chapter 2).

   a. Biopsy.

      i. *H&E*—broadly shave entire new vesicle/blister.

      ii. *DIF*—4 mm punch (or shave), perilesionally if there is a blister (not the blister where the immune reactants are chewed up), or lesionally if there is no blister.

      iii. *IIF*—BP (salt split skin), PV (monkey esophagus), paraneoplastic pemphigus (rat bladder).

      iv. *ELISA*—asking if antibodies are in blood; BP (BPAG2, kDa 180), PV (Dsg3, kDa 130), paraneoplastic pemphigus (BPAG2, kDa 180, and BPAG1, kDa 230), LABD (BPAG2, kDa 180, and BPAG1, kDa 230), pemphigus foliaceous (Dsg 1, kDA 160, and Dsg 3).

3.2.4 "Concern for Vasculitis"

3.2.4.1 Vasculitis

1. Get good social history, review of systems, maybe family history; figure out why LCV, and do they have IgA? The two main things to suss out (because IgA, particularly in adults, can have a much more fulminant course [particularly renal progression] than regular LCV).

2. Main categories (infectious, autoimmune, paraneoplastic, drug-induced, idiopathic).

   a. Not everyone gets the full work-up; should help narrow the work-up for the primary team (not everyone needs ANCAs and dsDNAs, etc.). For example, if think 2/2 bacterial infection, can go down that route vs. autoimmune route.

   b. Biopsy lesionally for DIF (not like bullous disorders).

   c. Levamisole vasculitis—impressive eruption; loves the face, commonly nose and ear.

      i. Not everyone who gets exposed to levamisole gets this (it's a common contaminant in majority of cocaine); only certain patients have a predilection to get it. They can also get positive ANCAs, or MPO, or high positive ANA.

      ii. Hard to test for levamisole, and cocaine washes out of UDS after 2 days.

3. Mimickers to consider: hemorrhagic bullae from heparin; urticarial vasculitis can be in setting of SLE; septic emboli, Degos, Langerhans cell histiocytosis, pressure-dependent accentuation of changes in exanthematous reactions (for example, if using crutches, their hands may look purpuric/dusky); pressure-related changes in patients with low platelets (traumatic purpura).

4. See vasculitis in Chapter 2.

3.2.4.2 Vasculopathy

1. Usually retiform purpura or livedo reticularis (sometimes nodules, ulcers, etc.).

2. Early vasculopathy = fixed purpura with surrounding hyperemia—basically penumbra of skin (at risk but salvageable).

3. Levamisole, calciphylaxis, autoimmune—all different patient populations, so take broad history.

4. Unusual in peds, but if it is a kid, then usually infectious (such as *Pseudomonas* bacteremia, etc.)

5. *Ddx*:

   a. Livedo reticularis (*FYI*: Is a clinical presentation [not an actual disease entity, unless it's idiopathic, which is a diagnosis of exclusion]).

      i. Common observation; usually people hone in on whether it comes/goes with cold (onsets in cold, goes away when warms back up).

      ii. However, what really matters is whether it's blanching vs. necrotizing.

         – If blanching, will probably never find an underlying reason, likely just that their connecting vessels are sensitive and the neurovascular functioning is just slightly off.

         – If necrotizing, probably has an underlying reason, possibly serious.

      iii. Other entities can present with LR: erythema marginatum, Still's, parvovirus.

   b. Retiform purpura (also a clinical finding, not a stand-alone entity).

      i. Usually on legs, but not always.

      ii. Ddx includes (more details on each follow):

         – Embolic (cholesterol embolus, septic embolus, etc.—usually all acral).

         – Thrombotic (protein C, protein S, levamisole toxicity, warfarin skin necrosis [soft], HIT [soft], calciphylaxis [hard], APLS, purpura fulminans [basically an acquired protein C/S deficiency—can come from strep, meningococcemia, variety of septic causes]).

         – Vasculitic (arteriolar side [not post-capillary venule side], includes PAN, ANCA-vasculitides, rheumatoid vasculitis, septic vasculitis, drug-induced [propylthiouracil, montelukast, etc.]).

- If think it's one of these, the occluded/involved vessel may be in an infarcted stellate purpuric area or a pale area (starved of blood), so need to biopsy both. Some of the red is just reactive hyperemia (shunting away from the blockade).

c. Purpura fulminans (*FYI*: It is a reaction pattern [not a stand-alone disease entity], so best to specify in setting of something such as Pseudomonas bacteremia, placental abruption [OB GYN], a malignancy [elderly]).

  i. May have bullae and denuded necrotic skin.

  - Wound care—can do SSD and Xeroform gauze QD.

  - If the denuded skin sticks to the bedding, can apply a generous amount of Aquaphor to chuck pads and place those under the patient.

  ii. Infectious work-up.

  iii. If altered mental status, consider MRI brain +/− neuro consult (for LP to rule out CNS infection).

  iv. Can do biopsy—would show vasculopathy.

d. Warfarin necrosis (usually within 1 week of starting warfarin).

  i. *FYI*: Even if has supratherapeutic INR, consider heparin (since it's a paradoxical hypercoagulable condition).

  ii. For initial work-up, probably should do hypercoagulable work-up:

  - CBC with peripheral smear, platelet function tests, cryoglobulins, CMP (Cr, LFTs), antiphospholipids, UDS (cocaine)

  iii. Tends to happen in people who weren't bridged from heparin first.

  iv. Don't have to stop the warfarin; just treat through.

  - Reason is that if you stop the warfarin and have to restart it, then you're starting from square one again (protein C/S are your anticoagulants, and they drop before clotting factors drop—so you get a window period where anticoagulation hasn't happened yet and proteins C/S are low/dropped).

  v. Heparin-induced thrombocytopenia (HIT).

  - Must stop the heparin, have thrombosis, but also risk of life-threatening cerebral hemorrhage because of the anti-platelet antibodies.

  vi. Cholesterol emboli (usually hours to weeks after cath or after thrombolytic treatment [or even if on prolonged anticoagulation], often have peripheral eosinophilia).

  - Most commonly affects skin and kidneys.

  vii. Also consider signs of bacterial endocarditis (Janeway lesions [non-tender stellate infarction related to acute bacterial endocarditis], Osler nodes [tender pink papules related to subacute bacterial endocarditis], splinter hemorrhages—will need echo).

- *FYI*: Splinter hemorrhages not specific.

- Dry gangrene of acral skin is concerning for embolic phenomenon.

viii. Type I cryoglobulinemia (cryoglobulin can act as both an immune complex [get LCV lesions] and as hyperviscosity state [get vasculopathy findings, such as LR]).

ix. Livedoid vasculopathy (atrophie blanche).

3.2.4.3 Calciphylaxis

1. Commonly ESRD, but not always (can be non-uremic).

a. Other risk factors: obesity, hypoalbuminemia (perhaps poor nutrition), vitamin K antagonists (via decreasing proteins that inhibit vascular calcifications).

2. *Early*: spiderweb of erythema and small ulcer (all the red tissue is at risk for ulcerating).

3. *Late*: obviously harder to treat; tends to affect LEs, pannus, breast, but can occur elsewhere. Ulcers are dry because of the calcium—basically infarction without much inflammation. You clean/debride the black eschar, then it's an ulcer (albeit hard to heal).

4. Dx with ultrasound (preferable [less-invasive, can scan huge area]) or biopsy (difficult histologic diagnosis and painful).

a. Vessels affected are at dermal–subQ junction—highly relevant for diagnosing via either US or biopsy.

i. *US*: best imaging modality for the smallest-caliber vessels (where it's relevant for calciphylaxis).

- Daunting, but don't need to be an expert to find calcium; start with basics.

- *How it works*:

- Probe sends and receives waves; the image is based on the waves it receives (brighter [hyperechoic] = more waves caught from dense stuff because waves bounce back to probe easily).

- So you basically need to **catch the sound waves.**

- *Picking the probe*: **essentially will only ever need a high-frequency probe** in dermatology (high-frequency probes have clear image and go ~6 cm deep, which is roughly the length of your thumb).

- Only need to see from like 0.5 cm–2 cm in derm.

- *Orienting probe*: **probe marker lines up with screen marker** (always **on L side** [only on R side if looking at heart], thus probably don't need to worry about this).

- Use gel to limit air between probe and skin (air is bad, interferes with image because slows down the waves [in other words, want all waves to get to the target and back]); thus, **impossible to use too much gel.**

- **Set the probe on the edge of the lesion—good place to start scanning.**

- *Settings*: then just decrease the **depth to 1.5 cm** (the **pathology in calciphylaxis is at ~0.5 cm deep).**

   - The most common mistake is probably setting the wrong depth (looking at the wrong area).

   - If probe doesn't seem to be working, make sure it hasn't frozen.

   - *Advanced stuff*: can use colored Doppler to find vessels (*FYI*: "Blue away," and red means moving toward probe; don't make mistake of thinking it tells you if the vessel is an artery or vein).

b. *Biopsy*: deep process, thus large punch, perhaps telescope punch; similar to biopsying for panniculitides.

   i. If in outpatient setting, can do this; request Von Kossa (VK) (path probably adds it on, anyway).

      - Even with VK stains, high false-negative rate.

   ii. Some think trauma can incite development of calciphylaxis (which is why common to get on legs [not a fatty area]).

      - Almost like rock candy, where you have a supersaturated solution of phosphorus, and just takes a little nidus to ignite precipitation of rocks (calcium) into the vessel walls; thus, early detection critical.

2. *Management*:

a. Usually sodium thiosulfate (STS) (dosing depends on if PD [25 mg QW] vs. HD [25 mg TIW after HD]; can't do if on continuous renal replacement therapy).

   i. Although STS chelates calcium (trades Na for Ca), once calcium is in the vessel walls, hard to get it out, so trying to prevent additional calcification and allow the body to regenerate blood vessels and heal the tissue on its own (same concept with anticoagulation for pulmonary emboli when mainly just trying to prevent further clots).

      - Issue with STS is nausea; have to give after dialysis because IV infusion (so they already feel terrible and have to have it at their infusion center).

         - Pretty predictably causes metabolic acidosis, so monitor for this.

         - If calciphylaxis is progressing on PD, usually appropriate to recommend switching to HD (STS works much better on HD than PD).

         - Pentoxifylline 400 mg TID (or 400 mg QD if on PD, since it's renally cleared).

3. *Other things to know/look at*:

a. Labs.

   i. Calcium and phos product.

      – Serum phos levels more important than serum calcium levels (thus, tighter control of phos a better goal than controlling calcium levels).

   ii. Serum albumin or pre-albumin.

   iii. PTH levels (*FYI*: If ESRD on HD, then OK [from calciphylaxis standpoint] for it to be 2–3× ULN, but if 10× ULN, then probably at higher risk for calciphylaxis).

b. Look at their meds (if on warfarin, get them on alternative AC, etc.).

c. Figure out when they started dialysis; often will be within first few months of transitioning onto dialysis (probably the highest-risk period).

d. Sometimes they get if they transition from HD to PD, or if they become non-adherent to HD.

e. Some get after abdominal surgeries (like gastric bypass) or serious illness (some physiologic insult that precipitates calciphylaxis).

- *FYI*: Sometimes patients can have painful subQ nodules without overlying skin change, and the classic skin changes can declare themselves later, so still have suspicion if classic demographic.

- *FYI*: If you get a CT or XR (which are not high-resolution enough to see calcium in the smallest-caliber vessels [where it's relevant for calciphylaxis]), you will often see large vessel calcification (which most patients on HD will have and does not mean they have calciphylaxis).

3.2.5 "Rule Out Child Abuse"

- Some pages you can field by yourself (especially as the year goes on), but regardless of your comfort levels with this topic, I would probably get your attending's input for these types of issues.

- Even injuries that are seemingly medically minor (such as bruises, abrasions, etc.) are objectively significant, because they are essentially foreshadowing for more severe abuse in the future (sentinel injuries).

3.2.5.1 Suspicious Things

- Bruising in infants who cannot mobilize is rare (in contrast to mobile children [cruisers and walkers], who commonly experience accidental bruising).

- Most babies can sit up without support at ~6 months old.

- Can crawl on hands/knees (cruise) at ~8 months old.

- Can stand unassisted at ~11 months old.

- Can walk at ~12 months old.

  • *FYI*: >50% of children >1 year old have accidental bruising (usually front of body, such as face, head, shins).

- Of course, mobile children can be victims of abuse, though, too, and bruises in certain locations are suspicious (torso, ear, neck, frenula, auricular area, angle of jaw, cheek, eyelid, sclera).

- Patterns of bruising can also be telling (clustered, bilateral, involving multiple planes, and of course, if they are uniform in shape and reminiscent of an object).

- *FYI*: Aging bruises is impossible, so don't try (color changes occur at variable rates from person to person).

■ Don't exclude the possibility of the patient having both an actual medical issue and being a victim of child abuse (and in fact, children with disabling conditions are at higher risk for mistreatment).

3.2.5.2 Obtaining History

■ The goal is to get enough info to triage (not to figure everything out).

■ Of course, need to separate the child and caregiver (should interview the caregiver alone first, then get permission to speak with the child alone [assuming they're older than 3 years old]). Consider having a chaperone present for both interviews.

■ Obviously, make sure you ask age-appropriate questions to the child; always best to keep things simple ("What happened here?").

■ Documentation should be descriptive and verbatim (use quotes). Need to include more details than regular notes (date/time/place, source of history, anyone else present during history-taking).

■ Take photographs.

3.2.5.3 Physical Exam

Need to be thorough. Don't just look at the lesions that are obvious and/or pointed out. Need to look at the genitals and inside the mouth (don't forget about the frenula).

3.2.5.4 Next Steps

■ If suspect it, should transfer to peds ED (if not already there) for the full evaluation (skeletal survey, imaging, etc.).

• When explaining the need, can say something along the lines of, "The lesions are not normal, could be a sign of a serious medical issue, and requires further evaluation at the ED. We will arrange for an ambulance to transport."

■ If have reasonable suspicion, legally obligated to report to child protective services (your only job here is to report facts; it's not to find proof of abuse, have all the answers).

• If unsure whether a report is warranted, it might be possible to triage the case via phone consultation with a child abuse pediatrician.

- In some cases, you might consider having a lower threshold to biopsy since, at the least, it may help you exclude other things (and add more objectivity to the case).

- If end up needing to report to child protective services, communicate to the caregivers, but keep it simple; can say something like, "When we see cases like this, we are obligated by law to report to child protective services. They may contact you if they feel a follow-up to our report is warranted."

- If they ask questions, you can just say you can't give a definitive answer because you don't know anything about how they run things, but you're available and happy to answer any questions related to the child's medical needs.

3.2.6 Erythroderma Differential Diagnosis

Erythema + scale >90% BSA (or technically >80% BSA for CTCL).

Dramatic epidermal turnover; diseased skin = poor temperature regulation, high-output heart failure, risk for infection, etc.

Most commonly exacerbation of pre-existing AD/psoriasis (especially after systemic steroid tapers, but also lithium in psoriasis or phototherapy burns, etc.).

This section is mainly for differentiating high-level categories.

See other sections for more granular details regarding each condition.

Ddx:

1. *Eczematous*

    a. Eczema (AD, contact, seb derm)

        i. Exfoliative dermatitis—associated with heavy drinking (EtOH-induced diuresis -> xerosis). Will see psoriasiform dermatitis on path, so don't get these presentations ("chronic skin failure") confused with psoriasis (see Section 2.1.2 about the worthlessness of biopsying crusty old plaques if trying to ddx eczema vs. psoriasis). Don't let a nonresponse make you think it's psoriasis either because may not necessarily have atopic dermatitis; could have CTCL or Sezary on ddx, though which is of course a reason to biopsy crusty old lesions.

            – Could potentially do phototherapy.

            – Also should rule out nutritional deficiencies if alcoholic as well.

2. *Papulosquamous*

    a. Psoriasis—particularly rebound from systemic corticosteroids or CsA

        i. Nail pitting

        ii. Scaly

        iii. Deeper red

    b. *PRP*

        i. PPK

        ii. Salmon-colored

        iii. Thick nails, subungual hyperkeratosis

3. *Vesiculobullous*

   a. BP

   b. Paraneoplastic pemphigus

   c. Pemphigus vulgaris/foliaceus

      i. Foliaceus tends to have moist, crusty lesions on face/upper trunk before becoming erythrodermic.

   d. Mucous membrane (cicatricial) pemphigoid

      i. Tends to involve GU tract and conjunctiva.

4. *Toxic erythemas*

   a. Drug reactions (particularly HIV)—exanthematous drug reactions, DRESS, TEN, etc.

      i. Usually exfoliate large skin sheets.

5. *Neoplasms*

   a. MF/CTCL (get broad shave—want a lot of epidermis)

      i. Palmoplantar keratoderma in Sezary.

      ii. Sezary is chronic, so thus may have TE (or frank diffuse alopecia), nail dystrophy, epiphora (excessive tearing) with blepharitis, ectropion (eyelids point outward).

   b. Hematologic and solid organ malignancies

6. *Hematologic disorders*

   a. Mastocytoses

   b. GVHD

      i. Tends to involve mouth (mucositis).

7. *AICTDs*

   a. SCLE

   b. DM

8. *Infections*

   a. Scabies

   b. Candida, tinea

   c. Staphylococcal scalded skin syndrome (SSSS)

9. *Broader ddx for kids*: congenital ichthyoses, SSSS, immunodeficiencies, etc.

MANAGEMENT

Depends on etiology. See other sections.

Of course, prevent/monitor for infection (usually staph), manage fluid imbalances, etc.

If idiopathic, then wet dressings and symptomatic treatment (TCSs + antihistamines).

If don't respond to TCSs, then systemics might be fine, but probably only if symptoms are severe.

SCSs probably make most sense because they're fast enough (days vs. weeks for something like MTX, MMF). Can start at 0.5–1 mg/kg per day for 10 days (max 60 mg QD), then slowly taper over several weeks (can institute MTX/MMF during taper if needed). Be careful about rebound in psoriasis, especially, and also other chronic stuff, like AD. MMF typically better for erythrodermic AD (vs. CsA more commonly used in erythrodermic psoriasis).

Can consider whirlpool for exfoliative erythroderma (see DIY section in Chapter 4 for instructions). *FYI*: Sometimes patients are not allowed if they have a port.

3.2.7 Acute Infections

Much of management for these is obviously antimicrobials, which primary teams are usually quick to start. However, important to promptly recognize and institute treatment, as some can progress quickly and extensively.

3.2.7.1 Angioinvasive Fungal Infections

Reasonable to suspect in cancer or BMT patients; leukemia and lymphoma patients are at highest risk (poor immune response). Histologic diagnostic challenge. Tissue cultures can take long time to speciate. *FYI*: Impossible to speciate based on H&E alone (and classic descriptions of hyphae, etc., are based on culture dishes, not the tissue specimen).

1. Most common: disseminated candidiasis.

2. Aspergillosis also common, at sites of IV/lines, skin breakdown.

3. Fusarium often presents as purple toe; issue is their platelets are like 10k, so any trauma to toe can cause hemorrhage. Difficult to differentiate, so oftentimes should biopsy with tissue culture.

    a. Echinocandins good for aspergillus and candida; but don't cover fusarium, which is the most important cause of fungal death in immuno-suppressed patients.

        i. Fusarium is in shower caps, so every time you shower, you're inhaling black mold and fusarium; so basically the only reason we don't die is that we have neutrophils. So if you're neutropenic and inhale these organisms, you'll eventually get fungal sepsis (thus why cancer patients on chemo should only take baths and avoid showers [because of the aerosolized fungus from showerheads]).

4. Mucormycosis, of course, known for its association with diabetes; may be related to iron overload.

5. For biopsy, punch (get subQ—sometimes the fungal elements may only be in the subQ).

3.2.7.2 Bacterial Infections

1. *Staphylococcal scalded skin syndrome (SSSS)*

    a. Usually kids <1 year old and ESRD patients.

    b. *FYI*: Need to take the culture specimen from where the bacteria/infection is (such as the nares [as far forward as you can, since it's anterior nares], oropharynx, conjunctiva, perianal, or blood (not the skin lesions [the peeling skin is secondary]).

   i. Wound cultures of blisters or peeling skin are unhelpful.

   ii. Looking for MRSA.

c. Management: anti-staph IV antibiotics (need to know which antibiotics get to the nose reliably; should think about strep too).

   i. PO antibiotics that do get to the nose:

     – Clindamycin (can clear staph carriage with clindamycin 150 mg QD for 1 month)

     – Rifampin (but don't want the bug to see rifampin alone, so need to pair it, possibly with topical mupirocin)

     – Minocycline

   ii. PO antibiotics for staph that don't get to the nose reliably: TMP-SMX, doxycycline, B-lactams (TMP-SMX and doxycycline don't work for strep, anyway).

2. *Necrotizing fasciitis*

a. Usually febrile, ill-appearing, very painful.

b. Spreads rapidly; cancer patients + diabetics most susceptible.

c. Usually polymicrobial (staph, strep, clostridium, bacteroides).

d. Management: Aggressive debridement, IV antibiotics—needs STAT surgery consult.

3. *Toxic shock syndrome*

a. High fever, HA, pharyngeal erythema, vomiting, hypoTN (look up diagnostic criteria).

b. Staph and strep; worse mortality in strep.

   i. Staph classically from tampon, but more realistically may see post-op, burn patients, nasal packings, etc.

     – Rash starts on trunk, spreads to arms/legs and palms/soles.

     – Desquamation (sheet-like peeling) is 1–3 weeks after rash onset, usually palms/soles.

     – Look at mucous membranes (strawberry tongue, hyperemic conjunctiva).

   ii. Strep can have a primary underlying strep infection; can also be from eating undercooked pork or bites/cuts.

     – Shock occurs 2–3 days after onset (vs. staph, which is longer); may not always have widespread rash.

   iii. Management obviously anti-staph/anti-strep antibiotics, aggressive IVFs; of course, should involve ID. Systemic steroids not recommended.

4. *Capnocytophaga canimorsus*

   a. Doesn't have to be stray dogs.

   b. Can cause vasculitis and vasculopathy at the same time (check feet under socks).

   c. Slow-growing bacteria, so if you don't have high suspicion, can get ugly.

   d. Management: Vanc (often what patients get put on) is OK, but not really treatment of choice; usually susceptible to amoxicillin (don't typically need anything crazy).

5. *Ecthyma gangrenosum*

   a. Pseudomonal ecthyma gangrenosum tends to affect high-blood-flow areas (axillae, anogenital/perineal); smear will show Gram-negatives.

   b. Has punched-out ulcers like a streptococcal ecthyma (but that tends to affect lower legs).

   c. In moist areas, you'd typically write off Gram-negatives as colonization, but this is a time you shouldn't write that off as colonization.

6. *Gonococcemia*

   a. Stereotypically acral hemorrhagic pustules and a septic knee or something on exams.

   b. Gunmetal gray in center of stellate purpura septic emboli.

   c. Remember, need SCSs in addition to gonococcal antibiotics (Waterhouse–Friderichsen syndrome—adrenal gland necrosis/acute Addisonian crisis).

7. *Cellulitis*

   a. Usually unilateral; ED may call about "bilateral cellulitis," which is usually actually stasis derm, especially if strikingly symmetric/been a chronic issue.

   b. Risk factors: eczema/fissured skin, lymphedema, injured skin (wounds, radiation, IV drug use, etc.), immunosuppressed, CKD, etc.

   c. Usually staph + strep.

      i. Mostly actually strep, which has a tendency to invade lymphatics and cause scarring of lymphatics (vs. staying in dermis), thus can cause lymphedema as sequelae (and in fact, a lot of lymphedema is post-strep).

        – *FYI*: The "SLANT" ddx is more in reference to chronic lymphangitis (vs. acute lymphangitis, which is usually strep).

   d. Not really contagious; affects deep dermis/subQ.

   e. Management depends on severity:

      i. If localized to skin -> PO antibiotics for 5–10 days; manage risk factors (eczema, tinea, etc.).

    ii. If systemically ill, IV antibiotics, IVF, involve ID (antibiotics choice), +/– surgery (if abscess or necrotic tissue to debride or if concerned for compartment syndrome, etc.).

  f. After treating, skin may flake off and be itchy as it heals.

3.2.7.3 Other

1. *Disseminated zoster* (20+ lesions outside primary dermatome).

  a. May not catch in vesicular stage (may just be really crusty—look hard for vesicles).

  b. Tzanck smear (the blister fluid)—if has multinucleated giant cells, then is either HSV or VZV (need PCR to distinguish the two).

  c. Have suspicion in cancer/immunosuppressed patients; can be rapidly fatal (more severe in immunosuppressed/transplant patients).

    i. Possible complication is stroke.

2. *Crusted scabies*—not as urgent/emergent as earlier entities, but you may see; has distinct clinical appearance (very heavy mite burden causes extreme crust), and startingly white/silver.

  a. Most often seen in unkept general medicine patients (even though you'd expect it more in cancer/immunosuppressed patients).

  b. Ivermectin safe in renal transplant (cleared by liver).

3.2.8 Pregnancy Dermatoses

1. *PUPPP (pruritic urticarial papules + plaques of pregnancy), AKA polymorphic eruption of pregnancy (PEP)*

  a. Common, mostly found within striae on abdomen (spares umbilicus) in third trimester or even immediate post-partum.

  b. Management: conservative, no threat to mom or baby; can moisturize +/– TCSs.

  c. Resolves spontaneously 3–4 weeks after delivery.

  d. Usually doesn't recur.

2. *Herpes (pemphigoid) gestationis*

  a. Misnomer; nothing to do with HSV.

  b. Very itchy, hives-like rash, second to third trimester.

  c. Tense fluid-filled blisters; starts around belly button, progresses to other parts of trunk, buttocks, extremities.

  d. Management:

    i. TCSs or PO corticosteroids

  e. Resolves days after delivery.

  f. *Risks for fetus*: SGA, prematurity; will often recur in subsequent pregnancies and often worse, with 10% chance baby will have bullae.

3. *Atopic eruption of pregnancy*

   a. Essentially AD, either new or worse/flaring (80% new onset, 20% flare).

   b. Management:

      i. TCSs, antihistamines

      ii. *No fetal risk*

   c. Might recur in future pregnancies.

4. *Intrahepatic cholestasis of pregnancy*

   a. No primary lesions (only excoriations/prurigo, etc.).

   b. Management: ursodeoxycholic acid (decrease serum bile acids).

      i. *Fetal risks*: stillbirth, fetal distress, prematurity

      ii. *Mom risks*: post-partum bleeding (low vitamin K from steatorrhea)

   c. Might recur in future pregnancies/OCPs.

5. *Pustular psoriasis of pregnancy* (*impetigo herpetiformis*)

   a. Usually third trimester; starts in flexures (groin).

   b. Associated with hypocalcemia, hypoVit D.

   c. Management:

      i. Correct hypocalcemia, if applicable

      ii. Prednisone 60–80 mg QD for few days, taper when improves

      iii. *Fetal risks*: stillbirth, placental insufficiency

      iv. *Mom risks*: heart/kidney failure

   d. Resolves with delivery.

   e. Recurs with future pregnancies/OCPs.

6. *Physiologic skin changes in pregnancy*

   a. Breasts enlarge, often 2–3× normal size.

      i. Areolae enlarge and darken.

   b. Moles darken, linea nigra, melasma of course (increased estrogen melanocyte stimulating hormone).

      i. Melasma usually fades 2–3 months after delivery. Best to avoid retinoids and probably hydroquinone, too; happens in 1/3 of pregnant women.

   c. Acne (hormonal)—avoid traditional acne meds (retinoids, etc.); can use azelaic acid (Finacea) or topical clindamycin/BPO.

   d. Palmar erythema (also related to estrogen).

   e. Bleeding gums, nosebleeds, varicose veins, hemorrhoids (increased blood volume).

   f. Striae—typically abdomen and breasts.

Consider also primary dermatoses not related to pregnancy:

1. *Nipple eczema*

   a. Common in breastfeeding (increased moisture from baby's saliva and minor trauma from baby) mothers, avid exercisers (constant chaffing from tight sports bras); itchy, red, scaly fissuring around areola.

   b. Classically bilateral; if just one nipple or doesn't respond to treatment, consider Paget's.

   c. Management: TCSs + moisturizer.

2. *Paget's disease*

   a. Looks eczematous; usually middle-aged women.

   b. Diagnose with skin biopsy + mammogram.

   c. Treat underlying breast cancer.

   d. Can have concomitant EMPD.

3. *Cutaneous breast CA*

   a. Breast cancer number 1 metastasis to skin in women.

   b. Variable presentation (Paget's vs. carcinoma erysipeloides, carcinoma en cuirasse, alopecia neoplastica, distant metastatic nodule).

   c. Skin lesions on breast can also be sign of metastatic cancer of non-breast origin.

4. *Mastitis*

   a. From breastfeeding, involves breast tissue + overlying skin.

   b. Blocked mammary gland + staph or strep.

   c. Acute onset of redness, swelling, warmth, pain; one section of breast.

   d. Management: warm compresses, frequent breastfeeding, PO antibiotics (cover staph, strep).

   e. If progresses to abscess (rare), needs I + D and better antibiotics.

3.2.9 Infantile and Neonatal Dermatoses

Neonates = younger than 1 month. Skin much more vulnerable, and presentations can be atypical. Most of the common stuff is benign.

Eval: overall appearance, size/growth, whether the skin issue resolving/worsening.

- *If diffuse and worrisome*, think broadly—infectious vs. inflammatory vs. genetic or related to something mother had (thus, get mother's past medical history, asking if had appropriate prenatal care [if so, likely had several labs you can check]/how pregnancy went, any concerns followed). May help to ask vaguely if mother had cold sores, etc.

- *For infectious*: get swabs; typically want to cover empirically. Usually bacterial or viral (more than fungal, though possible, of course).

- *AD doesn't* really start until ~2 months old at earliest, so if seeing a true neonate with something that looks like that, consider hyper-IgE syndrome, etc.

■ Diaper stuff: usually topical barrier (zinc oxide paste, etc.) is all you need; consider less-common conditions: acrodermatitis enteropathica (looks psoriasiform without satellite lesions; look around mouth too), Langerhans cell histiocytosis (accentuation in folds, more hemorrhagic-erosive look).

■ Some of the more common genetic stuff that would warrant a skin biopsy: mastocytosis, epidermolysis bullosa.

1. *Acute hemorrhagic edema of infancy*

   a. Not ill-appearing.

   b. Might have tender facial edema.

   c. Usually after illness or "antibiotics/analgesics" (meds people take after illness).

   d. Resolves in 1–3 weeks.

2. *SubQ fat necrosis of newborn*

   a. First few weeks of life; healthy and post-term neonates who receive hypothermic treatment.

   b. Fat-rich regions (back, cheeks, butt, thighs).

   c. Management: Supportive, manage hypercalcemia if needed (and avoid vitamin D supplements).

   d. Resolves in weeks to months; might scar.

3. *Transient neonatal pustular melanosis*

   a. Benign, more common in Black babies.

   b. Unclear etiology.

   c. Isn't bothersome to baby.

   d. Self-resolves in 4–6 weeks.

   e. Ddx neonatal HSV.

      i. Ask if mother had history of HSV.

      ii. Tzanck any vesicles.

4. *Acropustulosis of infancy*

   a. Infants and until age ~3.

   b. Start small red macules, then papules, vesicles/pustules.

   c. Itchy.

   d. Resolves in few months spontaneously.

5. *Neonatal cephalic pustulosis*

   a. Variant of acne, but no comedones.

   b. Usually third week of life.

c. Related to Malassezia (not hormones); can use ketoconazole cream.

d. Might have cradle cap.

6. *ETN (erythema toxicum neonatorum)*

   a. Common (usually primary teams will know), benign, well-appearing.

   b. Begin in first couple of weeks of life (usually first few days).

      i. Usually starts on face, spreads to trunk/limbs.

   c. Waxes/wanes (unusual for a single lesion to persist 1+ days).

   d. Exams emphasize the eosinophils on histology but is a clinical diagnosis.

7. *Dermal melanocytosis*

   a. Increased number of dermal melanocytes, very common in skin of color.

   b. Parents will often be most concerned about aesthetics.

      i. Patchy ones on body go away (peak ~1 year, fade by adulthood); ones on the buttocks tend to persist.

      ii. Can consider laser or excision in adulthood.

   c. Documentation important to avoid confusion with abuse.

8. *Miliaria*

   a. Usually crystallina (fragile small vesicles) in newborns, quite common.

   b. *FYI*: Not same as milia.

   c. From immature/weak/clogged eccrine sweat ducts at superficial epidermis, related to sweating or occlusion.

   d. Asymptomatic, self-resolves.

   e. Emollients may actually make worse.

9. *Palatal/gingival cysts of newborn*

   a. Benign, asymptomatic, regress within few weeks.

   b. Three major types:

      i. Epstein pearls—white-yellow, from epithelial remnants trapped along median palatal raphe (or hard/soft palate junction) when palates fuse.

      ii. Bohn nodules—soft, translucent, from heterotopic salivary gland tissue, found along facial and lingual surfaces of alveolar ridges and on palate.

      iii. Dental laminal cysts—from remnants of tooth bud; found on top of alveolar ridges, more common in maxilla and mandible.

3.2.10 Other Inpatient Entities
3.2.10.1 Graft vs. Host Disease (GVHD)

1. *Acute*: conventionally <100 days, but can happen after.

   a. Usually patients still in hospital after getting their transplant.

b. *FYI*: Can't get from an autologous transplant (those are the ones you get from yourself). But can get in allogeneic, so read the oncology/transplant notes; usually bone marrow or stem cell transplants.

c. Usually macular erythema on trunk, scalp, palms/soles; sometimes can almost look targetoid. Usually need biopsy to diagnose.

d. Graded 1–4; grade 4 are often erythrodermic, with secondary blister formation (such extensive vacuolar change and dyskeratosis, the epidermis becomes separated from dermis).

e. Skin manifestations are typically first, but patients also usually get GI involvement with diarrhea and hyperbilirubinemia too—so look for that (first sign of hyperbilirubinemia is under tongue, NOT the eyes!).

2. *Chronic*: conventionally >100 days post-transplant.

a. Usually skin-limited (not as much liver/GI tract involvement as acute).

b. Looks more chronic . . . lichenoid/sclerodermoid.

   i. When becomes sclerotic, gets a corrugated roof appearance (striated, like Ruffles potato chips) from the parallel rows of sclerosis.

   ii. Clinically tends to accentuate around acrosyringium and follicles (around all the adnexal structures), which can cause drop-like pigmentary changes.

c. Hard to treat; can try systemic immunosuppressives + phototherapy.

   i. Usually start with NBUVB (most are at least partially responsive).

   ii. Some may also need a systemic immunosuppressive; CsA works for anything lichenoid, but problem is, GVHD patients are often getting a good graft vs. tumor response as well, so hesitant to ablate that (thus, light therapy favorable to start with because it preserves this but also helps with the rash).

3.2.10.2 *Acute Generalized Exanthematous Pustulosis (AGEP)*

1. Almost always 2/2 drug (>90%); usually antibiotics (B-lactams, macrolides) or terbinafine, diltiazem, anti-malarials.

2. Quick onset <1 week (usually 1–2 days, like FDE) after exposure.

3. Usually starts on face + intertriginous sites, generalizes within hours.

a. AGEP is accentuated on the face, whereas ALEP (acute localized exanthematous pustulosis) is restricted to the face (usually after URI).

4. Usually starts as macular erythema or looks like morbilliform drug, so must RECHECK on them to see if they develop pustules.

5. Becomes papular, almost targetoid, annular, edematous lesions with thick neutrophilic scale; studded with sterile crusted-over pustules.

6. High fever.

7. Sometimes geographic tongue, not true mucositis.

8. Usually doesn't kill people; tend to do well on prednisone for a couple of weeks, and can also use CsA and TNFs.

9. Can get a transaminitis.

10. HCQ-induced cases tend to behave differently—more severe, and flaccid a lot longer; median time to rash 15 days (sometimes a month or longer) vs. calcium channel blockers and antibiotics, where onset is much sooner.

3.2.10.3 Generalized Pustular Psoriasis (GPP)

1. Impressive migration of neutrophils; can get leukocytosis, swollen joints, erosions in mouth, etc.

2. Resembles AGEP, but if GPP is drug-induced (which AGEP usually is), management is similar, anyway (prednisone/CsA might be OK only for GPP in the short term, but need a long-term plan like a biologic).

3. Can also use IM MTX for GPP (but don't do full dose at once, because will solve it all at once and can cause ulcerations).

   a. Can do 2.5 mg QoD until perfect, then 2.5 mg QW.

3.2.10.4 Localized Fixed Drug Eruption (FDE)

1. Pink lesions that are round to oval that fade to blue or brown (usually dusky).

2. Commonly mucosal sites (genitalia, mouth); also hands/feet.

3. Ask if had before (happens in same exact spot).

   a. Onsets 1–2 weeks after exposure, or 1–2 days after re-exposure.

4. Heals with hyperpigmentation; comes back with more hyperpigmentation and more lesions with repeated exposures.

5. *FYI*: Can be any ingestant like cashews, red soda, etc. (not necessarily a drug).

3.2.10.5 Leukemia Cutis

1. Look inside mouths (should do anyway for most inpatient cases, but especially cancer patients).

2. Variable clinically; can look like Kaposi, thus biopsy helpful.

3. Lesions should not be in various stages of evolution.

4. Tends to onset at time of cancer diagnosis (often helps make the diagnosis for previously undiagnosed cancer, or right when diagnosed, or at relapse after consolidation chemo).

3.2.10.6 Sweet Syndrome

1. Can start looking like purple bug bites, then becomes more edematous/bullous over time.

2. Look for reason (usually 2/2 infectious or paraneoplastic).

3. Med management tough for cancer patients.

   a. Sometimes onc is OK with SSKI; most don't like prednisone.

4. Also for cancer patients, look to see if recently treated with G-CSF (most common drug culprit—makes sense because is a neutrophil simulant).

5. See Sweet's section in Chapter 2.

3.2.10.7 Symmetrical Drug-Related Intertriginous and Flexural Exanthema (SDRIFE)

1. AKA baboon syndrome.

2. Intertriginous + buttocks rash.

3. Lacks systemic symptoms, no major complications.

4. Type 4 hypersensitivity reaction to systemic drug (usually B-lactam antibiotics).

   a. Hours to days after exposure (can be first exposure).

5. Management: TCSs + stop offending drug.

3.2.10.8 Chemotherapy Reactions

1. Grades 1–3 = oftentimes, drug holiday vs. grade 4 = usually change chemo and do not re-challenge.

2. Immunotherapy.

   a. Psoriasis and regular drug rashes usually early.

   b. BP- or LP-like reactions usually later.

      i. Immunotherapy-induced BP tends to escalate quickly and is very refractory to treatment; treat aggressively with IV steroids, IVIG, sometimes rituximab if onc is OK with it.

   c. SJS/DRESS can happen at any time in relation to chemo (can be after several months).

3.2.10.9 Severe Toxic Erythema of Chemotherapy

1. Often from enfortumab vedotin and brentuximab vedotin (vedotin is the key contributor).

2. Ddx early SCORCH.

3. Self-resolves, but can try high-dose vitamin D (50–100k IU ×1, and again in 1 week), which may accelerate symptom resolution.

3.2.10.10 Sudden Conjunctivitis, Lymphopenia, Rash, and Hemodynamic Changes (SCoRCH)

1. Newer entity—young people, mostly from TMP-SMX.

2. Rash looks like sunburn.

3. Hemodynamic changes examples include tachycardia, hypoTN, etc.

4. LFTs commonly elevated, possibly elevated ferritin.

5. Management: high-dose steroids, recover quickly.

3.2.10.11 Nutritional Dermatoses

Won't cover the various vitamin/mineral deficiencies here; would be quite voluminous, and the same as boards exam content—so know that stuff and it'll integrate well into your diagnostic instincts. Included here because worth considering on most ddx, especially for inpatients/ED patients.

3.2.10.12 Wounds

If asked for inputs regarding a chronic non-healing wound, first eval to determine if it's actually a wound. Consider other entities (SCC, melanoma, PG, oozing AD, etc.). For context, a normal wound (a healing wound) may heal ~50% in ~6 weeks. If not healing on that timeline (or obviously, if it's getting worse), then re-eval diagnosis.

Three most common ulcers:

1. *Venous leg ulcers*

   a. Typically lateral leg.

   b. Can do Doppler that looks for venous flow/reflux to show related to venous insufficiency (**FYI**: Different from the Doppler they use for DVTs).

   c. Can also just be due to gravitational edema (which we all get with age).

2. *Arterial ischemic*

   a. Can do ABIs with handheld Doppler.

      i. If ABI of posterior tibial artery is equivocal, can do toe branchial pressure with Doppler of digital arteries (good especially in diabetics who have artificially elevated ABIs due to calcium in vessels).

      ii. Will not heal well, so little more caution with biopsying if you think it's an arterial ulcer.

      iii. Vascular surgery likely won't do angioplasty, unless they suspect critical limb ischemia or if it's very significant (might not even get them to do an angiogram to eval), so anticipate having to manage on own.

      – Can do moist dressings above ankle or topicals if below ankle.

3. *Pressure* (such as diabetic foot ulcers, etc.)

   Biopsy can help rule out infection/inflammation/malignancy.

   Determine if healable. Sometimes can do tests to get an idea (such as ABIs, etc.). Sometimes have to trial treatment/compression to see if they improve. The longer it's been there, the longer it will take to heal (more scarring/fibrosis that inhibits healing process).

   If healable, then determine if suitable for moist wound healing (for example, occlusion).

   Purpose of moist dressings is to increase the time you can leave it on. Thus, wouldn't use moist dressings on an infected wound.

   The spectrum of organisms in a wound is essentially contamination, colonization, critical colonization, and infection. Infection is the only one that warrants systemic antibiotics. Others can do topicals. Thus, don't swab wounds.

Any necrotic tissue needs debrided (perpetuates the inflammatory phase and risks infection).

If exhausted all options and not healing/responding to anything, make sure their nutrition is on point (particularly protein), especially elderly. Ask what they eat. See if have albumin labs.

See Wound Care section in Chapter 4 for more.

4 Medications, Phototherapy, and Wound Care

Try to demonstrate how to apply topicals appropriately (show them a pea-sized amount for tretinoin [common misstep is that patients think more is better, put a bunch on, and get irritated and then don't like it; so show them how much to apply to the whole face], show them what it looks like to apply TCSs in the direction of the hair follicles [instead of rubbing it in back and forth, which can cause TCS-induced folliculitis]). Definitely do when asking them to apply to areas they might fear, like their eyelids, for example.

4.1 TOPICALS

Alleviate concerns/fears:

- Expiration dates exist mostly just because can't guarantee potency, but 10× -> 9× not a big deal; can probably use forever.

- A 2.5% hydrocortisone is safe for face; never been a reported ocular side effect in a 30-year database.

  - People use eye drops 1000× stronger for cornea transplants; ophtho uses all the time without increases in intraocular pressure.

- You can eat 60 g clobetasol QW and not get systemic side effects; the things written about TCSs in the 1960s are from lawyers and only relate to systemic cortisone; 99% of what is written on package insert is ridiculous.

- Tachyphylaxis debatable—is it a downregulation of steroid receptors? Or is it because patients don't consistently use it?

Prescription etiquette:

- Be mindful of how much they'll need.

  - Don't give them a 15 g tube if they have 60% BSA psoriasis (1 fingertip unit = 500 mg -> treats 2% BSA).

  - Give them at least enough refills to get to next appointment (probably better to slightly overshoot).

  - Good to be explicit about how much you expect them to use; for example, if expecting them to apply a 454 g jar of moisturizer to the entire body, nice to mention they should be going through half a jar per week if doing correctly.

    - It's nice to also ask them if they actually need refills (which can be telling as to whether they're actually using their meds, and also because the pharmacy may annoy them if a prescription is sent/filled but they never pick it up).

- Make sure the instructions are unambiguous. Probably wouldn't use the pre-populated stuff, especially if restricted to using on certain site (you don't want the instructions for clobetasol to read, "Apply once daily"; probably better if it says something like, "Apply once daily to active, thickest lesions only until clear; never apply to face/armpits/groin/genitals").

  - I like to put stuff we talk about too, such as taking isotretinoin with fatty meals, not lying down for 30+ minutes after taking doxycycline, etc.

- Better to print prescriptions with GoodRx coupons vs. sending to a pharmacy (they can take the printed one to any pharmacy—where it's cheapest).

- For Medicaid patients, look up CMS Medicaid preferred drug list.

- Be careful of blindly signing nursing home orders (especially because they're often on numerous meds); review your meds and write "derm only."

General info:

- Tell patients to not mix their topicals (unless intended) with anything, including other topical prescriptions; otherwise, will end up with half of both but have to pay full price (dilutes it by volume).

- Probably good to know relative strengths (ointment > cream > lotion > gel > spray > foam), etc., but the best and most effective topical is the one they will actually use. Ask them if they have a preference (and be aware most meds only come in a few vehicles).

  - Info for counseling/navigating the options:

    - Ointments—thick like Vaseline, greasy, don't burn usually; good for fissuring/breaks in skin integrity; otherwise, will hurt to apply; definitely be mindful for peds patients.

      - Most vehicles have at least one inactive ingredient: ointments and solutions are probably the cleanest in that sense, so if has a lot of skin allergies, might lean toward them.

    - Cream—thicker lotion, absorbs a little better than ointments; good for trunk or face, not really good for hairy areas for legs/arms; tend to be cheaper than lotions.

      - Cream stings, but less messy.

    - Lotion—more EtOH content (more potential burning if breaks in skin); spreads easy (so a lot of patients like them); tend to be pricier.

    - Gels—EtOH-based emulsion; easy application; more preservatives; can cause burning; some patients have sensitivities to preservatives; more irritating than creams.

    - Oils—good for scalp or inside ears; can't get in large quantities.

    - Foams—loose, dissolves easily; has burning.

    - Solutions—watery, good for scalp; pretty clean from preservative standpoint.

    - Spray—basically solution with special nozzle.

      - *FYI*: Can prescribe generic clobetasol solution and put it in spray bottle (cheaper than clobetasol spray).

- Often better to use generics, but sometimes brand names come in a better vehicle, and sometimes brands can actually be cheaper, depending on insurance/coupon card, and can be more convenient (combination topicals).

■ Probably should know about GoodRx, Skin Medicinals (make an account for this), Mark Cuban's pharmacy (Cost Plus Drugs), etc.

1. *Topical corticosteroids*

   a. Start with knowing one from each strength (high/med/low).

      i. For example: clobetasol 0.05%, TAC 0.1%, hydrocortisone 2.5%.

      ii. Explain OTC hydrocortisone is 1×; we give prescription hydrocortisone (2.5×), TAC (15×), clobetasol (1600×), etc.

   b. Consider site:

      i. Weaker TCSs on face, eyelid, genitals, neck, skin folds (occlusion increases potency 10×).

         – Desonide is strongest; can go on face (4×).

         – Medium: mild to moderate nonfacial and nonintertriginous sites.

         – Super high: scalp, palms, soles, thick plaques.

            – If has super thick active areas and want to apply with occlusion, tell the patient to apply the TCSs, then Aquaphor, then gauze, then wrap in Coban (this can have the dual benefit of increased potency and protection of the area from scratching [help break itch–scratch cycles]).

   c. Side effects: basically just skin thinning, but also can cause atrophy, telangiectasia, striae, acne/rosacea, ACD, hypopigmentation.

      i. Tell patients only apply to thick lesions (if it's thick, it won't thin the skin).

         – Will only thin normal skin if placed on normal skin QD for 3 weeks.

      ii. If have atrophy, can try tretinoin cream.

      iii. Lot of cross-reactivity between TCSs; would take a pic of the seven classes of steroids to reference. Also helpful to know the cross-reactivities in case patient says they're allergic to one.

      iv. A lot of fragrances in TCSs (which is pretty whack, but should be aware).

      v. Sometimes patients have actual allergies to steroid itself; can patch test for this.

2. *Topical calcineurin inhibitors*

   a. Ointments (tacrolimus, AKA Protopic) and creams (pimecrolimus, AKA Elidel) are expensive; can formulate mouthwash or gauze soaks for vulva:

      i. See tacrolimus swish/spit in DIY section in Chapter 4.

         – Cheaper, stings less, doesn't need lab monitoring; accidental ingestion is negligible and not clinically significant.

b. Can consider tacrolimus solution for scalp if need to wean off TCSs (usually ~$60 for 30 mL).

3. *JAKis*

a. Explain package inserts from sick RA population studying systemic tofacitinib (Xeljanz), not young healthy patients with vitiligo applying creams, etc.

b. Warn patients 20% will get acne; can treat with clindamycin or PO doxycycline, then resume; usually more mild if recurs.

c. Also approved for AD, but expensive, and many other options for AD.

d. Doesn't seem to work well for AA.

4. *Retinoids*

a. Tretinoin (Retin-A).

   i. Inactivated by sun; thus, use at night.

   ii. Flakiness/peeling is the epithelial surface renewing itself (vs. true dryness) but nonetheless can moisturize for the flaky appearance (fine to describe as dryness).

   iii. Recommend photoprotection. Don't use in pregnancy. Don't use at same time as BPO (can inactivate it).

   iv. Example instructions: Wash face gently. Apply mild cleanser. Pat dry. Apply moisturizer (such as CeraVe/Cetaphil). Wait few minutes, then apply pea-sized dab of tretinoin. Gently spread around face. In am, can wash with mild cleanser or just water if irritated. Start MWF. If not too dry after a couple of weeks, use every other night, then QHS as tolerated; 2–3 months to see benefit.

b. Adapalene (Differin): OTC now, and can give them the previous instructions.

c. Adapalene-BPO (Epiduo, Epiduo Forte).

d. Other OTCs: retinols and retinals.

e. Tazarotene—strongest topical retinoid, pretty irritating, use controversial; if using it as anti-neoplastic, probably best to use as adjunctive therapy (probably not good enough as monotherapy).

5. *Anti-neoplastics*—good for AKs, warts, superficial skin cancers. If immunosuppressed, might consider LN2 over topicals (since the topical chemo won't work as well). Good to outline the tumors (with desired margins) with a marker and take pics with the patient's phone so they know where to treat, because sometimes they can lose sense of where the tumor is/was when gets red/blotchy.

a. Imiquimod (FDA-approved for AKs + small superficial BCCs)

   i. Big molecule; might struggle to get through epidermal barrier for things like warts.

   ii. Tell them to poke holes in the packets and squeeze a little bit out to apply (then clip it closed and reuse, etc.).

iii. Works slower than 5-FU; can cause flu-like symptoms for some patients somehow. Can be pricey; comes in small packets.

b. 5-FU (FDA-approved for AKs + superficial BCCs, thus EMPD, SCCIS, all off-label)

    i. Probably more sun-sensitizing than imiquimod; comes in different concentrations.

        – Best to apply in the winter/fall.

    ii. Can get nonspecific irritation; would do 3× yearly max. If applied to mucosal sites, can cause crustiness/swelling/irritation.

    iii. Example instructions:

        – Apply thin layer to cancer area + small rim of normal skin surrounding site.

        – Wash hands thoroughly after applying.

        – In 1–2 weeks, you will notice redness/crusting/irritation (indicative of cream working). If too severe, can skip 1–2 applications but would continue (something is better than nothing).

        – Wash gently 1–2× daily with mild soap (Dove) and water. Do not scrub/rub.

        – Usually don't want to cover the area, but if clothing rubbing on it, can use piece of gauze and paper tape to cover it. Covering with Band-Aid will make more severe (occlusion).

        – After completing course, apply Vaseline/petrolatum QD to BID until heals; redness/swelling/discomfort will improve within 1–2 weeks but can take 4–8 weeks for redness to resolve.

c. Cantharidin

    i. Extract from blister beetle; causes blisters when applied to skin (disrupts desmosomes).

    ii. Tell patients to leave on with Band-Aid for 4–6 hours before rinsing with soap + water; then can apply Vaseline.

    iii. Some providers prefer to limit to palms/soles only because of blisters/scars.

    iv. Don't use it on the face; could get in eyes.

    v. Reasonable to try just one spot first for kids to see if they like it.

6. *Antimicrobials*

a. Topical antibiotics—usually combination (mindful of AAD appropriate use guidelines and antibiotic resistance, for example, don't do clindamycin alone).

    i. Clindamycin-BPO, some insurances prefer BenzaClin or Neuac.

b. SSD—has activity against yeast + bacteria, possibly also good for shingles blisters.

    i. Even if allergic to sulfa, can use SSD (it's used even in burn patients who don't even have an epithelium).

    ii. SSD has possible side effect of argyria (blue skin), thus probably should avoid SSD in nose/mouth, where they will absorb a lot of it; if burn patients apply excessive amounts, could get deposits into dermis, but otherwise, usually fine. Start with QW and, at most, QD.

  c. Miscellaneous OTCs:

    i. Interdry AG—silver.

    ii. Zeasorb = activity against yeast, not bacteria; more for adults with hyperhidrosis.

    iii. Theraworx Protect foam (has silver); can apply after bath if have overgrowth of anything (good for abrasions + diaper rash).

    iv. Lotrimin = butenafine.

    v. Compound W = salicylic acid.

7. *Other treatments*

  a. PDE-4 inhibitors: topical analogs of apremilast

    i. Crisaborole (Eucrisa)—approved for AD 3 months and older; supposed to be BID; stings on application, pricey, not super effective.

    ii. Roflumilast (Zoryve)—approved for psoriasis, QD; pricey.

      – PDE inhibitors supposedly work well for interface pathologies (for example, if ddx seb derm and DM on scalp, might try roflumilast)—of course, beneficial to be targeted even with topicals.

    iii. *FYI:* The various PDE-4 inhibitors are not exactly the same; roflumilast is stronger than both apremilast and crisaborole (25–300× higher binding affinity).

  b. Tapinarof (Vtama)—tar derivative; pricey.

    i. Brilliant for face stuff because can't go stronger than desonide on face.

    ii. Reportedly good for nail psoriasis (I've heard someone say want to avoid strong TCSs on fingertips because can lead to bone atrophy—though almost everyone I've asked after that has strongly disagreed this actually happens).

  c. Vit D analogs.

    i. Calcipotriol (Dovenox) = slow to work, slow to come back (vs. clobetasol—fast to work, fast to come back).

    ii. Can mix with 5-FU to make 5-FU work better.

4.2 SYSTEMICS

See Package Inserts in Section 1.3.3 in Chapter 1.

    Patients commonly ask whether a med will "suppress their immune system." I usually explain that most meds would suppress their immune system to some extent, but that it's all relative: chemo > prednisone > MTX > dupilumab > ibuprofen > sun > water, etc.

For biologics, can generally reassure they don't have to live in deep fear of infection and wear mask all day every day but might expect to take longer to recover from colds, for example.

If on systemic treatment, always ask if have HA, GI upset, N/V, diarrhea, new rashes.

Diseases will become labile if abruptly discontinuing systemic treatment (or even if just given less than duration of disease)—particularly fast-acting meds (corticosteroids + CsA).

4.2.1 Small Molecules

1. *Systemic corticosteroids*

   a. Should mostly be reserved for acute control/arresting acute processes.

      i. Relied on too much by non-dermatologists (some providers put polymyalgia rheumatica patients on 10 mg QD prednisone for life).

      ii. Patients often like the short-term effectiveness of SCSs, but should counsel them that unlike many meds, where there's only a chance of side effects, SCSs have guaranteed side effects if given long term (weak bones, high blood sugar, impaired vision, etc.)—talk to them about those things, and let them know you care about them now but also care about them 20 years from now and need to get them on a sustainable plan.

      iii. Unlike a lot of medicines where you titrate up to the desired effect, you typically will be titrating down SCSs.

   b. For context, the body makes 5–10 mg prednisone QD naturally.

   c. For IV methylprednisolone (Solumedrol), know weight for dosing.

   d. Bone damage most significant in first 6–12 months of therapy, especially in kids.

      i. Supplement with vitamin D + calcium.

2. *MTX (methotrexate)*

   a. Start 2.5 mg QW small kid or 10 mg QW in adult.

      i. Check Cr and CrCl before starting/refilling and for dosing.

   b. Baseline CBC CMP; recheck in 2 weeks (to see if anything crazy), at 4 weeks (to see if any side effects), then Q 3–4 months when stable.

   c. Don't forget:

      i. B9 supplementation (1–5 mg QD—except MTX days).

         – Let them know it will decrease side effects without impacting efficacy.

         – If they're kids and don't like pills, can do 800 mcg of a B9 gummy or can crush the pills.

         – Can increase B9 dose if experiencing MTX side effects.

       – Splitting the dose between 2 days also helps (for example, if on 12.5 mg QW, then can do 7.5 mg on Sundays and 5 mg on Mondays).

  ii. No EtOH (at least don't drink on MTX days; no alcoholics).

  iii. No TMP-SMX.

       – Tell them to make sure their doctor knows they're on MTX before given any antibiotics.

  iv. Must not get pregnant (and not good for family-planning males [decreases sperm count])—must be off MTX for 3 months before planning to conceive (men also need 3 months' washout).

d. Tell patients it takes 6–8 weeks to work (for most epidermal rashes; longer for PRP and dermal/granulomatous stuff, etc.).

  i. Can explain background for package insert fears: ~50 years ago, MTX was approved to treat psoriasis, up to 10 pills per *week* (whereas chemo was 20 pills per *day*). Package insert based on the chemo side effects. Basically, MTX has three side effects: must not get pregnant (men also get lower sperm counts), must not drink EtOH on days you take the med, and kidneys need to work to pee it out.

e. Pulmonologists don't like MTX because of its reported association with pulm fibrosis, but only very rarely (if ever) does it actually occur (especially with weekly dosing). Can pretty confidently tell them that if they don't have seropositive RA or DM, then probably won't get pulm fibrosis on weekly MTX.

  i. The reported pulm fibrosis cases were probably caused by under-treated/aggressive AICTDs that progressed to involve lungs.

  ii. Chemo doses can cause it, however.

f. GI doctors don't like MTX because of its "association with hepatic fibrosis."

  i. Might occur if heavy drinker (not good MTX candidates) and taking high doses; otherwise, shouldn't be an issue.

  ii. Elevated LFTs can also be from fatty liver in overweight patients.

       – Also ask patients if they had their labs drawn the day after their weekly dose.

g. IM MTX is 10× more expensive because they're pre-loaded syringes (used to be cheaper when wasn't pre-loaded).

  i. Harder to tolerate for patients; more side effects, such as the MTX-induced oral ulcers; also may feel more queasy (the "nausea," which is a dose-related central issue and not a true GI upset, thus why actually might be worse with IM than PO MTX).

       – If have GI upset/queasiness, can try to increase B9 to 3–5 mg QD or add leucovorin 12 hours after MTX dose (may help with fatigue too).

- Splitting the dose between 2 days also helps (for example, if on 12.5 mg QW, then can do 7.5 mg on Sundays and 5 mg on Mondays).

ii. If have to do IM, consider 2.5 mg QoD-QD, then QW when controlled.

iii. Rheum tends to do IM more routinely than derm.

h. Great for blocking antibody formation in infliximab and adalimumab; should definitely consider in kids with chronic diseases that will need infliximab (need it to work) for multiple years (like >2–3 years).

3. *MMF (mycophenolate mofetil)—stronger than MTX*

a. Start 500 mg BID, max 1500 mg BID.

b. Baseline CBC CMP and Q 3–6 months.

c. Tell patients of most common side effect: GI upset; 1/1000 get leukopenia.

i. Explain the package insert is based on data from transplant patients who are on Prograf, pred, and high-dose MMF (makes their immune system like AIDS patients), which is not the context we'll be using it in.

ii. Many supposed associations are also tied to CsA for the same reason.

iii. If have GI upset with CellCept, switch to Myfortic—enterically coated and shouldn't cause GI upset (but hard to get covered and more expensive).

d. Also should tell them they can ignore the pharmacist recommendation to take it an hour before and hour after and just take it 5 minutes before a meal (pharmacists just say that because you absorb a very small [likely clinically irrelevant] amount more doing it their way—but it's so impractical [patients will set alarms to wake up at 1 am or something] and doesn't matter because you'll be titrating the dose based on the way they take it, anyway).

e. Better for lungs than MTX.

4. *HCQ (hydroxychloroquine)—rational for UV and lymphocyte-mediated disorders*

a. Start 200 mg BID (except for PCT—200 mg TIW).

b. Baseline CBC CMP, then Q 6 months.

c. Baseline ophtho exam and Q 1 year.

d. Textbooks state that 25% get depigmentation as a side effect, though seems less than that; don't think I've actually ever seen it (vs. minocycline hyperpigmentation, which is for sure real).

e. Irreversible retinopathy more common with chloroquine, but higher risk when chloroquine combined with HCQ.

5. *AZA (azathioprine)*—really not a great drug for skin stuff; rheum seems to use it more than derm.

   a. Start 50 mg QD.

   b. Baseline CBC, CMP, Q 1 m for 3 months, then Q 3 months.

   c. Check TPMT (enzyme that breaks down the toxic products of AZA metabolism).

   d. Avoid allopurinol.

   e. Causes years of increased photosensitivity and skin cancer risk (up to 5 years after cessation).

6. *Thalidomide*

   a. Start 50 mg QD, max 100 mg QD.

   b. Always ask about peripheral neuropathy (hands/feet tingling).

   c. POCT pregnancy Q 1 month.

   d. RTC Q 28 days (regulation via REMS—nurses also have to get auth numbers for each fill).

   e. Miraculous for multiple myeloma and cutaneous lupus, but infamous because causes phocomelic babies.

   f. Weirdly good for apoptotic stuff, but also for neutrophilic processes (which is basically the opposite).

   g. May work for recalcitrant sarcoid (skin and organs), though not much published evidence yet.

   h. Also good for MGUS-related stuff and pruritus.

   i. Good because compendium approval (insurance has to pay).

7. *Colchicine*—good for neutrophilic processes + LCV + complex aphthosis

   a. Ancient drug with novel applications.

   b. Weak, tends to work well with concomitant dapsone.

   c. Usually 0.6 mg QD to TID.

   d. GI upset very common, often treatment-limiting.

   e. Neutropenia quite rare; when happens, tends to be in older women.

8. *CsA (cyclosporine)*

   a. Start 3–5 mg/kg in BID dosing.

   b. Baseline BP and Qvisit.

   c. Baseline CBC, CMP, Mg, lipids (repeat 2 weeks)—may not need if on for just a short stint (for instance, if arresting acute process and only using for 5–7 days).

   d. Rebound with CsA is worse than with prednisone.

   e. Also, get kidney fibrosis after 6 months (was in an ocular Behçet's study), analogous to high-dose MTX with concomitant EtOH (get a little hepatic fibrosis); thus, should probably reserve for only arresting acute issues or if has failed everything else.

    f. Gingival hyperplasia usually only occurs with high-dose CsA.

9. *Retinoids*

    a. Acitretin—essentially normalizes keratinocytes.

        i. Start 25 mg daily.

        ii. CBC, CMP, TGs at baseline; repeat in 1 month, then Q 3 months thereafter.

        iii. Potent teratogen, short half-life, but if taking cough medicine or drinking EtOH, etc., will esterify to etretinate, which has very long half-life; thus, must not get pregnant for 3 years after completing treatment. Red Cross also doesn't want your blood until off 3 years.

        iv. Decreases formation of NMSCs—good if constantly sprouting NMSCs, etc.; used in transplant patients for this.

    b. Isotretinoin

        i. Start 40–80 mg QD.

        ii. Baseline CMP, TG, repeat 1 month later.

          – Probably don't need to do in healthy kids.

            – CMP is for liver because it's a vitamin A derivative (could really just do LFTs).

            – TGs is a fasting blood test, and rarely are patients going to have actually fasted for the 9–14 hours; so if they're slightly elevated, not a huge deal. If above 800, you usually just reduce the dose.

        iii. POCT pregnancy Q 1 month (females).

        iv. Warn about photosensitivity (which lasts several months after completing therapy).

        v. Can't take doxycycline until 1 month after finishing (and of course not concomitantly) (pseudotumor cerebri).

        vi. See Acne section in Chapter 2 for more.

    c. Bexarotene

        i. Thyroid, TGs.

4.2.2 Biologics

Access:

- Prior auths typically are for 1 year, but sometimes insurance companies change it to 6 months and don't tell anyone; best to always document BSA, PGA, prurigo nodule count, itch score, etc. at all visits (usually, documentation needs to include past attempted treatments and/or severe disease [to warrant initiation] and a positive response [to stay on it]).

- If struggling to get access, look up validated scales (that incorporate quality of life impairment, etc.).

- Can also write letters of necessity stating all the things they need it for and how they're missing work, etc.

■ Manufacturer PAPs (patient assistance programs) often kick patients out if they change insurance (so may need to go through enrollment process again).

■ Be mindful of ICD code (if want psoriasis biologic, some insurances won't cover it, unless it's specifically plaque psoriasis; if want biologic on IBD dosing, then will need GI to use their ICD code).

Choosing:

■ Sometimes just based on availability, but good to be familiar with dosing schedules (for patient convenience) if there are options. Would also look at the injection volumes needed to get the dose (larger volumes tend to hurt more).

Safety/vaccinations:

■ Provider vs. insurance definitions of *immunodeficient* are often different (sometimes insurance won't pay for VZV vaccination, even if on immuno-suppressive therapy).

■ TNF inhibitors had case reports of VZV (so got on package inserts), but no increases in age-matched controls (further, not age-matched controls with same diseases, which would be ideal).

■ Usually, VZV vaccine is a two-dose series that's 2–6 months apart (50+ years old if healthy [can just walk in to pharmacy], 18+ if immunosup-pressed [needs a script]); can compress to 1–2 months when beneficial (being able to start the medicine); bear in mind even just getting the first dose provides significant protection.

■ Associate order for Shingrix vaccine with immunocompromised diagnosis (vs. psoriasis ICD, for example) if patient is <50 years old (helps with billing insurance and allowing pharmacist override it vs. needing a prior auth).

■ The VZV vaccine needs to be reconstituted and only good for 30 minutes, so let patient know they need to make an appointment usually.

■ For vaccine-hesitant patients, make sure you mention the risks; 1/100 Sotyktu patients got VZV (quite a bit).

■ If want to do a psoriasis biologic in HBV(+) patients, refer to ID for eval (to essentially get their blessing); if patient refuses, then should get HBV viral load Q 3 months.

■ Realize a lot of patients think pills are safer than shots even though they're less targeted; so make sure to have discussion with patient (because indus-try loves to ride on this misconception).

1. *TNFs*—can't use in CHF/MS; should get baseline and Q 1 year TB-QuantiFERON. Baseline hep panel (only problem is HBV reactivation).

   a. Adalimumab (Humira)

      i. Psoriasis: 80 mg on day 1, then 40 mg on day 8, then 40 mg every 2 weeks.

- QW for HS, QoW for psoriasis, off-label for PG, so depends on what insurance approves it for PG.

b. Etanercept (Enbrel)

  i. At 25 mg subQ twice weekly (doses 72–96 hours apart).

c. Certolizumab pegol (Cimzia)

  i. Doesn't cross placenta—good for women who are family planning (safest for pregnancy).

  ii. At 400 mg on weeks 0, 2, 4, then 200 mg Q 2 weeks.

d. Infliximab (Remicade)

  i. Infusions (not at home).

  ii. Consider concomitant MTX to block antibodies from forming.

  iii. At 5 mg/kg at weeks 0, 2, 6, then Q 8 weeks.

2. *IL12/23*—get baseline TB-QuantiFERON and Q 1 year (guidelines also state CBC with diff, CMP).

a. Ustekinumab (Stelara)

  i. IL23s approved for IBD; good for PG and HS.

  ii. Psoriasis and HS:

    - <100 kg: 45 mg at week 0, 4, then Q 12 weeks.

    - >100 kg: 90 mg at week 0, 4, then Q 12 weeks.

  iii. Sometimes actually harder to get because older and doesn't have PAPs, but nice to use if patient has sacroiliitis and has you wondering whether they have occult bowel disease (when you'd want to avoid 17s).

3. *IL17s*—fast relief, good for peds, great for joints; TB reactivation not as big an issue as TNFs; nonetheless, guidelines still recommend TB test at baseline and Q 1 year + CBC with diff + CMP.

a. Secukinumab (Cosentyx)

  i. Even though approved for HS, IL17s potentially not good for PG/HS because of their association with IBD (should avoid 17s in colitis).

  ii. At 300 mg QW weeks 1–5, then 300 mg Q 4 weeks (consider Q 2 weeks for HS if not controlled Q 4 weeks).

b. Ixekizumab (Taltz)

  i. Good for genital psoriasis.

  ii. At 160 mg week 0, 80 mg Q 2 weeks at weeks 2–12, then 80 mg Q 4 weeks.

c. Brodalumab (Siliq)

  i. At 210 mg QW from weeks 0 to 2, then Q 2 weeks.

d. Bimekizumab (Bimzelx)

    i. At 320 mg Q 4 weeks from weeks 0 to 16, then Q 8 weeks.

    ii. Oral candidiasis.

4. *IL23s*—many pros: work for IBD, better for skin than IL17s (but slightly not as good [at least not as fast] for joints), convenient (less-frequent) dosing, safety, but per usual: guidelines rec baseline TB-QuantiFERON and Q 1 year, CBC with diff + CMP.

    a. Guselkumab (Tremfya)

        i. At 100 mg at weeks 0 and 4, then 100 mg Q 8 weeks (or Q 16 weeks if they're super responders).

        ii. Good for palmoplantar pustulosis.

        iii. Baseline CBC, CMP, TB-QuantiFERON, viral hep panel.

    b. Tildrakizumab (Ilumya)

        i. At 100 mg at week 0 and 4, then Q 12 weeks.

        ii. Needs administered in-office.

    c. Risankizumab (Skyrizi)

        i. At 150 mg at weeks 0 and 4, then Q 12 weeks.

5. *IL4/13*

    a. Dupilumab (Dupixent): very safe and selective; essentially only person wouldn't want to give it to someone with a hookworm

        i. No lab monitoring.

          – Can get conjunctivitis—if really bad, should refer to ophtho.

              – Alternatives would probably be MTX, MMF, or maybe JAKi (tralokinumab also can cause conjunctivitis).

        ii. Adults: 600 mg load, then 300 mg Q 2 weeks.

        iii. Peds:

          – For 15–30 kg: 600 mg load, then 300 mg Q 4 weeks.

          – For 30–60 kg: 400 mg load, then 200 mg Q 2 weeks.

          – For 60+ kg: 600 mg load, then 300 mg Q 2 weeks.

6. *IL13*

    a. Tralokinumab (Adbry)

        i. Similar to dupilumab—no lab monitoring and shouldn't give to people with hookworms; similarly can get conjunctivitis.

        ii. At 600 mg load at week 0, then 300 mg Q 2 weeks (can stretch to Q 4 weeks if <100 kg, and clear after 16 weeks of treatment).

7. *CD20*

    a. Rituximab (Rituxan)

        i. Baseline CBC CMP hep panel, TB-QuantiFERON (and yearly), +/– HIV.

    ii. Dosing depends on indication.

8. *IVIG*

   a. Check IgA (if deficient, risk anaphylaxis).

   b. Lots of volume; be aware in heart/kidney patients.

   c. Nice because can be administered at home.

9. *Biosimilars*

   a. Used more often in rheum.

   b. Unclear why not more widespread adoption in derm, though now seem to be gaining at least some traction.

   c. Will be interesting to see to what extent results are sustained in biologic-experienced patients who switch to biosimilars.

4.2.3 Newer Therapies

1. *JAKi*

   a. Exciting and popular; was a big fad 15 years ago, with doing trials with JAKis for RA and IBD (GI and rheum loved JAKis because they were oral, though seemingly a drift back toward targeted therapies in rheum and GI).

   b. Potential issues:

      i. They aren't really targeted therapies for most conditions (oddly targeted for dermatomyositis); they block cancer genes, herpes genes, etc.

        – Be careful in atopics; takes 8 weeks to kick in, and because you're suppressing the immune system, can get disseminated herpes before the eczema clears, so should give acyclovir prophylaxis (why dupilumab overall more favorable).

      ii. They cost just as much as targeted injections.

      iii. Don't seem to yield durable responses off treatment, so basically have to stay on it for chronic diseases, which is not sustainable (might cost $60k per year, which no one will pay for/insurance won't continue to cover).

        – So have to ask if worth $60k for 1 year of hair in AA (probably even less since takes long to grow), 1 year of color in vitiligo, etc.

        – Exemplifies why it's important to come up with treatment plans that match the duration of the problem.

      iv. Patients don't seem as smoothly controlled compared to targeted treatments (especially for reactive dermatoses, like PG, Sweets, etc.).

   c. Baseline CBC, CMP, TB, hep panel, lipids (~12 weeks after initiation and periodically thereafter).

Nonetheless, they work well initially and many patients are on them.

- Ritlecitinib good for peds AA; start 50 mg QD.
- Baricitinib good for adult AA; start 2 mg QD, up to 4 mg QD.

- Topical JAKis don't work well for AA.

- If history of cancer, consider alternatives.

2. *Deucravacitinib (Sotyktu)*

   a. Pharma loves to frame it as "not a JAKi" (and it doesn't come with the same black box warning as JAKis), because technically doesn't block JAK1–3, but Tyk2 is selective JAK enzyme so can essentially think of it as "JAK4" [and really should've been called JAK1, since it was discovered first]; still get herpes because it blocks interferon response.

      i. Sidenote: anifrolumab not referred to as a JAKi either, but it inhibits IFN receptor (with JAK-STAT intracytosolic signaling), so basically same thing (can still get VZV, etc.).

   b. Good for scalp psoriasis (other PO options aren't very good).

   c. Basically 2× as effective as Otezla.

   d. Start 6 mg QD.

   e. TB-QuantiFERON screen, shingles vaccine—see earlier (safety/vaccinations).

   f. Main side effects: URIs, acne/folliculitis (topicals).

3. *Antibiotics*

   a. When using antibiotics to treat infections, should know the pharmacokinetics/dynamics.

      i. Most antibiotics we use are time-dependent (bind reversibly and only work when they're around—thus have to be at twice the MUD for half the dosing interval for them to work); thus, treatment failure is more often non-adherence to time-dependent antibiotics than it is true antibiotic resistance.

         – For example, cephalosporins (have to take cephalexin QID for it to work [levels are quick to rise and quick to fall]—how many patients do you think can take a pill QID for 10 days?).

            – Cefadroxil is an alternative first-gen cephalosporin that is a truly QD antibiotic (and is actually slightly cheaper than cephalexin).

         – There are time-dependent antibiotics that have residual effects (damage ribosomes)—this is how you can get away with something like a Z-Pak (because inflicts enough damage on the ribosome during a short course).

   b. In contrast to concentration-dependent antibiotics, which bind irreversibly, the question is, "Can you achieve adequate concentration in the tissue so it can bind to the organism?"

   c. Obviously, know the coverages. TMP-SMX doesn't cover *Pseudomonas*; most penicillins cover Gram-positive, third-gen penicillins get more Gram-negative and less Gram-positive.

      i. Any B-lactam works for strep.

     ii. Doxycycline, TMP-SMX do not work for strep.

d. Also, be mindful of cultures and when they don't tell you what you need; if you culture anything perioral, perirectal, HS lesion, etc., it's the stuff you don't culture (anaerobes) that are the pathogens.

      i. For anaerobes:

- Clindamycin and B-lactams above diaphragm.

- Metronidazole below diaphragm is only reliable option but doesn't have much of a spectrum beyond anaerobes. Has some coverage of C diff (which you will inevitably give someone at some point—and in fact, cephalexin is the most common cause because so commonly prescribed and so broad [not clindamycin, the step 1 board answer]).

e. Doxycycline—inhibits lymphocyte and neutrophil migration (albeit somewhat weakly).

      i. Better than minocycline (which causes guaranteed irreversible hyperpigmentation if used too long; half melanin, half minocycline, not evenly black, and no cure/treatment).

     ii. Don't use if <8 years old.

    iii. GI-excreted (OK if kidneys don't work, unlike other tetracyclines).

    iv. Take after eating and with a large glass of water to avoid nausea and GI upset.

     v. Don't lay down for at least 30 minutes (pill esophagitis).

    vi. Probably best to use 3 months at a time, then re-evaluate (concern for bacterial resistance), 4–6 months max.

f. Dapsone—good for neutrophilic processes, IgA diseases, LCV.

      i. Start 50 mg QD, max 150 mg QD.

     ii. Baseline CBC, G6PD.

    iii. Repeat CBC 1–2 weeks, then Q 3 months once stable.

    iv. Dapsone makes RBCs fragile but don't become iron-deficient because body just recycles the iron that spills out.

- Used to have/use sulfapyridine if received too much hematologic toxicity from dapsone, but no longer available.

g. Rifampin.

      i. Orange body fluids.

     ii. Used in HS.

    iii. Also used in triple-antibiotic therapy (rifampin, ofloxacin, minocycline—given Q 1 month).

h. Macrolides—can try if cannot do tetracyclines (such as young children).

    i. Azithromycin usually 250 mg TIW. Can cause GI upset. Look at med list—can interact with other medications (QT prolong).

    i. TMP-SMX—for young patients and those that cannot tolerate other antibiotics. Make sure not on MTX.

  j. Cephalosporins and penicillins (cephalexin, etc.)—good for pregnant patients.

    i. If want to use a first-gen cephalosporin, cefadroxil is a good option that has QD or BID dosing (good for kids and those who don't like taking pills).

4. *Anti-fungal*s

  a. Terbinafine: careful about SCLE, alcohol.

    i. Consider checking LFTs (baseline and 4–6 weeks into treatment).

    ii. At 250 mg QD for 12 weeks for adult onychomycosis.

Other miscellaneous meds:

5. *Pentoxifylline (Trental)*

  a. Usually 400 mg BID to TID.

  b. FDA-approved vasodilator for PAD; also used in granulomatous conditions, like pulm sarcoid and skin granulomas.

  c. Makes RBCs more squishy/deformable (after 8 weeks of treatment), so also rational for calciphylaxis, etc.

  d. Also has weak impact on neutrophil migration.

6. *Apremilast (Otezla)*

  a. Systemic version of crisaborole—and similarly doesn't really work very well in majority.

  b. One-third as effective as MTX.

  c. Start 30 mg BID; discuss diarrhea/weight loss, depression.

  d. Main pro is no lab monitoring.

  e. Might be useful for mouth stuff like oral LP or complex aphthosis (could try swish/spit—see tacrolimus in DIY meds section in Chapter 4).

7. *SSKI (saturated solution of potassium iodide)*

  a. Solution doses in drops, not mL (so they have to assume 20 drops = 1 mL); usually $500 for a 30 mL bottle. Tastes bad. Mix with orange juice or something.

  b. Can get SSKI tablets OTC, but they're small tablets ($8 on Amazon for 60 30 mg tablets).

  c. Good at breaking up granulomas but doesn't work for GA.

  d. Not many side effects (other than tasting bad), but can flare DH and impact thyroid.

8. *Glycopyrrolate (Robinul)*

   a. Anticholinergic; used for hyperhidrosis and conditions exacerbated by hyperhidrosis (Hailey–Hailey, etc.).

   b. Typically start 1 mg BID.

   c. May get dry elsewhere (dry mouth, constipation); some patients also say they get palpitations.

9. *Gabapentin*

   a. Good for itch, neuropathic, dysesthesia type of stuff, burning tongue, etc.

   b. Can potentiate SSRIs.

   c. Mindful of dose in older folks on many meds. Probably start 100 mg QHS and stay low-dose; don't want to sedate especially if fall risk.

   d. Makes sleepy—tell patients first couple mornings after starting, they will feel hungover but then will get used to it.

4.3 PHOTOTHERAPY AND PHOTODYNAMIC THERAPY (PDT)
4.3.1 Phototherapy

Should try to administer a phototherapy treatment before end of residency.

Good for psoriasis, eczema, pruritic disorders, vitiligo (works because turns off skin's immune system and makes melanocytes want to repigment [encourages them to migrate]).

Effect can be generalized, but also at least partly localized (could shine a laser through psoriasis plaque and only the laser spots will resolve).

Basics of basic science:

- Joules = amount of energy.

- UVB photons are higher energy (shorter wavelength) than UVA; longer wavelengths (UVA) go deeper into skin (UVB only gets to the papillary dermis).

- UVA causes immediate darkening because of oxidative reaction and also associated with more chronic collagen changes (aging).

Cancer risk:

1. PUVA great for CTCL but not supposed to be used for benign stuff like psoriasis (increases risk for SCC and probably melanoma).

   a. UVB probably increases risk for malignancy too, though probably very small (studies haven't been adequately powered—but if it takes that much power, then it's probably such a small risk); also consider the face naturally gets the most UV (so giving UVB to the body probably not going to cause an insanely higher risk).

   b. Adding systemic retinoid encourages free radical formation and oxidative damage similar to PUVA (so UVB + retinoid probably same end result as PUVA).

The dogma is, UVA isn't effective for psoriasis (board answer).

■ This is because UVB is 100× more effective at clearing psoriasis than UVA on a per-joule basis; however, UVB is also 100× more effective at burning people than UVA.

• So they're actually equally effective for psoriasis relative to how likely you are to burn the patient (though maybe UVB is a little better as far as aging since doesn't go as far into skin and impact the collagen/cause photoaging).

Some people say tanning beds don't work for psoriasis (because they're usually primarily UVA).

■ But standard tanning bed light bulbs are 5% UVB, so if you give a joule of UVA, you're getting 50 mJ of UVB (which is plenty), even if it isn't a UVB bed; they seem to work well for psoriasis (more on this in *the psoriasis section 2.1.1.1.1*).

Boards answer: NBUVB is more effective than BBUVB (but if you give enough BBUVB to get them close to burning, then probably will be just as effective as NBUVB).

Practical things:

1. Might be cheaper or more convenient to go to tanning bed (probably couple hundred bucks a year).

   a. Practical and easy; don't need materials.

   b. Every bed is different so can't tell them a time, but the tanning bed people will know their beds and suggest a safe time (can tell patient to start at half that to just be extra safe).

      i. Use the same tanning bed for added consistency (facilities probably have several beds).

   c. Tell them to get the unlimited tanning plan; try for QD to get money's worth.

   d. Don't add acitretin after already been on light treatments (better to do it at beginning), or if you do add later, cut the light time in half.

   e. Do NOT give psoralen + have them go to a tanning bed (people have died!).

      i. If want it to be more effective, can put thin layer mineral oil on the psoriasis or TAC ointment to make light penetrate better.

2. Can prescribe home light unit (probably preferable to coming in for office light [may have to copay for office visit and procedure visit]).

   a. There are a few options: full-body surround unit, flat panel, or flat panel with wings.

      i. Best to get flat panel with wings (we usually prescribe Panasol 3D).

         – Convenient; can close wings and fold it up, so better for storage.

         – Also best for reimbursement because it still falls under the reimbursement code for a 3D panel even though it's much cheaper than the full-body surround 3D panel.

ii. Even if the whole-body light unit might cost $2–3k, that is far less than the lifetime cost of MTX, which is far less than lifetime cost of any biologic (which might be $70k per year).

iii. Can cover face with towel to avoid the photoaging on face.

b. *FYI*: There's no dial to control how much comes out of each bulb; it's either on or it's not. But the number of bulbs may differ if the light box has a mix of UVA and UVB bulbs vs. just UVB bulbs, for instance (which is probably fine for most patients); the variability in treatment strength is primarily dictated by how much time the bulbs are on.

c. UVB dose schedules based on skin type; should look up initial dose and incrementally dose.

d. If doing a minimal erythema dose (MED) test, you can just start there and it'll be fewer treatments.

e. When in doubt, start with 15 seconds, increase by 15 seconds each day, and do QD (if NBUVB can tell them every other day); do until slightest sign of sunburn, then hold at that dose.

i. If they miss a week of doses, then cut in half.

ii. If they miss 3–4 weeks, then start over with dosing (body builds up immunity to light [skin gets darker]).

iii. If phototherapy not working well enough and want to add acitretin, should decrease the light dose in half (otherwise will burn).

iv. If achieve remission, should taper by one day over a few weeks; if had refractory disease to start, then may need maintenance. Some only need in winter when there is no sun; some can taper off completely.

3. Legs tend to be resistant.

a. Have them stand so they're closer to the middle of the box (want to get contributions from the entire length of the unit [top, bottom, middle]— in other words, if at foot level, they're missing everything below from a symmetry standpoint).

b. Legs probably inherently more resistant, too, to an extent; can just leave them in the light box longer if they'd rather sit in a chair in front of the light.

4.3.2 Blue Light Therapy (AKA PDT)

Conversions in PDT are temperature-dependent (destroys where the porphyrin is).

Hot areas get increased blood flow (erythema), which is where the porphyrin goes (thus, these are the areas that get killed). Patients with hot red faces are going to say it hurts; patients with cool gray faces are going to say the treatment did nothing. So have to adjust the temperature. Can be pretty painful. Concept also applies when considering the lesions you're treating; works well for AKs because they're hotter at their inflammatory base. For DSAP, usually need to do under-occlusion and heating pad.

You basically apply a cream, occlude for 3 hours, wipe off, then get light for 16 minutes, which activates the cream and kills the cells, then just have to heal (painful for a couple of days, but results are good for 1 year). Good for patients with extensive damage or those who fail/don't like 5-FU (which requires routine application and not good when hot/sweaty). Better during fall months, when sun is gone.

If trying to treat a cancer, best to have them come in the same day before treatment and almost do like a superficial EDC (to give the light better access to tumor, and also to numb them up). Can also decrust with sterile sandpaper.

Probably shouldn't do broad-field treatments before PDT (high-concentration TCA peels can be harsh for legs with extensive actinic damage and/or eruptive KAs, etc.).

PDT has better clearance than LN2, which is better than 5-FU at 3 months; response not durable for any of them (but expected since patients are likely making more—field effect), so probably need repeated treatments.

Poorly differentiated keratinocytes are less sensitive to PDT, so probably not good for moderately to poorly differentiated SCCs or signs of histologically aggressive tumors, like infiltrative, etc.

4.4 DIY FORMULATIONS INSTRUCTIONS

1. *TAC wet wraps*

   a. Soak hand towel in warm water, rinse so not drippy, lay out chuck, apply TCSs, then put towel over it. Leave applied for 30 minutes to 1 hour. This typically works better than cream alone.

2. *Tacrolimus swish/spit and gauze soaks*

   a. Open a 1 mg capsule, dissolve contents in 0.5 L of water, swish for 2 minutes, then spit out once to twice daily (QD if controlled, BID if flaring). Each time they compound solution, should last 1–2 weeks; store in refrigerator.

   b. Can use the same solution to soak gauze in and apply to vulvar lesions or PG ulcers, etc.

3. *Home chemical peel*

   a. St. Ives 2% salicylic acid QD for 3 minutes max on face when shower (can use for epidermal discoloration issues).

4. *Dakin's solution*

   a. A 32 oz. boiled water.

   b. Add 1/2 teaspoon of baking soda.

   c. Add 3 tablespoons of household bleach.

   d. Soak for 5–10 minutes TIW.

5. *Bleach bath*

   a. Dilute 1/2 capful of bleach in 1/4 tub of water.

   b. Sit in for 10 minutes.

6. *Inpatient whirlpool therapy* (removes toxic debris, improves circulation, aids in dressing removal—all accelerate wound healing).

a. Provide these instructions to primary team: Take patient to whirlpool tub. Clean tub with bleach cleaner. Rinse tub. Add liquid dial soap to tub. Fill tub 1/2 with tepid water (not hot, not cold). Submerge patient. Add warm or cool water to comfort to full with patient in tub. OK to use jets with patient in tub if comfortable. If jets uncomfortable, OK to just soak for minimum 5 minutes as tolerated. Remove patient from tub, then try to remove the patient's remaining adherent dressings. Then replace dressings.

4.5 WOUND CARE AND WOUND HEALING

Wound care is what we do. Wound healing is what patients do. If you only think about the wound care part, you may end up doing that forever. Nutrition in chronic wound patients is underappreciated.

Most wounds you see will be clean, so don't chase every culture positivity. Would only treat with antibiotics if they clinically have lymphangitic or cellulitic change. Or consider based on symptoms (they may say feels stingy/burning pain when it didn't before).

Major question is differentiating inflammatory vs. non-inflammatory wound.

Will never heal if inflammation is uncontrolled, but also don't want high immunosuppression if inflammation isn't the problem (if it's just a healing wound).

For ulcers:

1. If raw, paint on gentian violet (GV) QW.

   a. GV helps cleanse, doesn't help debride. Can dry things out. Apply Vaseline over it.

   b. Tell patients to wear cotton gloves to prevent purple stains on clothes.

2. If tendons are exposed in ulcers, they never heal, because tendon is always moving; control the inflammation (if inflammatory ulcer), then send to plastics for graft.

3. Unna boots work well (they basically look like ACE wrap on outside but have calamine medication wrap underneath [soothing, stops itching, stiff and inelastic bandage; great for venous stasis]).

   a. Unna boots are ~35 mmHg (pretty high compression).

   b. So good to document an ABI: patients need to lie flat for 5–10 minutes before measuring.

      i. Need ABI because this is what the guidelines refer to, although it's somewhat irrational (for example, could have a brachial artery pressure of 180 and an ankle pressure of 90 [in other words, ABI is 0.5, but the ankle pressure is 90, so no way you're going to collapse arterial perfusion with 40 mmHg compression garments]).

Things you don't want:

1. Swelling -> less circulation of nutrients.

2. Scabs/dryness (like a boulder sitting on top of growing grass; edges will struggle to approximate which may cause depressed areas).

a. Keep wounds sterile and greasy with Vaseline. Cover with Band-Aid when wound is still wet and trying to lay epithelium down (don't let "air out" like conventional [outdated] wisdom).

i. Keeping a wound covered while re-epithelializing is helpful because moisture allows keratinocytes to slide more easily over wound bed, local factors are better kept in place when occluded, and has lower oxygen tension than if you had it exposed to ambient air (want the wound base to have low O_2 tension because signals to cells that you need angiogenesis).

– Especially important for ulcers (will really struggle to epithelialize if dry).

3. Dressings that stick/adhere -> rips off new skin, thus replace frequently.

a. Issue is, some dressings like alginate are $500 and can still stick; might be feasible/worth it if inpatient and just need for short period of time, but if managing a chronic wound as outpatient, probably more realistic for patient to keep up with cost of Vaseline gauze or gentian violet or Theraworx Protect.

4. *FYI*: New skin (fibrinous slough) looks yellow and white; hamburger meat–colored stuff is granulation tissue.

a. If there's too much granulation tissue (to the point where it's higher than the edges of the wound [like a mound]), some people use silver nitrate sticks to destroy the excess granulation tissue and give the fibrinous slough a chance to catch up.

i. They roll the sticks (which look like matches almost) over the granulation tissue to chemically cauterize the vessels [basically turns the hamburger meat black instantly]).

5. Crusty, scaly stuff is where they should focus on applying antiseptics—such as SSD or Theraworx Protect.

Dressings selection is a big industry and great exam material, but in practice, essentially the only thing you need to know is one basic principle: if it's too wet, then dry it; if it's too dry, then wet it (want to optimize the moisture balance). There are tons of foams, sponges, films, but if you spend all your time memorizing that stuff, I don't anticipate it being very fruitful (might be a "hot take," but just my opinion. And all said, I included some of that info in the following since it's still helpful to know the basics of it). You can adjust the moisture balance by changing the type of dressing, or by changing how frequently you change whatever you have. For instance, alginate will be fine in ~70% of patients; just need to know whether to change it QD vs. QW, etc.

For wound cleaning, plain soap and tap water are best. Can also wash with saline or vinegar (dilute vinegar good for malodor; topical metronidazole also good for Gram-negative malodorous stuff associated with wounds).

FYI: Betadine fine for cleaning incision area, but not good for chronic use (cytotoxic). If patients are using it chronically, then sometimes all you have to do is have patients stop using it and they'll heal.

Dakin's: pharmacy usually prescribes 0.5% and 0.25%, but the best is 0.025% (diluted Dakin's). Sometimes the hospital can get it. Diluted better because still has antibacterial effects (good at controlling odor) but doesn't have cytotoxicity. It's basically 4 cups of water, teaspoon of Clorox, and a little bit of baking soda to neutralize the pH (makes it less stingy).

Hydrogen peroxide fine for a couple of uses (should rinse off shortly afterward), but not great to use repeatedly. Helps get bloody gunk off wounds, but not meant for saturating a wound and should try to avoid wound edges (cytotoxic to keratinocytes).

When you change the dressings, skin will tell you if you struck a good moisture balance.

If see crust on edges, it's too dry. If dressing is sticking to wound and pulling off the new skin, too dry.

If edges are macerated (looks like white soggy skin after sitting in water for too long), it's too wet.

Don't want to air-dry—will desiccate tissue and have slower turnover.

Don't wash fresh surgical scars.

Three main categories of chronic wounds:

- *Diabetic foot*

- *Vascular*

  - Venous ulcers = a lot of edema, so a lot of exudate (will also often require compression so has even more for ~4–5 days).

  - Arterial ulcers have less exudate because of poor blood supply.

- *Atypical (PG, calciphylaxis, etc.)*—most overlap between derm and wound care

All wounds will heal if given an environment to do so (so non-healing wound probably more appropriately framed as "chronic wound"). If wound is chronic, probably means you're not getting to the proliferative phase (stuck in inflammatory phase and will stay there until you address whatever is driving the inflammation) or you don't have enough building blocks (poor nutrition). All about angiogenesis and collagen deposition (which patient's body has to do and thus need a lot of things to be functioning right; need normal appetite and a good diet, functional gut to absorb it, need it taken to liver to make albumin and growth factors, etc., then need blood flow to deliver to site, etc.). Albumin is not a nutrition marker, more so a metabolic marker. Drainage from wounds is albumin (so need to account for losses, too, on top of whatever poor intake they may have). Low albumin causes third spacing (fluid shifts into tissues), skin elasticity decreases, and dermis essentially becomes a sponge (so need compression).

Some injuries (like lacerations from coffee tables, etc.) shouldn't be sutured (more foreign bodies, etc.); should just manage conservatively with compression, elevation, optimized nutrition. For healthy, active people, they get hypermetabolic/anabolic when get injured (think about freak accident horrific injuries like car crashes—they can have organ failure, but they still eventually heal; it's because they have good anabolic response). In contrast to acute wound patients, chronic wound patients have a lot of comorbidities (age only really a factor when they accumulate comorbidities; somewhat shockingly, 70 year olds with diabetic foot ulcers probably heal better than, say, a 40 year old with a diabetic foot ulcer, because they're usually more adherent to what you say).

Debridement = take a chronic wound, excise it, and now have a fresh new wound.

FYI: "Wet-to-dry" is generally an old technique (where they put wet gauze on wound, leave until dried out, then tear off). It's fine to do that for a few days but would be wrong to do it forever (helps clean via mechanical debridement but doesn't maintain good moisture balance). Since multiple teams are often involved, can sometimes get conflicting recommendations. Can explain wet-to-dry is a painful debridement technique, and there are alternative techniques that are less painful.

Anything below the knee essentially has a stasis component. Even if just broken ankle or laceration, there is still swelling and a stasis component. So think of compression.

Moist wound healing always give better scar outcome than dry wound healing. Once epithelialized, can improve remodeling phase with silicone creams or pads (can buy OTC, cut into strips 2–3× size of scar, apply overnight, wash it with water, then can apply again). Good if developing hypertrophic scar. Massaging helps with scar tissue (so some of the stuff that's marketed to help might just help because they're rubbing it in).

See Scars section in Chapter 7 for more.

As promised, some of the basics of the conventional content that may be helpful to know:

■ Non-occlusive stuff like dry gauze, Telfa pads, ABD pads, etc. are good for moist wounds (basically lay them on and let them absorb the exudate).

■ Films (such as Tegaderm [the stuff they put over IV dressings]—occlusive, prevents water and air, but doesn't manage moisture).

■ Hydrocolloids (manage minimal amounts of moisture—thus probably best when wound has progressed through proliferation phase [when granulation tissue is more mature and the cells are more tightly together]).

■ Foams (absorb moderate amounts of moisture).

• Underneath foams can place things that suck up moisture (calcium alginates [seaweed, looks like pieces of felt, sucks up moisture], hydrofibers [desiccated carboxymethylcellulose, basically sucks up moisture and turns it to a gel]). So if taking dressing off and it's macerated, could use a different dressing or place either calcium alginate or hydrofibers, under the existing dressing (to make more absorptive).

Common dressings:

1. *Aquacel AG*—for infected (or high risk for infection) wounds (such as diabetic foot ulcers, leg ulcers, exudative pressure ulcers); highly absorbent, 1.2% ionic silver.

2. *DuoDERM (the original hydrocolloid)*—protects bony prominences for stage 1/2 ulcers.

3. *Mepilex*—for shallow exudative wounds, painful wounds, fragile surrounding skin; absorbent foam pad; needs to be wet to be active; good for large surface area.

4. *Sorbsan*—wounds with a lot of exudate; calcium alginate, highly absorbent.

5. *Vigilon*—wounds with sparse exudate.

6. *Xeroform (yellow gauze stuff)*—for burns, lacerations, abrasions, skin tears, shallow wounds; nonadherent gauze impregnated in petrolatum; good if in stages of healing + superficial.

Common topicals used for wounds:

1. *Aquaphor*—moisture barrier, protects skin.

2. *Baza*—protects skin from incontinence; inhibits fungal growth (treats candidiasis); zinc oxide–based cream + 2% miconazole.

3. *Collagenase/Santyl*—to debride necrotic/sloughing wounds, use QD; an enzymatic debriding ointment.

4. *Dakin's (antimicrobial solution)*—for wounds with necrotic tissue, malodorous + infected wounds.

5. *SSD*—removes eschar tissue; prevents infection.

5 Procedures

5.1 GENERAL PRINCIPLES

- There are many different ways to do things well; recommend learning it the way your attendings do things (same for clinic).

- Learn what makes a helpful assistant; this will help you in guiding your eventual assistant.

- Usually, the light is best on the left side of the surgeon (assuming right-handed); if the light is behind your head, you'll get the "surgeon's eclipse," and if it's on the dominant-hand side, then the surgeon's hand will block it.

- Have thorough plan for all parts of the procedure; if something feels off, slow down. Should know why everything is the way it is. Always consider possibility of a misdiagnosis.

- Obviously, always be careful about what you say (never say "Oops," joke around, or say stuff that could be misconstrued).

- Creating a perfect wound is the best way to create a perfect closure (more on this later).

- Obviously, know the anatomy (not only the structures and things you should avoid but also the plan for how you will maneuver the tissue).

  - For example, if working on the back of an ear, consider suturing the ear to the preauricular area of the face (which you need to numb, of course) so you don't have to use your hand to hold it down during the whole procedure.

  - Consider utilizing a traction stitch for mobile skin, like labia, tongue, lip—helps shape into straight line for easier approximation.

    - Though will say that for labial and scrotal skin, it's not as big of a deal if have dog ear (like not in a straight line), because skin is baggy, so it comes together well.

  - If on elbow, don't get into the bursa—will have stiff elbow; if do get into bursa, then suture it (consider figure of eight), otherwise will scar + get sticky.

  - Know the blood supply—not just the names of the arteries/veins and where they are, but also where you can pinch to minimize bleeding (for example, if working on upper lip, then pinch where the superior labial arteries are on either side of where you're working—this can literally be game-changing).

    - This also helps limit cautery in areas where it's super unfavorable to use (eyelids, lips, etc.).

  - If you're struggling to finesse instruments that are seemingly too large for a small area (so if the headrest is getting in your way), then rotate your hands 180 degrees.

- For instance, if you're putting in tops from the right to the left side of the wound bed from superior to inferior, you can just put in the tops from the

DOI: 10.1201/9781003537946-5

left to the right side of the wound bed from inferior to superior (without having to backhand everything).

Counseling patient pre-procedure:

- Patients must understand that they are trading their lesion for a scar (and your goal is to make as imperceptible as possible).

- Always chance of recurrence.

- Talk through what to expect and recovery timeline (sometimes patients will have upcoming golf tournaments, or family events, etc., so make sure they know all that before starting the procedure).

- Usually, patients are excited for procedures to be done, but some can be nervous/anxious. Try to get a read on their comfort level, and consider what you're going to be doing. For instance, locally anesthetizing genitals hurts a lot and will bleed (especially if they're already anxious about it at baseline [higher blood pressure = more bleeding]). Be mindful of possible abuse/trauma. If they're not enthusiastically on board about a lesion on their genitals being removed and/or if it's a big lesion or something, might be better to just have them get it removed in OR under sedation with plastics.

Positioning patient:

- Be very picky about positioning; find one that works best for you, then find one that works well for the patient.

  - For perspective, you'll likely be doing procedures for 30 years; the patient will be there for 30 minutes.

    – For example, for a back excision, probably better for your posture to have patient sit up vs. lie down like getting a massage (though patient has higher chance of vagal-ing sitting up—has already happened to me a couple of times).

5.1.1 Numbing

Best to do yourself (vs. someone else), because you will lose a lot of valuable info by not doing the numbing (such as getting a sense of how deep their skin is; hydrodissecting cysts, which makes the cutting way easier; limiting bleeding to improve vision).

The nerves are in the dermis, so aim pretty superficial (same as biopsy).

Want to see the skin balloon up/turn whitish, but realize it can still balloon up if you inject in fat (thus, always test whether they're numb before cutting).

When testing if they're numb, just inject small amounts while doing this— will save time (if they say it hurts, you're already in and can just inject more).

Injecting some extra local in the middle of the lesion after numbing the periphery can also help reduce bleeding further. Sometimes, should consider waiting a few minutes (until the pinpoint bleeding stops) to really let the epinephrine work if the patient is on a blood thinner or if you're working on a really vascular area.

If anticipating cutting deep (where different nerves are), warn that patient may require extra anesthetic and proactively ask them to let you know if they feel sharp pains at any point.

Also warn patients extra when numbing areas like the lips that can hurt pretty bad.

5.1.2 Cutting

Will re-emphasize that good closures start with good incisions.

- Draw things out perfect—be picky, and do it before numbing, or it will be hard to see the tumor/lesion (skin will get pale and you won't be able to palpate anything).
  - If working in a very small area, you can use a blade to file down the marker tip to make it finer (set yourself up for success).
  - You can also pull the marker tip out if you're in a small area that's tough to finesse a long marker.
- Want to orient in a low-tension area/direction.
- Draw it out in the proportions it's supposed to be, particularly in the beginning (length should be 3× the diameter of the lesion); this helps avoid the standing soft tissue cone deformities (dog ears) that happen when it's too wide at the ends (which look worse than longer scars).
  - Might be able to get away with doing less than 3× diameter in length (being more diamond-shaped) and not getting cones on places like the face (since the dermis is thinner).
  - Include the size of the marker tip in the margin (because you should be cutting outside of the marker for tissue specimens).
  - I like to press the alcohol pad (or chlorhexidine, etc.) down instead of doing a scrubbing motion, so the marker doesn't get blurry—unless there's impetigo-like crusty stuff, then you should scrub that off and redraw it. Chlorhexidine great except for eyes/ears.
- Get good tension, and try to get to subQ in one cut (don't want to cut, readjust, cut, readjust, etc.).
  - Harder for the back because dermis is so thick (thus, probably should use a 10 blade for the back).
  - If need to recut to get to fat or release tethers, hug the non-tumor side of the skin with your scalpel when re-cutting to avoid shelving.
  - Shelves (look like staircase) can occur if:
    - Retraction not equal (epidermis/dermis slides around).
    - Too much cutting and looking (moving skin, etc., and blade doesn't stay straight).
- Don't bevel (cut straight up and down [90-degree angle to skin]; only time bevel potentially is in the hair [in direction of hair follicles], and for Mohs, of course).
  - Ideally, when you cut the ellipse out, it will have squared-off walls (90-degree walls) and a flat bottom (all same depth) (in other words, you should only see epidermis and subQ if looking straight down).

- If you do bevel (common tendency), you can reverse it with the scalpel.

- Sometimes, beveling can also happen if you pull traction to the sides (in other words, if you're going to cut with manual traction, best to pull the tissue in the same direction you're cutting [up and down, not side to side]).

■ Want to free the tips and get the "island" of tumor before grabbing pickups.

• After getting the island, better to maintain the natural orientation/ direction of the specimen when taking it (don't flap the specimen down, because will obscure the depth and make harder to cut at same depth across entire specimen).

• If you're assisting, release traction when surgeon is taking the specimen.

■ After removing the lesion, you'll usually want/need to undermine (loosen the skin to help it come together better).

• You should undermine in even plane (usually at level of subQ; one exception is the scalp: want to undermine at subgalea because that area is avascular [less bleeding] and because the dermis down there is more fibrous [easier for sutures to grab onto vs. thinner dermis, where all the hair follicles are]—need to grab subgalea with sutures or won't come together well/will slide apart).

• Look up the undermining planes before you operate obviously; this should be part of your prep/planning. Knowing the planes for various anatomic sites is worth knowing for exams too.

– Other planes that aren't subQ: nose (submuscular), periorbital (above orbicularis oculi), ear (just superficial to perichondrium).

■ Always anticipate things; if you accidentally cut a vessel, put pressure on it immediately.

• If not done cutting, hold pressure and finish cutting, then cauterize (more time under pressure + specimen won't get inadvertently mis-handled while handling something else).

• Holding pressure and having plentiful gauze within reach on the sterile field are perfect jobs for an assistant—so if there's bleeding and you're not operating, make yourself useful.

■ Generally better to not cut fat if don't have to; risk fat necrosis -> infection risk.

5.1.3 Suturing
5.1.3.1 General Things

■ Be mindful of where you lay the sutures, especially when handing them to attending if you're assisting (sterile field).

■ *FYI*: The straight scissors are for cutting suture (whereas the curved scissors are for cutting tissue—if trying to create a tunnel/tissue plane to make easier to dissect around, helps to turn the scissors to the side so you don't get too superficial or too deep).

■ Don't leave tails on deeps (cut sutures close to the knot); only leave tails on tops (shorter tails for face compared to the trunk or legs, etc.).

• If scissors aren't cutting well, turn them slightly or push with thumb (to make the blades come closer together); you can also try cutting further up the scissors, but it's probably better to be precise and use the ends of the blades when possible.

■ Try to avoid leaving long tails to cut (wasting suture); pull it further through before knotting/trimming the tails.

• If pulling it through too far (almost all the way through—which is easier than you think, especially when the tissue is moving), push the suture from the long side instead of trying to grab and pull the really short tail.

■ Be very gentle with the forceps (only use it to move skin [basically as a skin hook], not gripping it).

• Should use them as close to epidermis as possible (want to maximize visibility of dermis to give yourself a full view for suturing).

■ If you don't like a stitch, take it out and re-do it (especially on a location that needs to be perfect, like a lip or eyelid)—perfection is better than speed (speed will come with time/experience).

5.1.3.2 Nomenclature Basics and Choosing Appropriate Sutures

Possible hot take, but in my opinion, learning a lot of the basic testable content (like pliability, coefficient of friction, etc.) is not a great use of your time (particularly in the beginning) (although it's still worthwhile learning/knowing eventually). Same with learning all the different wound dressings and their properties/nuances (another big industry). Doing that would be like spending hours reading about how to hit a golf ball (better to just go do it). The more you practice with sutures (and the more you see them being used), the more you'll start to develop an intuition (which also gives the properties clinical context).

Needle:

■ Higher numbers = smaller (and weaker/more susceptible to being bent).

• For example, PS-4 needle is a smaller curved than PS-3.

■ Conventional PC cutters vs. reverse cutters.

• The way you steer needle is different (with conventional cutters, you enter flatter).

– Thus, PC needles don't require the use of pickups as much, because can rest on tissue without it cutting it.

• Reverse cutters are good when something tight and want to pull; harder to get eversion right because have to enter at 90-degree angle.

Suture:

■ Higher numbers = smaller (applies to both suture diameter and needle size; for example, 3–0 is smaller diameter than 2–0 suture).

- Also depends on material.

  - A 4–0 Prolene is smaller than 4–0 gut (because Prolene is stronger, so takes less diameter relatively to offer same strength).

■ Monofilament (such as Monocryl) = moves through tissue easily, less inflammation, but decreased knot security; easier for it to snap (may struggle with high-tension areas, like the scalp).

  - Monocryl's T50 (loses 50% tensile strength) is 7 days (most likely to dehisce at 10 days); Vicryl's T50 is 21 days (in other words, its suture material lasts longer).

■ Multifilament (braided, such as Vicryl) = strong, secure, but more infections + inflammation (higher risk of spitting—but still, if it occurs, it's because you're not putting them deep enough).

  - Vicryl better than Monocryl for tight spots (snaps less because it's braided); recommend pulling the suture all the way through after each bite (probably for all suture types, but especially for braided).

Overall, choosing sutures depends on location (how much tension and how much suture the location can tolerate).

■ For example, scalp is high-tension (will probably snap with 2–0 Vicryl, for instance; 3–0 Vicryl PS-2 is a good choice for scalp).

■ For example, thin atrophic sun-damaged elderly arms won't tolerate a huge needle.

■ Good place to start: 4–0 Monocryl anywhere on head/neck (unless around eyelids or somewhere really low tension, can use 5–0); trunk, 3–0 Vicryl (usually thick dermis under high tension).

  - Be mindful of patient characteristics that vary, such as habitus.

    - Heavy breasts need stronger sutures.

    - Obese people need deeper dermal sutures or will fall apart.

5.1.3.3 Closing (Primary)

■ Control bleeding first (see Hemostasis section in Chapter 5).

■ Best to stand perpendicular to closure line.

■ Always close with patient in position of maximal tension (full extension of arm, bending over a pillow for back/scapula, etc.).

■ Start suturing from the highest point so you don't have to contend with blood (gravity).

■ Similarly, consider starting cutting from the lowest point (for same reason).

5.1.3.3.1 Deeps

■ The more dermis you grab (bigger bites), the less suture used, the less gaps, and the more eversion (usually good, but *FYI*: Still possible to grab too much dermis).

- The perceived purpose of eversion is to take tension off epidermis as skin contracts when it heals. So if working on a location where skin is already loose/lax, the eversion isn't going to have enough tension to pull it back down, anyway (in other words, there's no tension on the epidermis by nature of the location—for example, might be better just putting tops in on the ears, eyelids, glabella, etc.). Would also avoid hyper-eversion on neck + chest (prone to keloid); most everywhere else, eversion is generally good.

- If space is small, don't need to bite much dermis (so no need to struggle trying to take a big bite in small opening).

■ Close dead space (usually need to do when removing a large space-occupying lesion, like a big cyst or lipoma, etc.).

- Basically, grab deep dermis (but above the level of the bottom of the defect) and do a deep stitch; should look like you can just glue the top, because the epithelial edges should basically be sitting together/touching each other.

- If you don't, will get crater (depressed scar), and possibly seromas/infections; don't trade bumps for holes.

- Can do plicating sutures (like a horizontal mattress, grabbing fascia, muscle, etc. and pulling together), which also reduce tension for the dermal sutures (good for backs and older people's sun-damaged arms).

■ Need to enter and exit at the same levels or will get step-off (uneven heights).

- To correct (minor) step-offs, can do high-to-low stitch (which is basically just evening it out by compensating in other direction; lift up the deeper side with the pickups to make the bite on that side deeper), but overall, it's best to just take out the stitch and make sure it's done right.

- Enter and exit perpendicular to the wound edge (helps make the scar straight); you should almost have to curve it a little bit to stay true to this, especially for fatter ellipses.

  – This is particularly true for areas that absolutely need to be perfect, such as lips, eyelids, etc. (because it's so easy to notice small imperfections).

■ You want the sutures to be heart-shaped when the knot is tied; so basically want to enter the side of the wound closest to you via undermined surface, move the needle up (almost until you can see it through the skin), then point the needle back down so you exit via the reticular dermis (basically with the needle pointing away from the epidermis); then mirror that path on the other side of wound. Helps if you manipulate the skin (with your forceps hand) rather than trying to do all that with the needle driver hand alone (can almost evert the skin when taking the far bite so you enter deeper than the DEJ, but the skin is positioned so that you just have to push the needle straight forward to get the arced path).

- Grab the needle at a consistent place (because want the same arc/path) to get the mirror image.

- Traditionally, you'll be taught to grab the needle ~1/3 the way down with your drivers, and take your bites at a distance (from the wound) equal to half the remaining ~2/3 of the needle.
  - If you grab the needle too high, the suture has higher chance of coming off the hook, but if you grab too low, you won't have as much needle to work with.
- Simulate the approximation via the sutures by pushing skin together—this will help you determine where to take your bites.
  - Can stick forceps in wound and open them up to find widest point (to help identify where to take bites).
- If sutures cross the wound bed too superficially, they can spit.

■ Want suture tails to be on the same side (relative to the part of the suture that went through each side of the wound bed) before tying the knots.

■ Everyone seems to do their knot sequence differently. Just do whatever ones your attending does and see which ones you like.

- Granny knots = basically a string wrapped around a straight string (unravels, but easier to move to where you want).
- Square knots = looks like first knot in shoelace.
- I personally like 2 grannies, then 2 squares; works well if struggle with knot slipping in high-tension areas like back or scalp (can pull only the shorter end [only pull on the side that doesn't have the needle] to push the second granny knot down and approximate skin without "locking the knot" above the wound).
  - If the knot slips, can also have assistant pinch the knot (or push and hold skin together).
  - If the suture keeps snapping because the wound is too high tension, undermine more.
- Good to practice on large strings (like drawer strings on your scrubs), so you can see what the knots are actually doing.

■ If struggle with wide areas, go to narrow areas (more closely approximated areas).

- Some people start on the ends, anyway (to help avoid soft tissue cones).

■ Pull knots parallel to wound.

- Make sure the first knot is pretty tight (deep) on deeps (whereas on tops, don't need the first knot to be super tight).

■ Closures shouldn't have any room to stick instruments through.

- If have open areas, put simple interrupted on top at the end (if you leave it open, Dermabond/bacteria will get in and will likely get infected + open sutures).

■ After finishing putting in deeps, make sure to check that there is no epidermis overhanging (loupes help); if there is overhanging tissue, trim it off with tissue scissors; otherwise, won't heal as well (overhanging exposed dermis also tends to bleed).

Knot Techniques

So many. These are the ones I'd learned to start with. To be honest, though, it's more effective/efficient to watch videos than me trying to explain via text.

Deeps:

■ Simple buried

　• Minimal eversion, high spitting rate.

■ Running subQ.

　• Running them in superficial dermis (not epidermal surface).

　• Less track marks, but spitting suture risk, usually used with buried vertical mattress.

　• Don't overlap (always stay in front); otherwise, will be hard to pull out when heals (and will hurt for the patient).

■ Purse string

　• Makes the scar a small dot instead of a line

　• Faster to heal, more to take care of for patient, though

　• Small superficial bites, overlap the last bite; only for cheeks/lips (not temple/nose). Let patient know will be bumpy, circular scar.

5.1.3.3.2 Tops

Top sutures don't matter as much if everything has gone perfect, but one should strive to make them look perfect regardless (it's obviously what the patient sees).

Can do dissolvable vs. non-dissolvable—most patients prefer dissolvable, and that way, you don't have to worry about track marks.

Obviously, try to avoid cutting the deeps when you put in the tops, but if you do, make sure you correct it and/or say something (feels like resistance when trimming the sutures, so the assistant is usually best positioned to notice, unless they're cut by the needle by the person suturing [you can sometimes almost see where the deeps are if you look closely at the sides of the wound—loupes help]).

Consider interrupted tops (vs. running) for super-tight places.

Bites should also be wider on forearms/back than on face (enter and exit further from wound).

Take really small bites on eyelids, because heals fast and don't want it to heal everted. Can stay pretty superficial.

Don't catch fat in top sutures -> fat will die, necrose, get infected.

Knot techniques that are good to start with:

■ *Simple interrupted*

　• For moderate- to high-tension wounds; pointing needle away from wound -> more eversion (less sunken scars).

- I almost curve my hand the other way to get 90-degree angle entry.
  - Except on the neck or chest, where I enter much flatter, almost like a scooping motion (because don't want much if any eversion on these sites).

- *Simple running*—looks like baseball stitch.
  - For minimal tension, dehiscence risk.
  - Faster because don't have to cut every stitch.
  - Shouldn't be too tight, just enough to slide instrument underneath.

- *Running locked* (intentionally loop it through previous stitch).
  - Provides hemostasis, strangulation risk.

- *Vertical mattress*
  - Strongly everts, eliminates dead space, decreases wound edge tension.

- *Horizontal mattress*
  - Provides hemostasis, eliminates dead space, decreases wound edge tension, better eversion; high strangulation risk (thus use mostly in highly vascular areas—such as scalp).

Dermabond is another option but in general makes worse scars than dissolvable sutures on face (not really the body, except hands [use nylon because hands move so much] and perineum [can use chromic because train tracks aren't as big a deal]).

Good for older people (they don't have to come back in for suture removal, and they have less dermis, so less scarring).

5.1.4 Hemostasis

Proactivity >> reactivity. Let the lidocaine with epinephrine help you (see earlier text). Know the anatomy.

Don't just rely on the Bovie for everything.

Should know the differences between the electrosurgery terms (*electrocautery* vs. *electrodesiccation*, etc.). Here I'm referring to stopping the bleeding (so either electrocautery [handheld thing for patients with pacemakers] or electrocoagulation [the Bovie]).

Make sure you understand how the instruments actually work.

- If using Bovie and it's not stopping the bleeding (and you're convinced you're aiming correctly), make sure you're pushing the correct button (coag vs. cut).

- If you're using the bipolar cautery (no grounding pad, has two forceps tips), then the circuit is between the two tips (in other words, it won't do anything if the tips are touching or if they're too far apart).

- "Measure twice, cut once" mentality—look where bleeding is coming from, and only get that part. Be very precise. Drawbacks of cautery: necrosis -> infection risk, scar burden, cost.
  - Can pinch the bleeding vessels with forceps and touch the cautery to the forceps.

- A little oozing of dermal walls is probably fine—will likely stop via tamponade with sutures and pressure.

- Just don't want high-pressure stuff or really deep bleeding/pooling of blood.

In general, it's best to limit the cautery. Placing dissolvable sutures is an alternative option (pressure slows the bleeding, allowing it to clot). For mid-procedure bleeding, can place figure of eight stitch (basically like two simple interrupted without cutting after the first).

When holding pressure to stop oozing, wet gauze is more effective than dry gauze (dry gauze basically rips the platelets off).

5.1.5 Peri-Operative Considerations

- If sutures burst <24 hours, restitch, unless infected (can be the reason the sutures burst sometimes); still give antibiotics.

- If >24 hours, assume infected, do secondary intention; of course, give antibiotics.

- If concerned for infection on ear, should probably give ciprofloxacin (higher risk for *Pseudomonas*).

  - Almost everywhere else, doxycycline or clindamycin would probably be fine.

5.1.6 Bandaging + Post-Care

- Do pressure dressing for patients on AC (leave on for 48 hours, or if complex, then can leave bandage on for 1 week).

  - Basically, apply Vaseline then Telfa pad (or some non-adherent pad) on top of wound, then gauze (to add pressure), then MedFix tape or similar.

- For legs, use Coban (or Unna boot [basically a zinc paste bandage] if poor healer).

- Combo of Tylenol and ibuprofen (or naproxen) is better than opioids (make sure no liver or kidney issues before recommending).

- No topical antibiotics (don't work).

- Pain peaks 4–6 hours after surgery.

  - If extended or excruciating pain, not likely normal -> might have infection or hematoma

- Sutures (if non-absorbable) should be removed 5–7 days on face, or 10–14 days on trunk/extremities.

5.2 ELECTRODESICCATION AND CURETTAGE (EDC)

Commonly oversimplified. Highest risk for failure due to the user (you), because remember, you're not checking path, so in some ways they take more skill/acumen to successfully clear than an excision, where the margins/planes are well-defined and the specimen is checked histologically. Technically are really more like "curettage and hyfrecation" (because you scrape first and it's best to not actually make contact [which would be desiccation]).

Get a good outline of the tumor and margin before you numb (it's really easy to lose sight of tumor after you numb/start scraping). *FYI*: If your curette is 3 mm (a reasonable margin for a low-risk BCC), just scrape a donut to a good depth right outside the pen marking first—accomplishes the margin (recurrences tend to occur on the periphery) and preserves the outline of the tumor. Then continue scraping from the outside inward (if you scrape from the middle outward, you may lose track of your margins once you scrape through the marker). Be precise with scraping margins (both peripherally and deep).

Most curettes only cut in one direction.

- Sharp side is opposite of the rough-textured marking (point the rough texture end from you, and it will cut as you move it towards you).

- Scrape with curette relatively flat (maybe like 30 degrees or so relative to skin).

- Stay oriented to the skin plane; otherwise, will get shreds.

- The rotten apple stuff is the tumor. Scrape until all that is gone and feels like you're scraping normal skin (the texture will change, and the sound it makes changes too [sounds like you're scraping something rough vs. smooth rotten apple stuff]).

- Don't scrape into fat—will not heal well (so be mindful of site). If scrape too deep, then convert to excision.

Hyfrecate the entire base. Do the scrape and burn twice each.

5.3 INCISION & DRAINAGE (I&D)

1. Wipe with EtOH pad.

2. Drape.

3. Numb (will re-iterate staying superficial when numbing; if you inject the anesthesia into the actual cyst, you could rupture the cyst if it's too much volume).

4. Make incision (doesn't necessarily need to be that long but may need to be deeper than you think, especially if on the back); 11 blades are nice because they're pointy.

5. Push (may need to push pretty hard).

6. Watch out (the pus might come flying out in unpredictable directions)—wear goggles/gown/hat, especially if wearing nice clothes and/or have long hair.

Milial cyst extractions are similar, but on a much smaller scale, obviously. Don't really need to drape or numb, because only superficially nicking the cyst (18 blades are good unless they're big milia, then could use an 11). Using comedone extractors to get the contents out can be game-changing (vs. trying to squeeze it out with your fingers). Let patient know may cause bruising (generally heals within ~10 days) and be mindful of direction/orientation of incision (for example, if on lip, make the incision vertically—heals better).

5.4 EXCISIONS

See cutting/suturing sections. Need to know all that stuff. The following pertains more to specific stuff about things you'll be excising.

I find malignant lesions more straightforward to excise than some benign lesions (like cysts, lipomas). Know the margins, get good at estimating mm (should probably measure everything out with a ruler in the beginning—and obviously no shame in doing that even if you're already experienced).

Sometimes patients will show up with no visible tumor (all removed from biopsy or something). You can consider monitoring (usually if recurs, it recurs quickly) vs. EDC, though you should consider site (hard to self-monitor lesion on back; excision makes more sense than EDC on a sun-damaged forearm since going to fat, anyway).

Backs are good to learn on because not many structures you have to worry about but can be tight (harder to approximate if you don't undermine enough). Arms are also good for learning.

5.4.1 Benign Lesions

Most of the following details are in reference to EICs, though many of the concepts will help you with pilar cysts and lipomas as well (will briefly cover some specifics of these at the end of the section).

5.4.1.1 Epidermal Inclusion Cysts (EICs)

Few options:

1. Can inject ILK to shrink them first and have them RTC later for excision.

   a. Want to inject the ILK into the cyst, not around it.

2. Can cut around the cyst and take the surrounding tissue (like a regular elliptical excision).

   a. Quick, but may not have the luxury if really big on the face.

3. Can find the cyst capsule and dissect around the capsule—probably the best way.

   a. One advantage is if you stay along the capsule, you will never cut into important stuff like nerves.

To determine the best approach, get idea for what condition the lesion is in:

■ If infected: treat with antibiotics, and don't cut for at least 3 months, maybe even 6–12 months (if you try to cut it out when still in fibrosis phase 2 weeks after finishing antibiotics, you'll be frustrated—it will be sticky, tears easily, fibrotic, etc.).

   • If patient wants removed, then you should cut around the cyst and take the surrounding tissue (like a regular elliptical excision).

■ If inflamed cyst -> likely scarred -> do wider excisions.

■ If neither infected nor inflamed, then the dissecting around the capsule is probably the best method.

No matter the approach, you need to make sure the punctum from the skin surface is included in what you cut out. This is another advantage to dissecting around the cyst, because you can dissect from one side only first, then pull on the capsule to help dimple the punctum (sometimes it's not super visible without doing this). Cut from side, you can see best with scalpel aimed away from cyst (almost like reverse bevel).

Dissecting around capsule:

■ First, draw the borders of the cyst (by feeling it), and outline the overall size; then draw the ellipse inside of that circle to mark where you'll be cutting, then numb outside the overall cyst outline you drew (for bleeding control), then numb over top the cyst (for hydrodissection)—need to inject very superficial, should see the skin turn pale and will see tiny little pops as it dissects through; this is how you know you're not in the cyst.

  • If the lidocaine squirts out of the punctum, it means you're injecting into the cyst (don't want because could rupture the cyst if injecting too much in it).

  • Tempting to want all the glory to come from the cutting, but hydrodissection can make the cutting/dissecting so much easier (helps you get in the right plane).

■ First cut is pretty superficial, obviously want to avoid cutting into the cyst (need to ensure in right plane—this is where you'll notice how big a help hydrodissection is).

■ Need great vision (make sure you cut a long enough superficial incision); need enough space to manipulate the position of the cyst.

■ Traction and countertraction are key—utilize hooks, and use the skin surface as a handle to the capsule.

  • Best to grab the triangle of skin that the cyst is attached to in order to manipulate the cyst, but if you choose to handle the actual cyst, then better to do so with blunter pickups (take big bites where it's most robust [don't grab small bites near the top, where the pore comes out to the skin because the capsule is weaker there]).

    – Pilar cysts (moderately hardier than EICs) and lipomas (much hardier than EICs) can usually withstand manipulation with the forceps without ripping; can also tolerate pushing on the surrounding skin when trying to squeeze them out.

    – Don't try to push on skin to squeeze out an EIC (it'll likely burst, and you'll end up with malodorous purulence on yourself).

    – When you do try to squeeze out lipomas/pilar cysts, make sure your incision is big enough (they can obviously still rupture), and that you dissect it out enough (the pushing on surrounding skin/ squeezing them out is more of a final step than a key step).

    – For pilar cysts, have to dissect out ~50% before trying to pop them out.

  • Use gauze to hold slippery stuff (such as cyst, lipoma, etc.).

■ Scalpel is good for dissecting tight stuff.

  • Try touching blade on soft skin without tension—it won't cut/cause damage; thus, perfect for working on scarred cyst (if it was inflamed, infected, if they picked at it, attempted to self-extract, been there for multiple years, etc.—thus important to ask these questions before starting).

■ Want to paint the blade against the spiderweb stuff around the capsule (begging fibers).

- Take advantage of the sharpness of the blade (never stab into tissue).

- Can also use a Q-tip to bluntly dissect.

■ Scissors good for dissecting soft stuff (pulling soft stuff from hard stuff), so NOT good for scarred cyst because will rupture the cyst; want it full so you can see the sack and make sure you get it all.

- Can also turn scissors sideways to help dissect the spiderweb stuff.

■ Want to get underneath the red shiny, filmy stuff when dissecting (it's scarier to be right on the cyst, but it's actually safer and will make for a better dissection).

- If you dissect between the red shiny, filmy stuff and the surrounding tissue, it'll be too hard to cleanly separate, and it'll bleed more (so want to be as close to the cyst as possible).

  – Same concept for lipomas, although it is more a whitish, filmy capsule stuff than red.

- Once you're in the right plane (right against the cyst), you can do more snipping (vs. scissor spreading), but make sure you orient the scissors away from the cyst.

■ If you rupture the cyst and lose tension, then can cut around cyst and stay in dermis; probably should irrigate with saline.

- Obviously, ideally never pop the cyst, but if you do pop the cyst, try to at least not do it before getting around it some (because it's going to be a lot harder to differentiate the cyst from surrounding tissue).

- Also, if you pop the cyst, the best plane is no longer right on the cyst (you'll have to go a little bit wider around it [leave the red filmy stuff on it] to ensure not leaving any behind).

5.4.1.2 Lipomas

The preceding passage applies to lipomas, too, for the most part. Make sure you excise the tumor and its fibrous capsule fully. Be careful of lipomas on scalp—tend to sit below or above nerves (so be suspicious if complaining of pain), and be extra cautious with cutting (make sure to discuss with patient, too, before operating). These can be tough to remove correctly from the scalp (much harder than pilar cysts and EICs). Harder to misdiagnose superficial lipomas, but if you think something is a cyst and don't see a capsule, think what else it might be; go straight down where you feel it. If you get to the fat without seeing a capsule, then it's probably a lipoma.

5.4.1.3 Pilar Cysts

Pilar cysts are hardier and even more superficial than EICs, so much easier because can just pop them out (these sometimes only take ~5–10 minutes).

Same process as the earlier benign lesions: outline the cyst via feel, numb around the cyst, and then over top of it, very superficially hydrodissect (again, use this as an opportunity to get a sense for skin thickness—if the pilar cyst is very small, you should maybe anticipate that you'll need to make a slightly deeper incision than a large pilar cyst, since a large one will essentially stretch out the skin). The incision will be a straight line (vs. an ellipse-shaped in EICs, since no punctum to cut out) and very superficial (let the weight of the blade do the cutting and only hold it tight enough so that it doesn't move—this will help keep you up against the cyst [which is obviously curved]; if you hold with a death grip, then you're essentially just guessing the plane of the cyst and have much higher risk of cutting through it). Need to dissect them ~50% before popping them out (spread the scissors more aggressively at the corners of the incision since you know there won't be any cyst there [based on your outline]). Want to dissect right on the cyst just like EICs (under the red filmy stuff, which you can grab with the forceps to help get under them). You shouldn't really ever have to cut around these/do regular elliptical excisions that include surrounding tissue. Staples are good for the scalp (obviously, explain to patients that you're not doing it out of laziness but because staples are gentler on hair follicles than sutures [lower risk of localized scarring alopecia]). Helps to put a deep stitch in the middle before stapling so you can line it up better (easier to leave longer tails in the hair [before cutting] so you don't lose them in their hair [obviously, still cut at the same place, as always do, at the knot for deeps, and leave small tails if decided to put in tops]). Other things I recommend when suturing the scalp: pull the short-tail suture (needleless side) straight up (like 90 degrees with respect to the scalp surface) before you let go of it, so it doesn't get lost in the hair; keep your hands high and pull the knots straight down to avoid catching hairs (the body hates keratin products [just look at the histology of a ruptured cyst—will allow you to appreciate how good surgical technique can avoid a lot of unnecessary inflammation]); try to limit blotting (for the same reason, since it will basically be pushing hairs into the wound), try to avoid catching follicles when you put in tops (otherwise will cause more scarring alopecia). If doing a primary closure on the scalp and it's tight and fatty (which is hard because doesn't bite very well), you might have to put in vertical mattresses in the middle to give you any hope of getting deeps in. Just get as many as you can in, and warn them about the possibility of scarring alopecia in that area.

5.5 MOHS

Mostly for NMSCs (some melanoma and rarer tumors, like DFSPs, etc.). Of course, different from regular excisions. Layers are processed differently (flattened), so see 100% of peripheral and deep margins (vs. regular excisions—only see a slice of bread loaf; so *FYI*: When margins are clear in a regular excision, there is still a decent chance there is residual tumor that just wasn't seen [albeit *FYI*: That doesn't mean has a high chance of recurrence]).

The layers are frozen sections (not sectioned permanently like excisions/ biopsy specimens [which take much longer to process]).

The best thing to do to truly understand how the tissue is processed is probably to watch the histotechnicians do what they do in person (vs. trying to figure it out from visualizing a diagram).

General things:

■ Debulk tumor before taking first Mohs layer, because need full histologic characterization to know if there are high-risk features.

  • Use unbroken double-edge blade (or whatever you use for shave biopsy) for larger tumors to make this easier.

■ Bevel 45 degrees when taking the layers (different from excisions)—needed for histotechnicians to lay down epidermis so 100% of the margins can be seen (basically looking at the wrapper of a Reese's peanut butter cup).

  • Most will recommend undoing the bevel before closing (though some people say you don't have to).

■ After making the incisions around the periphery of the layer, you should score it (make orientation marks).

  • Most do the double score toward the superior helix, but the important thing is that you stay consistent in the way you do it (in case you lose your scores or if the marker disappears, etc., which shouldn't happen but still need contingencies).

    – Obviously, maintaining orientation is crucial, as the process basically fails without it.

  • Want to make scoring marks on both the specimen and the peri-wound epidermis (slightly more on the tissue specimen side).

  • After scoring, you can take the deep part of the layer (just like you take a regular excision).

■ Taking more layers has higher risk of recurrence (risks becoming more disoriented and probably also inherently a tough tumor if needing many layers).

■ Floater tumors—tumor cells that are dislodged during processing (can confound interpretation).

■ A "take and close" = when pretty confident you can get the tumor out with one more stage and close it up before confirming (before the tissue is processed and viewed).

5.5.1 Closures and Basics of Flaps/Grafts

Should first think: Appropriate to second intent? If not, then appropriate to do a primary closure? If not, then do a graft/flap.

5.5.1.1 Second Intent

Good areas for second intent = shallow, concave areas (nose [but not the tip], alar crease [but not where it bulges out], medial canthus [books say best when half defect is above and half is below a perpendicular line from the medial canthus], scalp [unless they have hair, because will get bald spot], temples if not close to eyebrow [if too close, will contract and pull eyebrow], ear might be OK but often gets tender/infected [definitely don't second intent when involves cartilage; in that case, you'd need to graft]). Also not good on free margins (will pull and distort the free margin).

Mucosal lip does well second-intenting if shallow (if above muscle). If into muscle, then have to stitch; otherwise, will drool and won't be able to purse lips together. Older people do especially well on mucosal lip (they don't have great vermillion borders vs. younger people, who have more well-defined ones).

Bad areas: deep, convex areas, near free margins.

Also depends on patient.

Pros: no restriction of activity (except first day, because don't want them to bleed), minimal pain.

Cons: can bleed (don't want to cauterize because won't second-intent nicely if damaging dermal structures, so need good pressure dressing).

Second-intenters should probably RTC Q 1 week; if re-epithelializing faster than filling in, then can curette the edges (to delay it again and let it fill in more)—but will have to numb it again. Some people dermabrade the edges before letting them second intent (instead of curetting).

5.5.1.2 *Primary Closures*

Mostly covered earlier in the Suturing section. Will obviously be doing more on face in Mohs than regular excisions, though.

5.5.1.3 *Grafts*

- More post-op restrictions for the patient.

- When preparing to take a full thickness graft, use the blood in the defect as ink to mark the size (press a Telfa pad or something white [such as the paper that the suture comes in] on the wound you're looking to graft).

  - Then cut around the blood markings on the Telfa pad or whatever you used.

  - Set that wherever you're taking the donor site, and circle it with a marker (can draw out the full ellipse after that if planning to close the donor site that way).

  - Then cut the negative margin (inside of the marker lines) to get your graft, before carefully placing it in sterile saline and getting hemostasis at the donor site.

- Thinner grafts are more likely to survive (if doing a large graft especially, then want it to be thinner)—but looks worse (will look white and thin because not getting the dermal structures that give skin it's normal look).

- Cut off all the fat to reduce metabolic demand of graft, fenestrate it (poke holes in it) to make more stretchy (and lets blood spill over the graft instead of collecting under it, which would reduce contact with the wound bed and increase failure risk).

  - Always hold graft over sterile field (in case it falls out of your hand when you're prepping it).

- Conventionally should suture "ship to shore" (from the graft tissue to the peri-wound tissue, and take slightly smaller bite on graft and slightly bigger bite on peri-wound tissue), but as long as the dermis is lined up, then the direction you suture may not matter.

- Helps to put in a couple interrupted sutures on opposite sides of the graft to hold/position it before running it around the graft.

- After running it around the graft, can place an interrupted stitch in the middle to improve contact with wound bed (like anchoring it down).

- Should probably give antibiotics for most (or even all) grafts since, if gets infected, will fail.

- If graft fails, then have to second-intent and do dermabrasion or laser later.

FTSG (full-thickness skin graft): higher nutritional requirement (more structures) so higher risk of failure (thus pin graft down to bed, shave off fat, etc.).

STSG (split-thickness skin graft): need a machine (Zimmer Dermatome) which only takes a little bit of dermis; mostly for really big defects.

- *Cons*: hard to take (need several people to hold skin taut for it to run smooth); patients have a lot of pain, from where you take it for about 1 month (feels like road burn—because transecting so shallow mid-dermis, so nerves are right there).

- *Care*: Xeroform over the graft and Tegaderm; leave it on for months, then take Tegaderm off, and Xeroform will basically be stuck on, then when they grow new skin, the Xeroform falls off on its own.

- *Composite*: cartilage + skin; high risk of failing, only for tiny spots on rim of nose; cutout spots on ear (skin with cartilage attached), and don't fenestrate (don't want to poke holes in cartilage).

- *Free cartilage*: only taking cartilage, possibly second intent, or do a flap over it.

- *Good sites for grafts*: eyelids, nose, ears, big defects.

For nose, take from pre- or postauricular; same with ear. If eyelid, can sometimes take from upper eyelid or postauricular.

Smokers have higher risk of failed grafts since tissue is so tenuous; flaps sometimes do OK (except banners, which don't do well even in non-smokers), bilobed and nasalis slings generally do well (just ask them to cut down on smoking for a week), forehead flaps do fine, and cartilage ones likely would fail in smoker.

FYI: Dipping/chewing tobacco also problematic because still getting systemic vasoconstriction.

If graft sites are painful after the wound healing process, always consider SCC on ddx.

5.5.1.4 Flaps

Consider age of patient. Younger patients heal more robustly, so scars have more potential to look worse. If they're <55 years old, should be careful doing geometric flaps (such as rhombic, V-Y flaps, etc.). Better to do straight lines in these patients. Younger patients also have more stretchy elastic tissue so don't need to cut as much/far to advance tissues.

Local skin flap is where you have a hole, make an incision beside the hole, then slide the tissue into that hole (without cutting the tissue all the way out).

Interpolation flap = taking skin and attaching to defect, but there's a pedicle that's over normal skin (which needs to be removed a couple of weeks later).

Best to look up pictures and videos. A good amount of the technical specifics are oriented mostly for exams, but should still at least know the common ones and some basic principles to start:

- Purple skin = a good sign on flaps—means good blood supply.
- Too much fat with flaps can cause edema and festooning.
- Bilobed (usually lower nose or big cheeks).
- Rhombic (upper nose or big cheeks or medial canthal if deep [like if you can see tendon or something]).
- Banner (basically a long rhombic flap—thus, higher risk of failing [usually distal necrosis]).
- Interpolated (staged ones): leave bridge of connected skin for 3 weeks, then go back and cut it down; paramedian forehead, nasolabial, retroauricular, etc.
- Sliding flaps (not cutting them out, lifting them up, and turning them in like bilobed and transposition; essentially just scooching them in).
- Advancement flaps (sliding in one direction, no twisting); A->L, etc.
- Rotation flaps (twisting).

6 Cosmetics

6.1 BOTOX

For wrinkles, also good for hyperhidrosis, maybe Hailey–Hailey (probably more so hyperhidrosis in setting of Hailey–Hailey).

Usually, insurance wants you to state in note where it will be administered, the dose, and indication (if using it for hyperhidrosis, for instance; of course, insurance not relevant if for cosmetic purposes).

General Things

■ Fill the syringes half way vs. all the way (the needles dull pretty quickly).

■ Use wrench to pull off cap so can get all the residual Botox in the vial (it's very dense in value, so try to avoid wasting any, even if it's just a little bit).

■ Need the bacteriostatic normal saline (NS) (NOT sterile water, which would be super painful).

- Bacteriostatic NS has preservatives (benzyl alcohol, which has anesthetic properties) in it, so it hurts less.

  – Bacteriostatic NS is also multiple-dose (vs. preservative free NS, which is single-dose).

  – Use bacteriostatic also when injecting NS for ILK atrophy.

■ Try to avoid the leaky dripping (wasteful); inject, then pull out.

■ Takes 1–3 days for initial response, 2 weeks for full response, which lasts 3–4 months.

6.2 LASERS AND ENERGY-BASED DEVICES

Lasers work by targeting something (such as melanin, hemoglobin, water, ink particles, etc.).

6.2.1 Basic Principles

Basic science background.

Lasers are one wavelength, coherent (peaks and troughs are synchronized), and collimated (parallel).

Need something to excite the atoms that will release the photons (solid, liquid, gas, semiconductor, etc.), something doing the exciting (flash lamp), and something to harvest the photons you create (a cavity).

■ For example, a ruby laser has a ruby rod, a flash lamp, and a cavity that collects the photons.

- First, the flash lamp turns on, electrons get excited to higher energy state, then they return to normal energy state by releasing photons (this is what stimulated emission of radiation [the "SER" in laSER] is, which allows for light amplification).

Basic terminology:

1. *Continuous:* keeping on (vs. flickering it on and off).

2. *Pulse duration:* how long stays on.

 DOI: 10.1201/9781003537946-6

3. *Thermal relaxation time:* how long it takes to cool by 50% of the max temp it achieved compared to its baseline temp.

    a. Same concepts apply with LN2; pulsing helps limit collateral damage, especially for smaller lesions.

4. They refer to it as energy, but it's actually energy per cm².

    a. Higher energy = more pain.

    b. Should use a machine in which wavelengths are optimized well for targets so don't have to use as much energy (less painful for patient).

General principles:

When you hit the button, the slit opens and sends the photons to the target, which can either reflect (come back to you), transmit (go through the target), absorb (what you want—damage the target).

- So basically you want your laser to get absorbed by your target structure and transmit through surrounding structures (selective thermolysis).

  - To achieve this, each target has an absorption spectrum (which never changes) with certain peaks (absorbs stronger at certain wavelengths).

  - To destroy target, need correct wavelength, sufficient energy, and pulse duration < thermal relaxation time (don't want to pulse so long that it can't cool down and is forced to pass off [damage] surrounding tissue).

    - Smaller targets heat up faster than larger targets, so only need short pulses to heat small targets up.

    - However, sometimes you want to manipulate this concept to intentionally cause collateral damage when you want to destroy something that can't be targeted. For example:

      - Blood vessel (nothing can target the endothelium), thus want to heat RBC enough that it causes collateral damage to the blood vessel.

      - Hair shafts: nothing targets the hair shaft, so target melanin in hair bulb to destroy the follicle (thus why can't remove white depigmented hairs).

      - Don't wear sunscreen before laser—laser will see if has pigment in it.

  - Cooling skin before laser helps (because laser has to pass via surface of skin, which can heat it up, and surface of skin is, of course, usually not the target).

    - Direct contact cooling (sapphire window)—cools well.

    - Spray—need to keep laser perpendicular to skin so the mist hits it correctly (otherwise, will only cool a portion of it and can get crescent-shaped burns).

- When wavelength, pulse duration, fluence are not correct, can get complications.

- Look at pics of complications to gain appreciation of what lasers are capable of—if you develop an intuition for this, the rest should fall into place.
- Consider location, too, when adjusting settings.
  - For example, the neck doesn't have as many pilosebaceous units as the face (can blast face harder because has enough stem cells to regenerate skin).

COMPLICATIONS

For operators:

1. Make sure wearing the correct goggles for the machine.

   a. OD = optical density (want 4–6, ideally at least 5)—measure of how protected you are at the wavelength listed.

   b. Cannot just turn around during pulse; if it hits your lens, radiance can be magnified 100k-fold; if hits fovea, you can go blind.

2. Can get plumes with laser hair removal—do in well-ventilated room (and/or wear mask, use smoke evacuator, etc.). Sometimes chemicals that are released can be harmful.

3. Put into standby mode after using (not doing is most common cause of fire).

For patients:

4. Trying to get too much done per treatment, carrying over settings from one device to the next, poor understanding of laser or skin, poor post-care, etc. are all potential missteps.

5. Know if they have baseline skin issues.

   a. For example, aggressive resurfacing contraindicated in vitiligo because don't know how they'll react to it (Koebnerization), though excimer can actually be used to treat vitiligo (is in UV range).

   b. Always consider ACD; may be allergic to lanolin (in Aquaphor).

   c. Not just rashes, but skin cancers too.

      i. If patient presents with a lesion after multiple removal treatments with recurrence, might want to biopsy (could be a melanoma or something); another reason patients shouldn't go to med spas.

6. Understand their skin type.

   a. Probably good idea to pre-treat skin of color (although somewhat unclear if actually prevents hyperpigmentation).

      i. For example, hydroquinone before (maybe PO TXA); something occlusive that's not reactive (no preservatives, such as Vanicream, etc.).

   b. Should definitely do post-treatment in all patients.

      i. Lysteda (TXA) for time window at beginning, when can't put topical on (tretinoin, hydroquinone, etc.), and then betamethasone or clobetasol immediately after (to get redness/inflammation down, which is what causes issues) for 1 week (some start after resurfacing 1 day after).

7. Obviously understand the device you're using/procedure you're doing to anticipate issues.

   a. 1064 Nd:YAG: long pulsed is probably the most dangerous, penetrates deep and has high energy—can cause punched-out ulcers if not careful.

   b. Infection risk higher in ablative treatments because leaving skin exposed.

8. Realize tattoos aren't regulated—ink contents differ from shop to shop.

   a. Granulomatous reactions: little bumps.

      i. Most common color of tattoo for granulomatous reactions = red (cinnabar).

9. Encourage protein intake to assist with healing.

Endpoints:

  Skin is always talking to you about your settings (under vs. overtreating); different endpoints, depending on what you're targeting.

- Skin of color throws curveball for endpoints.

- Bad stuff: Nikolsky sign, stamping (if debris collects on the window of your device—basically will burn that stuff on your skin; especially in hair removal; thus, tell people to shave it all the way down, because we're going after their bulge center, not the hair shaft), puckering (means you're desiccating the skin), charring, Chrysiasis (if have gold, which they used to use for RA, can darken), reduction process of tattoos (can darken); anything that has white in it—such as if patient has pink tone (red mixed with white) in tattoo, be careful. If happens, then just immediately stop. Maybe YAG pulsing can get it out, though.

6.2.2 Intense Pulsed Light (IPL)

1. Broadband visible light (almost like a very strong light bulb).

   a. Not a laser (not collimated, not coherent).

   b. Emits light at different wavelengths (400–1,200 nm) but has filters (so can optimize absorption peaks and filter out everything else).

      i. For example, if you put a 515 nm filter on IPL, it will leave out from 400–515 and put out 515–1,200.

      ii. Thus, choose filter based on what you're trying to treat.

      iii. DNA is not a chromophore at any IPL wavelength; thus, no risk of NMSC and is fine for lupus, DM, etc. (vs. phototherapy, which would flare these).

         – DNA is a chromophore (strands break + get mutations) at 290–320 nm (UVB); thus, devices that emit these wavelengths (such as excimer) are technically carcinogenic to skin.

2. Glasses are usually dark for IPL because have to cover a lot of wavelengths (but there are lighter ones and ones with shutters, etc.).

    a. Important obviously because you need to see where you're pulsing (especially for IPL, because it builds up heat quickly [don't want to pulse in the same space; otherwise, will get ulcer]).

3. Treats red and brown—lentiginous brown and telangiectatic red and maculopapular erythema from rosacea.

    a. Can wipe out hair, so if treating men for rosacea, tell them to shave and stay out of bearded area (centrofacial/nose probably fine).

    b. May get redness, purpura, crusting; if patients get tan 3 days before, can injure them (so tell them avoid the sun before treatment).

        i. Smokers, sun worshippers, nonadherent patients, etc.—consider denying treatment.

4. Basically want hemoglobin heated so that vessel wall is heated and vessel is destroyed (so technically secondarily treating the vessel by "treating" the hemoglobin).

5. If have vessels, can see them coagulating (same with PDL)—but end point for IPL vessels is more like blurring (if heat vessel wall, endothelial cells shrink up -> vessels become porous, start to get edema, which is a good thing).

6. Keeping the epidermis cool is the best way to prevent thermal injury (soaks up heat that escapes from chromophore).

    a. Usually, the tip is cold (can see the condensation).

    b. Put bottle of gel on ice, so if heat escapes, then gel can absorb it.

        i. Gel also facilitates penetration into skin via acting as interface (more even penetration) since going from gas to solid.

    c. You can adjust the energy, the number of pulses (slight delay between pulses allows surrounding tissue to cool down while the target heats up).

7. If treating brown, background ideally stays normal (so skin shouldn't turn red); ideally, brown will turn darker within a few minutes, with a little bit of erythema around it.

8. If seeing a lot of background erythema after treating, can give post-op TAC (for the night and maybe the day after; can do clobetasol for skin of color or if have very intense reaction or had reaction due to sun in the past week) and sunscreen.

    a. If rosacea, tell them they will swell for maybe 1 day.

        i. Can consider PO prednisone (40 mg QD for 3 days, or 20 mg QD for 3 days—if you're really worried about swelling), ice packs when getting home, or all these.

        ii. Sometimes people are vasoactive at baseline (for example, patients with sensitive rosacea or dermatographism or flushed easily, etc.).

        iii. Can also get red from the topical anesthetic.

9. Harder to use than PDL but much less maintenance (PDL requires dye changes, constant maintenance, etc.).

a. If treating full face, IPL with vascular settings preferred over PDL, but if treating focal areas, like cheeks, PDL is fine.

b. IPL probably also better for poikiloderma of Civatte than PDL, but still not really that effective; very hard to treat.

6.2.3 PDL (Vbeam)—585 nm for Vascular Lesions

1. Can work for rosacea, angiomas, erythema from newly formed acne scars, port-wine stains, bruising after filler, etc.

2. Usually requires 3–4 treatments, spread out by 4–6 weeks; 70–80% chance they go away (genetics + sun exposure play a part).

3. For vascular erythema, want roughly 20% overlap (think Olympic rings).

   a. Stacked pulses are fine in PDL because can dissipate heat quickly (common to stack pulses in PDL V-beam); however, if you stack pulses with YAG, diode, etc., you will cause an ulcer.

4. Redness/swelling = endpoint for rosacea.

5. Angioma won't respond to vascular erythema settings (need to decrease pulse duration).

   a. Angiomas look bigger, but the vessel size is actually smaller than vascular/rosacea erythema (it's the same chromophore, but the chromophore is within a smaller vessel in an angioma).

      i. Since spot size is smaller, need higher fluence (higher energy per cm^2).

   b. After zapping angiomas, the color changes immediately from red to dusky (purple-black) after one zap (coagulants form, then falls off in 1–2 weeks).

      i. The next day will be more swollen; swelling/redness persists 3–5 days, then improves.

6. Port-wine stains: targets so small need such a small pulse duration that it causes purpura; don't want grayish blanching stuff (skin burn).

6.2.4 Nd:YAG—532 nm for Black Ink

1. If don't have, then use alexandrite; if don't have that, then use ruby.

   a. Think of it as photomechanical—firing so fast it's hitting the pigment mechanically vs. IPL (photothermal—gradually treating via heat).

   b. Yellow, pink, orange are hard to treat because don't have complementary colors, but picosec lasers fire so fast that they treat the particle (so maybe can get away with 532—wouldn't do with 1064, though).

   c. Black is usually easy because usually single color.

      i. If have dark skin and dark ink, need to be very precise more so than in light skin (because it's targeting the dark).

      ii. Don't want gaps, but don't want to stack pulses; bear in mind there is a little lateral spread from where you pulse.

- If you stack pulses, higher risk for dyschromia (most common complication with picosecond lasers) because of bulk heating, disrupt melanocytes (thus hypopigmentation).

- When the laser hits black ink particle, it causes a mini explosion -> N2 gas forms (frosty stuff that bubbles between ink and epidermis), which dissipates over time (~20 minutes the frosting is gone) -> tattoo turns red.

  - Thus, don't treat through the frosty stuff (the LN2 would block ability to get to the pigment, and all you would do is damage the epidermis).

  d. Faded tattoos = old (macrophages take it away—good thing, because less pigment).

  i. Nowadays, tattoos have higher density and depth (they pack them so high it's basically raised—which are hard to treat, so tell patient it's going to take many treatments and has risk disrupting epidermis because pigment so high).

  e. Tattoos have different permutations (such as lip shadowing, tattooing freckles and eyebrows, etc.) and vary in ink size.

  i. Asphalt tattoos are fine to treat, tricky to treat, probably start with Q-switch (asphalt particle is bigger; basically going from rocks to pebbles, to grains of sand, and the 532 Nd:YAG is good for grains of sand).

  ii. Can treat radiation tattoos—but check with rad oncologist first.

  iii. Probably shouldn't treat gunpowder tattoos.

  f. One of the best uses for the 532 laser is to treat lentigos and macular SKs (532 treats red but also gets absorbed by melanin).

  i. The frost for this is mostly pigment color change, but maybe a little LN2 from DEJ, since they are epidermal lesions (vs. tattoos, which are dermal).

  ii. They'll turn dark and fall away.

  iii. If used, regular LN2 can get hypopigmentation, which won't happen with 532 if you're careful.

  g. After treatment, put on sunscreen and Vaseline.

  i. Will turn dark in 1–2 days, will peel away in 1 week, then normal skin appears.

2. A 532-long pulse (instead of short bursts, doing over longer bursts, going after melanin, melanin heats up, and by collateral damage destroys DPNs).

  a. Basically using the collateral damage that melanin will cause if exposed to a long pulse to our advantage.

  b. Works great for flat DPNs (heat dissipates over them).

  i. Not good for superthick DPNs (532 doesn't go very deep into the skin).

ii. If broad and flat, then track along them.

c. DPNs turn grayish immediately after zapping (cell death).

  i. Look like scabs about 1 week later.

  ii. Look great at 6 weeks.

  iii. If hazy hypopigmentation (like P versicolor look) at 2–3 months, then pigment will come back.

  iv. If pure white at 2–3 months, then might be long term.

d. Different from 532 earlier (not long pulse), which was good for lentigines and macular SKs (wanted shorter pulse to avoid collateral heating—similar to pulsing vs. continuous LN2 that you do in clinic).

6.2.5 Non-Ablative Fractional Infrared—1927 nm

1. Chromophore = water (anything infrared is water).

a. When treating fractionally, you have concurrent areas of normal spared skin (in other words, 100% is fully ablative, which would have a lot of downtime and patient discomfort; so you minimize this the same way they do radiation—in fractions).

  i. Should give HSV prophylaxis if doing fully ablative or even full-faced fractional, and full chemical peels/TCA, and if perioral, etc.

b. Erbium glass 1927: Good for epidermal pigment (lentigos, etc.).

  i. Targets water, but pigment is a bystander (water absorption is so high it peels off part of the epidermis—the pigment is at the basal layer so comes off the pigment does too).

  ii. Because epidermal treatment and generating heat, air cooling (blow cold air on patient) will help minimize pain—can be used for chemical peels too.

c. CO_2 is 10,600 also water but differs by how much loves water (CO_2 loves water so much it heats it up so fast it vaporizes the skin; has long downtime, so not great for sunny places like Florida).

  i. Some lasers are mirrors (CO_2), some fiber-optic (Erbium glass).

  ii. If vaporizing tissue (as in Erbium + CO_2, etc.), should wear mask + have smoke evacuator.

d. Erbium and CO_2 don't cause primary hair loss, but they vaporize hair and takes time for it to come back; so nice to do RF microneedling first over hairs, then Vaseline over hairs, and go all over it with ablative laser.

6.2.6 Radiofrequency (RF) Microneedling

1. Basically, small needles on an array are pushed into skin, and energy is delivered in dermis (thermal injury).

a. Needles usually have an insulated coating to localize energy to the exposed tip only (more control where energy is delivered).

      i. If no coating, can cause damage all the way down the needle (which is usually not desirable, especially for skin of color).

  b. RF useful because can shut on/off very quickly.

  c. Can adjust pulse widths.

      i. Ultrashort pulses can impact melanocytes or vasculature around melanocytes (for melasma).

        – Melasma can be vascular as much as pigmentary (so look for underlying redness [which PDL can address]).

        – Can combine microneedling with PDL.

        – Long-pulse microneedling likely better for skin of color because not stimulating melanocytes or inflammation (so less risk of PIH).

          – For skin of color don't want to be too close to epidermis because still a little bit of heat comes up (can get drift and get damage).

2. Resurfacing for acne scars.

  a. Have to get to mid dermis (where defects are).

      i. Microdermabrasion and microneedling might help, but adding energy stimulates healing cascade better (collagen remodeling, heat shock proteins, etc.)

        – However, the addition of heat also higher risk of hyperpigmentation; type 4 probably the scariest.

     ii. Should have a fair amount of pinpoint bleeding.

    iii. PRP after resurfacing seems to help; some people rub it on after doing the microneedling, and some inject it under the skin with a cannula (probably does better).

  b. Skin first turns white, starts to repigment ~1 week (around hair follicles), then over 2–3 weeks, becomes hyperpigmented, then it normalizes (would avoid lightening creams until you know they've completely repigmented); if stalling with repigmenting, can add TCSs, TCIs, Fraxel laser, excimer laser, etc.

7 Post-Procedure Counseling

7.1 POST-OPERATIVE CARE INSTRUCTIONS

- *Pain prevention*: alternate Tylenol and ibuprofen after excisions/Mohs (schedule it to stay ahead of the pain).
  - First 1–2 days post-op are the worst with pain.
  - Also, alert them of things they may experience further out in healing process (as nerve fibers begin to reform/reconnect, occasionally patients will complain of pins-and-needles sensations or occasional sharp bursts of pain; can reassure them this decreases over time and eventually goes away after several months).
- *Preventing infection*: probably give PO antibiotics for any flap/graft. Consider PO antibiotics for arms, etc. (sweaty), or if something happened during procedure, like ruptured a cyst or something. Don't necessarily need antibiotics empirically for scalp procedures.
- *Suture removal timeline*:
  - Head/neck, 5–7 days
  - Extremities/torso, 10–14 days
- *Spitting sutures*:
  - Usually happens ~4–6 weeks post-op (typically red spot over one spot—not the entire length of wound).
    - Versus infection (odd to get infected 1 month post-op, though is possible, particularly if the entire length of wound is red/inflamed, etc.; can sometimes start as a suture abscess that becomes an open wound and becomes secondarily infected).
  - Might see sterile pus (usually takes 2 weeks to do its thing, then feels better and less bumpy; OK to pull stitch out if sticking out [redness may improve if removing the stitch]).
- *Suture abscesses*:
  - Typically just one spot (not the entire length of wound).
  - Can usually just take out the suture (though some people do mupirocin; some people do PO antibiotics).
- *Wound healing*:
  - Keep greasy with Vaseline; avoid Neosporin.
  - Diabetics and especially smokers have increased risk for wound healing complications.

The best resources are probably the handouts your attendings give patients for post-procedure care.

Examples of general things:

1. *Post-LN2*

DOI: 10.1201/9781003537946-7

a. Wash skin QD; keep clean to minimize discoloration/scarring/ infection.

    i. Apply hydrogen peroxide in shower (dab with cotton ball), wash off the bubbles, then place Vaseline on when out of shower.

b. Do not pull scabs or blister roofs off; just clean with mild soap + tap water BID. Pat dry and apply plain Vaseline (warn them ~6% people are allergic to Neosporin).

    i. Blisters usually resolve within several days.

c. If oozes, can bandage.

d. If stays sore, red all around, draining, call or RTC.

e. Anticipate SKs to fall off in 1–2 weeks.

2. *Post-biopsy*

a. Clean with soap + water 2–3× daily.

b. Apply Vaseline after washing; keep greasy.

c. Mild pain + itching are normal.

d. OTC aspirin/Tylenol/ibuprofen are fine, unless doctor said they're not (such as if the patient has bleeding issues, liver/kidney issues).

e. For punches, sutures need removed in 1–2 weeks.

3. *Post-EDC*

a. Keep bandage dry for 24 hours; after removing, can shower.

b. Keep wound covered for 1 week.

4. *Post-excision*

a. Avoid strenuous activity (mowing, vacuuming, etc.) until sutures removed.

b. For primary closures, keep bandage dry for 24 hours; can shower after.

c. Clean with mild antibacterial soap + water; apply Vaseline/petrolatum, both BID. Avoid Neosporin (6% of Americans allergic to it).

d. Soreness, redness, bruising, swelling, and some drainage are normal.

    i. Bruising can last ~1 week.

    ii. Swelling increases for 1–2 days, then improves.

       – Can use ice pack for first 1–2 days (10 minutes on, 20 minutes off).

    iii. Best to cover wound with clean non-stick gauze for several days for the drainage.

    iv. If very sore, red, firm/hot to touch, draining pus, smells bad, or fever, then may be infected.

5. *If bleeding*, apply continuous firm pressure with cloth or gauze for 15–20 minutes (first with bandage on; if still bleeding, then try again without bandage).

7.2 PHYSICIAN'S ACCESS LINE (PAL) CALLS FROM PATIENTS

1. *Concern for infection*

   a. Patients are commonly concerned about regular peri-incisional erythema (actual infections usually have significant pain after a period of improvement).

   b. Nonetheless, if they are very concerned, can send them PO antibiotics (cephalexin 500 mg TID for 5–7 days if no allergy/renal impairment, or doxycycline 100 mg BID for 7 days for MRSA coverage and anti-inflammatory properties).

2. *Pain*

   a. Rest, ice, elevation.

   b. OTC NSAIDs, Tylenol—can alternate (assuming no contraindications—make sure no liver, kidney, or bleeding issues) and emphasize scheduling them to stay ahead of the pain (proactive vs. reactive).

3. *Bleeding*

   a. Advise patient to remove dressing and visualize bleeding area (hard to stop small leak in a hose through four soaked fluffy pillows).

   b. Hold firm, focused pressure (using 1–2 fingers) for 20 minutes. Set timer. No peaking. Watch a TV show. Stops 99% of bleeding. Tell them to call back if still bleeding.

   c. If controlled, can recommend OTC wound seal to help maintain the stability.

   d. If still bleeding, may have to meet them back at clinic. Probably better than them going to ED (who knows what they'll do there).

7.3 SCARS

Moist wound healing always gives a better scar outcome than dry wound healing.

Once epithelialized, can consider topical things to improve remodeling phase:

- Silicone creams/pads/sheets (can buy OTC, cut into strips 2–3× size of scar, apply overnight, wash with water, then apply again)—good if developing a hypertrophic scar or if excising in a patient with history of keloids/hypertrophic scars; better as prophylactic measure than treatment.

- Tretinoin good if atrophic, red, hyperpigmented scar tissue.

- Mederma—good for redder components.

- Hypopigmented flat scars are hardest to address.

- General things that might help: massage (will help soften scar, though may hurt a little if deep sutures still present, since will basically be in there pulling tissue apart); moisturize with Aquaphor or Eucerin.

  - Some of the stuff that's marketed to help might just help because they're rubbing it in (massaging).

Wait until 6 weeks after a procedure to do ILK for scars (otherwise, can depress the scar because it's still forming; for keloids, can be more aggressive and do earlier).

Can do laser if scar doesn't look good. Typically, scar revisions best done early because softens out the scar tissue and can reduce pull of structures (if, for instance, a free margin or something has deviated).

Takes 9–10 months for scars to mature (thus, if they ask if anything will change 5 years after scar formed, then probably not).

8 Miscellaneous Doctoring

8.1 DOCUMENTATION

It's all about being concise, comprehensive, and accurate. Include everything that happened, exclude anything that didn't happen, and don't drown people in info/starve them for wisdom.

1. Avoid unnecessary info; if it doesn't change anything, it can probably be deleted.

   a. *Example*: "I had the pleasure of seeing and evaluating this 45-year-old female who presented as a new patient to our outpatient dermatology clinic today for evaluation and treatment recommendations regarding a new rash. Upon questioning, she admits that she is not entirely sure when or where the current rash of question exactly started. She reports that the rash is sometimes itchy and sometimes it is not. She mentions that she has never experienced anything like this before and this is her first time at the dermatologist."

      i. That is a lot to basically say, "NPV, 45 F, no derm hx, p/w intermittently itchy rash of unclear duration." Clearly, I exaggerated to illustrate a point, but I have seen notes that really haven't been that far from that.

   b. *Another example*: "The patient is not really sure what prescription topical treatments they have tried but can remember reading the package insert about the potential side effects of corticosteroids and ended up only applying the creams for a day and then stopped. More recently, they tried applying creams they got from the drugstore, but nothing they got over the counter seemed to work. They went to another dermatologist in their home state of Virginia and tried a pill that they say they took once per week and weren't supposed to drink alcohol or get pregnant on. They brought the container in today to the clinic, and it appears this was methotrexate. Unfortunately, this made their stomach hurt, and they didn't like having to get their blood drawn, so they stopped taking it."

      i. Basically saying, "Failed rx: unspecified TCSs (steroid phobia), OTCs (no improvement), MTX (GI upset, didn't like lab draws)."

         – Ideally, you would also mention where they applied the topicals, how frequently they applied them, and how long they tried treating for (similar levels of detail, of course, help with PO or injectable meds too).

2. Don't omit relevant info.

   a. *Example*: "Hx melanoma + NMSCs."

      i. Big difference whether it was an MIS 25 years ago vs. a malignant melanoma 6 months ago currently undergoing immunotherapy.

   b. *Better examples:*

      i. "Hx melanoma s/p WLE (surgeon's name, 3/2023)"

      ii. "Hx BCC R forehead s/p Mohs (surgeon's name, 11/2019)"

    iii. Best to list it in a way that never changes, so if it's a patient who has had numerous skin cancers, can just add to the list.

3. None of this is to say that notes shouldn't ever be long, because complex patients sometimes need longer notes, but it helps if you strive to make them dense in terms of insight.

    a. For complicated patients, it's nice to have forward-looking plans (for example, RTC 12 weeks; if not much improved with MTX, can consider submitting PA for Humira; needs labs either way—or something similar); understand you may not always have time (or know what the next steps might be), but it's helpful for co-residents who may see them at next visit (especially if it's stuff that was discussed with the attending).

    b. Would also try to organize it in a way that makes it easy to follow their course (in the subjective write the date with the interval history [instead of saying stuff like last visit, etc.] and make sure to keep any relevant history [they shouldn't have to tell the resident they had GI upset with MTX at every visit, or that it worked but they've failed tapers]).

    c. Take time to explain the thought process/impression in the assessment (especially if diagnosis unclear), even if brief.

4. Some fluff is fine if it's specific/relevant (such as small talk with patient about their hobbies/life, etc. [for rapport, etc.]). But if you automate voluminous templates that have a lot of uninformative bloat, it's helpful to delete that stuff, in my opinion.

    a. The other (perhaps bigger) problem with templates is that it oftentimes includes a lot of stuff that might not have even happened or be true. For instance, a note shouldn't say you encouraged the patient to read the package insert if there wasn't even a prescription sent.

    b. How many times have you read a note for a patient that was referred for a rash and the skin exam says "warm and dry" or, better yet, "no rashes"?

5. Frame things in ways that won't change, if possible (specify a disease onset date rather than saying, "It started 1 week ago," etc.). I never understood why people put "at last visit." I find it so confusing, especially when it gets copy-forwarded and you have to dig through their records to determine when the "last visit" in reference actually was. Takes just as much time to write "started MTX 5/2023" as "started MTX last visit" but saves a lot of time in future visits to frame it as the former. Helpful things to include:

    a. Disease start

        i. *For example*: "Rash onset 1/2020."

    b. Disease course

        i. *For example*: "Waxes/wanes, never completely clears, flares ~Q 2 weeks, most recently yesterday."

    c. Meds (dosing and result)

        i. *For example*: "Current regimen: MTX 10 mg QW (helps with itch + redness), started 3/2020."

ii. For topicals, ideal to quantify how often and specify where.

- *For example*: "Applying Protopic QD to eyebrows (stable)."

d. Past meds (result and/or discontinuation reason)

i. *For example*: "Skyrizi (nearly cleared but dc'd 2/2 insurance change), clobetasol ointment (too greasy, lesions too diffuse)," etc.

e. Side effects

i. *For example*: "Tolerating well."

f. Also nice to quantify disease severity—helps for insurance approvals, and also for retrospective research.

i. *For example*: "BSA 10%, PGA 3 or TNTC/20+ prurigo nodules," etc.

ii. Usually have to mention somewhere how it compares to prior visits/before starting treatment.

iii. Would also include when the prior auth expires for meds that require it (which you should always be looking up, anyway).

- *For example*: "AD clear on Dupixent (PA exp 12/2024)."

8.2 WRITING MANUSCRIPTS

■ For project ideation, it's typically better to have a "measure twice, cut once" approach.

• Einstein said, "I spend 95% of the time thinking about the problem, and 5% of the time working on the solution" (or something like that).

- In other words, have a clear vision for what your proposed contribution to the literature is before diving into the granular details of the project.

- One way you can help hold yourself accountable to this is by drafting the cover letter to the target journal before even submitting the IRB proposal/designing the project.

- Look up papers that have been published in top journals to get an idea for their methods; this will save you mistakes/regrets.

- For instance, if you're doing a survey study, it helps to have attention check questions included in the survey.

- Also helps to use validated survey instruments when trying to measure something.

- The more literature you read, the more your project design instincts will improve (my opinion).

■ For writing, similar principles as writing notes (earlier).

• Be crisp/concise/clear; you'd be surprised at how much can be crammed into 500-word limit submissions (and even abstracts).

• Be very careful with how you word things; avoid ambiguity, don't overstretch things.

- It's usually fine to speculate, but just be very clear what is speculation and what is not.
- Typically best to avoid telling doctors what they should do (preferable to let them come to those conclusions themselves).

- Avoid "notably," "interestingly," etc. Everything you say should be notable/interesting, etc.

- Don't say "our results show," "it has been shown that," etc.; if it's been shown, then it just "is."

- Don't say "As previously mentioned," etc.; it adds nothing of value and is redundant.

- Avoid words like "extremely," "dramatic," etc.; they are subjective, at best, and very rarely does something actually deserve those words.

- If seeing word "significant," odds are you can cross it out; it's ambiguous. If the $p = 0.000001$ but you went from 140 to 160 scalp hairs in MPHL, then it's really not significant at all; be objective and just state the p-value.

- Try not to start sentences with numbers or percents (if you have to, then better to spell them out).

- When citing figures/tables, just put in parentheses at the end of the relevant sentence (don't waste words saying, "Which can be seen in Table 1," etc.).

  - Leverage figures and tables to trim word count.
    - Imagine the difference between "Our patients reported various side effects (Table 1)" and "Two patients reported gastrointestinal upset, another patient reported subjective hair loss, another patient self-discontinued their medication due to reported anxiety and cost barriers" (let alone if you waste words saying all this and then proceed to repeat the same info in a table).
    - Tables should almost have stand-alone value; use the title/caption to summarize the main takeaway and the table to show it.

- Don't conclude with "future studies are needed"; future studies are always needed; you can suggest specific future directions if you want (or better yet—do them).

■ Revision requests

- Have great gratitude and respect for reviewers' time and insights; they invest a lot in improving your manuscript.

- Embrace seemingly harsh constructive feedback; this is oftentimes the best feedback and a sign that they care (and see potential)—you will thank them later (same principle applies to anything in life, really).

- Make it as easy as possible for the reviewers to follow your changes and your thought process.

  - Craft a well-organized cover letter that clearly and comprehensively responds to their comments; while you don't necessarily need to implement all their suggestions, if you opt to not incorporate any of their suggestions, make sure you clearly communicate why (and nicely!).

- If there are areas that aren't addressable, take the next step and mention them in the limitations section; you want the reviewer to feel that every single comment they offered was "heard."

- Obviously, never argue; if something wasn't clear to them, then it probably won't be clear to other readers; take ownership of that and challenge yourself to make modifications that improve clarity.

• Obviously, pay close attention to deadlines (usually shouldn't be an issue)—best to turn it around ASAP, same day/week if feasible.

■ Rejections

• Every manuscript has a home somewhere, so don't worry about it too much; but make sure to take advantage of any/all feedback you collect along the way.

8.3 REVIEWING MANUSCRIPTS

Unlikely that any resident is going to be a true expert on a topic. However, you still may be asked to review manuscripts (maybe on topics you've published on, or you might've been recommended by another invitee, or know the editor). If you have solid knowledge of the topic, that's great. But in general, regardless of your knowledge base, I recommend always accepting these invitations (unless you have a conflict of interest or aren't confident you can provide a fair review or something). It's a good opportunity to stay up-to-date with literature and will improve your own research; you'll pretty much have to do a literature review to ensure accuracy and to assess how novel/original a manuscript is (don't worry—definitely doesn't take as much time as being an author of a literature review). At the very least, you can critique basic stuff, like how well written/organized it is, whether the methods are clearly explained and reproducible, whether the results are important/interesting and likely to impact clinical practices, whether the conclusions are justified, whether it fits the aims/scope of the journal, etc.

You should read the advice for reviewers on the JAAD website. They also have examples of strong reviews to give you an idea what is helpful and what is not.

Some thoughts to consider:

■ For treatment outcomes data papers.

• Relatively straightforward, but should include all (or at least enough) parameters to fully appreciate whether the meds were convincingly responsible for the outcomes reported.

- Some of these include pre-treatment disease duration, pre-treatment treatment failures, duration on treatment, concomitant treatments (especially systemics), time to achieve outcomes (and how outcomes were categorized), whether responses were durable (and when/whether flares were temporally related to dose reductions/discontinuations), side effects experienced, etc.

• Also consider whether they had biopsy-proven disease (which is more relevant for some diseases than others).

- For proposed associations:
  - Be careful of blindly accepting stuff being associated with "underlying malignancies, etc." Malignancies are common (for example, bullous pemphigoid was originally thought to be related to cancer because it affected people >70 years old).
  - Things that potentially make things more convincingly suggestive appear to have temporal relationship, same or similar cancers, if when you cure the cancer the rash gets better, etc.
    - For instance, can't just be that they have diabetes and have skin lesions; therefore, they're associated.
  - Also consider the practical takeaways; if a condition is statistically significantly associated with a particular condition, is it enough to impact how we work those patients up? The number needed to treat is a helpful way to quantify this question.
- For drug-induced papers, should ask yourself:
  - What was stopped when the proposed culprit drug was started, and how long does it take for the new drug to work?
    - Remember, other specialties sometimes have a tendency to start and stop meds (instead of overlapping them).
  - Is it a manifestation of the disease?
    - For example, weekly MTX "causing" pulm fibrosis in an AICTD that can involve the lungs.

Although associations don't prove causation (which I've admittedly somewhat heavily harped on throughout the book), just want to be clear: there are many things legitimately associated with drugs that are important to report. So don't blindly discount proposed associations either (otherwise, we would never find out about them).

General things for essentially all papers:

- While nice to have background info for context, the purpose of it should primarily be to set the stage; the main emphasis should be on the novel content (not a bunch of basic stuff we already know and then one sentence about the actual study).
  - Similarly, always ask yourself if the manuscript could be made more succinct (not only are concise manuscripts more time-efficient for the reader, but they are also more effective because the interesting contents won't be diluted out by a bunch of fluff).
- Should be intuitively organized (introduction, methods, results, discussion, limitations, conclusion, or similar)—and contents should be in their appropriate sections (sometimes people have results in their methods).
  - Hypothesis/aims should be clear.
    - Consider the practical value, and strive to see both the big picture and the granular details (something could be really cool but also impractical—for example, using ultrasound to characterize outcomes in rosacea).

- Methods should be adequately and clearly described (reproducible).
- Results should be clear and not obfuscated.
  - Ideally presented efficiently/effectively with tables/figures.
    - Images need to be high-quality and representative.
    - Assess for patient anonymity—see if patient consent form attached.
    - Legends should be succinct and accurate.
    - Be vigilant about numbers; are the authors showing you the whole y-axis? If not, they may be trying to blow up the difference.
- Discussion should have a clear conclusion regarding whether the aims of the study were met.
  - Conclusions obviously need to be justified.
    - Weigh clinical meaningfulness vs. statistical significance.
    - If risk of heart attack increases 2–3× in psoriasis, is that dramatic? If you're referring to a 20 year old, then it's almost nothing (and frankly, meaningless). Still fine to point out, but the value of the insight needs to be clear, and the conclusions need to be appropriately framed (a reasonable conclusion is probably something like psoriasis patients don't need specific cardiovascular screening but should probably follow PCP and get age-appropriate screening and stop smoking/have an appropriate BMI, etc.).
    - Point being, always ask yourself what the baseline risk is before RRs catch your eye.
- Make sure references are up-to-date, accurate, and ideally from credible journals (don't want outdated or incorrect info to live on)—it's OK to suggest citations if authors miss important ones.
- Every study has limitations; make sure they're clearly/explicitly stated and appropriately framed.
  - Generalizability of the data is something you should consider.
    - For example, if a group that specializes in high-risk SCCs reports their data on SCCs, this will inevitably consist of a disproportionate number of high-risk tumors that may not be representative of all practices, and their findings may reflect that.
    - Obviously doesn't mean it shouldn't be published (a lot of academic activity, of course, comes from tertiary care centers), but it should probably at least be stated, since a lot of readerships are likely comprised of dermatologists around the world in various practice settings.
- Confidential comments to editor are for basically anything you don't want authors to see, such as if you suspect misconducts like plagiarism, inappropriate or undeclared COI, falsification of results, etc.

- Submissions may be from other non-English-speaking countries; fine to suggest review by an English speaker if many grammatical errors, etc.

- Obviously, your ultimate recommendation should correlate with your comments. I usually don't say definitive stuff like, "This paper is ready for publication," in the comments to authors, because (1) who knows if the other reviewers will agree (you will often be blinded to other reviewers' reviews, at least until you submit yours), and (2) it would be redundant, anyway, if your recommendation is to accept; sometimes it's fine if they were just straightforward minor revisions that have been addressed and there's nothing to say (but even then I would be considerate of the opinions of the other reviewers that you may not necessarily want to contradict).

  - Obviously best to give specific comments that are corroborated (avoid saying vague/ambiguous stuff like, "The results are not robust"—or if you do say something like this, explain specifically why they are not robust).

  - If asking for revisions, the comments should be clear what needs revised.

  - Overall, would say it's relatively uncommon for initial submissions to merit an "accept" without revision, but it definitely happens.

8.4 BEING A RESIDENT

Thanks to the Wake Forest residents who came before me and lent some of this advice.

Aside from the obvious generic stuff (working hard, being a team player, being humble, recognizing limitations, embracing mistakes, etc.), some advice and perspectives.

Appreciate the unique situation you're in:

- You have everyday direct access to field leaders in multiple areas and get to compare your impression/plans with theirs. It's essentially like learning on your attending's credit card; you only get this for 3 years and will never have it this good again.

- Patients travel from far away, take time off work, pay a lot of money to see you to get answers, etc., and oftentimes we are only able to reciprocate a fraction of that due to the inherently busy nature of the derm clinic; try to keep this in perspective, especially when the going gets tough.

- It's good to mentally simulate being on your own, as you soon will be (take full ownership and don't just passively wait for them to take over). This helps you identify what your knowledge dead ends are, and also how to deal with tough patients.

- Embrace the hard/complex patients (one of the plastic surgeons I work with framed this concept well: "You gotta take the hard cases or your easy cases will become hard. Don't have a passive mindset or your scope will shrink"). Thinking this way will also cause you to ask better, more meaningful questions (allowing you to get the most out of every day).

  - At this stage in training, focusing efforts at becoming clinically and procedurally competent is probably more of a priority than acing tests (though performing well on exams is obviously still important and, in some ways, related).

As far as explicit suggestions go (and of course, everyone's best learning method is different, but these are just things that work well for me):

- I wish I'd saved patients on lists earlier on—this allows you to track how they actually did in the long term (it's pretty crazy the absolute max follow-up you could get for a patient in residency is 3 years).

The best thing to do would be to keep a spreadsheet of patients you want to follow (for example, make an Excel sheet with one tab for diagnostic dilemmas [or patients you weren't sure what they had or curious what their course might be], another tab for procedures you've done [so you can track their long-term results and see whether they recurred, etc.—will give you a better idea how much is too little or too much for an EDC, for instance, etc.], another tab for treatment responses [perhaps all patients for a particular condition that you're trying novel medications for or something], etc.—you get the point).

You could even keep columns that record the date you saw them and the date they're next scheduled for follow-up, and then just sort by follow-up date.

- Try to look at your own biopsies, especially in the beginning; it'll give you much better context about what you're giving the pathologist to work with, and it'll improve your sense of what is too superficial or too deep, etc.

Maybe you're shaving deeper than necessary for stuff like BCCs, or shaving too superficially for inflammatory stuff, or perhaps you're not handling punch specimens well and you're unknowingly crushing the tissue; it's also possible your biopsies are perfect and you should continue doing what you're doing, but in any case, it's good to have feedback.

- Take advantage of biopsy site pics and pics of rashes—there is nothing better (that I can think of) than real-life photographs.

It's also nice because you can check your answer with a real-life histologic report.

I would also take as many pics as possible in clinic and use them when you present photos to your co-residents; this helps tell more of a practical story (rather than just quizzing your co-residents on the same boards factoids/obvious pictures) and stimulates more productive discussion.

- Similarly, try to look at a lot of pics of the same conditions, and read up on the same topics in different books (or other resources, such as podcasts [some include Dermasphere, Dermalogues, Grenz Zone], VisualDx [which has patient handouts that come in Spanish as well], DermNet, JAAD CMEs [all of which I would be remiss to not acknowledge], etc.).

- Ask the same questions to different attendings—this will help you get an idea for how you'll shape your own style.

- Don't mistake activity for achievement. While you can passively go through the motions and still learn a good amount from sheer volume, it's much more effective/productive to have a clearly defined "thing" that you're actively working on (for instance, if you're in an excision clinic, make it a goal to put perfectly spaced tops in that day or something; if you're in hair clinic, make it a goal to give good trichoscopy descriptions, etc. [generally, the more specific the goal, the better]).

■ It's obvious, but I have learned a tremendous amount by listening closely to what my attendings say during patient encounters (and how they counsel them, etc.). From day 1, I made it a goal to never miss anything they taught me. I'm sure my memory has failed me to an extent, but I tried to write down as much as I could (which is actually where all this originated). I prioritized this over finishing notes so I could devote all my attention to them (even though I know it's nice to get notes done). It also helps you learn what you don't know. That way, you can read up on things later with an intent. I find this much more fruitful than just reading for the sake of just getting through a chapter. And if you can't find answers after doing that, then write it down, and ask the next time you're in clinic.

If you've made it this far, thanks for reading! Hopefully, you enjoyed it and found it useful. There are probably so many more things I haven't realized yet or forgot to include, and I don't think something like this could really ever feel complete, anyway. Nonetheless, I hope it accomplishes what I initially intended it to (which was to give you a good head start). Best of luck, and don't hesitate to reach out with any questions!